BASIC TOXICOLOGY
Fundamentals, Target Organs, and Risk Assessment

Third Edition

Frank C. Lu
Consulting Toxicologist
Miami, Florida

Taylor & Francis
Publishers since 1798

USA	Publishing Office:	Taylor & Francis 1101 Vermont Avenue, NW, Suite 200 Washington, DC 20005-3521 Tel: (202) 289-2174 Fax: (202) 289-3665
	Distribution Center:	Taylor & Francis 1900 Frost Road, Suite 101 Bristol, PA 19007-1598 Tel: (215) 785-5800 Fax: (215) 785-55154
UK		Taylor & Francis Ltd. 1 Gunpowder Square London EC4A 3DE Tel: 0171 583 0490 Fax: 0171 583 0581

BASIC TOXICOLOGY: Fundamentals, Target Organs, and Risk Assessment, Third Edition

1 2 3 4 5 6 7 8 9 0 BRBR 9 8 7 6

This book was set in Times Roman by Pro Image Corporation. The editors were Catherine Simon and Elizabeth Dugger. Cover design by Michelle Fleitz. Printing and binding by Braun-Brumfield, Inc.

A CIP catalog record for this book is available from the British Library.
⊚ The paper in this publication meets the requirements of the ANSI Standard Z39.48-1984 (Permanence of Paper)

Library of Congress Cataloging-in-Publication Data
Lu, Frank C.
  Basic toxicology: fundamentals, target organs, and risk
assessment/by Frank C. Lu.—3rd ed.
        p.   cm.
  Includes bibliographical references and indexes.

  1. Toxicology.   I. Title.
  [DNLM: 1. Toxicology.   2. Poisoning.   3. Poisons—
pharmacokinetics.   4. Toxicity Tests—methods.   QV 600 L926b 1996]
RA1211.L8   1996
615.9—dc20
DNLM/DLC
for Library of Congress   96-12505
                                                                                          CIP

ISBN 1-56032-379-5 (case)
ISBN 1-56032-380-9 (paper)

Contents

PART II TESTING PROCEDURES FOR CONVENTIONAL AND NONTARGET ORGAN TOXICITIES

PART III   TARGET ORGANS AND SYSTEMS

PART IV   TOXIC SUBSTANCES AND RISK ASSESSMENT

Preface

This introductory book is intended for students taking toxicology courses and for scientists of allied disciplines who require a background in toxicology. The book was first published in 1985. Apart from updating, the second edition, published in 1991, was expanded by the inclusion of discussions on four groups of important chemicals and toxicants. The additional material was intended to provide not only a general knowledge of these substances, but also a better appreciation of the broad scope of toxicology as well as the great variety of toxic effects.

The book has received worldwide acceptance, as evidenced by the availability of five foreign language versions.

In recent years, toxicology has made great strides in understanding the mode of action underlying various toxic effects. This knowledge is valuable in predicting certain toxic effects, ascertaining the seriousness of exposure to certain toxicants, and facilitating rational assessment of "safe" intakes or the risks associated with specified levels of exposure. Consequently, a variety of mechanisms of action, along with examples of toxicants, is provided. In addition, more detailed descriptions of a number of important/ typical toxicants are included in the relevant chapters.

Better understanding of the mode of action of the differences among carcinogens in terms of weight of evidence, as well as the mode of action, including the role of oncogenes and oncosuppressor genes, is more fully described. Other topics that have been updated and expanded include the section on receptors; their importance in toxicology is becoming more widely recognized. Furthermore, many host and environmental factors may alter the nature and/or severity of toxicity. The major underlying mode is attributable to differences in the detoxication of the toxicant. However, a variety of other factors have been shown to play important roles; for emphasis, these factors have therefore been compiled in a list.

Because of the importance of the subject of toxicological evaluation, the chapter dealing with this subject has also been expanded. In addition to descriptions of procedures commonly used for this purpose, their advantages and limitations, as well as brief descriptions of alternative procedures, have been added. Other chapters have also been updated, notably the chapters on the nervous, reproductive, and cardiovascular systems, as well as the one on mutagenesis.

Brief descriptions of testing procedures have been an integral part of the book since its first edition. They assist the readers in visualizing the toxic manifestations and in deciphering the way they are elicited and detected. However, to make room for the additional material mentioned earlier, some details of the testing procedures have been abbreviated. To compensate for this shortage, up-to-date references have been added for those keenly interested in these topics.

A considerable amount of information on metals and pesticides, as well as on indoor and environmental pollutants, is included.

To facilitate the acquisition of a broad knowledge of toxicology, this book is divided into four major areas. General topics related to absorption, distribution, and excretion of toxicants, their transformation in the body, the various types of toxic effects they exert, and the host and environmental factors that modify these effects are covered in Part I. Procedures used to discover the general and nontarget organ, adverse health effects (i.e., carcinogenicity, mutagenicity and teratogenicity), and organs/systems that are the targets of the toxicants are elaborated in Parts II and III within the broad areas of testing procedures and target organs, respectively. A number of important toxic substances are briefly discussed in Part IV to illustrate the diverse nature of toxicity. The last chapter outlines the widely adopted approaches to the assessment of safety/risk of noncarcinogenic chemicals. In addition, two indexes are appended, listing chemicals and subjects, respectively, to assist the reader in retrieving relevant parts of the text.

It is hoped that these alterations and additions will enhance the usefulness of the book. In making these changes, the author has kept in mind the broad aims of the first edition, namely, relatively comprehensive coverage of the subjects and brevity, thereby continuing to serve as an updated introductory text for toxicology students and for those involved in allied sciences who require a background in toxicology.

Preface to
the Second Edition

As noted in the Preface to the First Edition, this book is intended as an introductory text for students taking toxicology courses and for those involved in allied sciences who require a background in toxicology. Since its publication in 1985, this book has been favorably accepted in the United States as well as in many other parts of the world. The wide acceptance is evidenced by the fact that the hardcover edition has been reprinted twice and the paperback edition has been reprinted five times. In addition, there are several foreign language versions.

However, a number of important developments have occurred in toxicology in the past few years. Furthermore, several colleagues and students have suggested that discussions on a few groups of important chemicals and toxicants would provide a general knowledge of these substances. More importantly, such discussions would facilitate a deeper appreciation of the various aspects of toxicology, thereby enhancing the value of the book in the field of basic toxicology.

Taking into account these considerations, many chapters have been updated and expanded, notably the chapter dealing with carcinogenesis, immunotoxicology, and assessment of risk/safety. Four chapters have been added to briefly discuss the toxicological aspects of food additives and contaminants, pesticides, metals, and a number of other toxicants of occupational and environmental concern.

The book is now divided into four parts: (1) general principles of toxicology, (2) testing procedures, (3) target organs, and (4) toxic substances and safety/risk assessment.

It is hoped that these alterations and additions will enhance the usefulness of the book. In making these changes, the author has kept in mind the broad aims of the first edition, namely, relatively comprehensive coverage of the subjects and brevity, thereby continuing to serve as an updated introductory text for toxicology students and for those involved in allied sciences who require a background in toxicology.

Preface to the First Edition

Toxicology is an important science. It provides a sound basis for formulating measures to protect the health of workers against toxicants in factories, farms, mines, and other occupational environments. It is also valuable in the protection of public health against hazards associated with toxic substances in food, air, and water. Toxicology has played and will continue to play a significant role in the health and welfare of the world.

Cognizant of the importance of toxicology, the World Health Organization (WHO) organized a toxicology training course in China in 1982, as part of the ongoing China–WHO collaborative program on medical sciences. The course consisted of two parts. The author was invited to lecture on basic toxicology, and lectures on occupational toxicology were given by others. This book originated from the author's lecture notes.

The subjects covered in the book are divided into three parts; they are general principles, testing procedures, and target organs. The first part deals with absorption, distribution, and excretion of toxicants; their biotransformation (detoxication and bioactivation); their adverse effects; and factors that modify their effects. It also includes chapters dealing with various approaches to toxicologic evaluation, including risk assessment, and the type and amount of data required to carry out such evaluations.

Part II covers topics related to conventional toxicity studies of different durations. It also deals with the nature of and tests for such specific effects as carcinogenesis, mutagenesis, and teratogenesis. Part III deals with toxic effects on specific target organs: the respiratory system, liver, kidney, skin, eye, nervous system, and a number of others. The effects of toxicants are not described systematically, but they are used in illustrating various categories of toxic effects and the underlying mode of action. Knowledge of general toxicology in its diverse field will promote better understanding of toxicologic data on specific toxic substances and their interactions.

This book is intended as an introductory text for students taking toxicology courses and for those involved in allied sciences who require a background in toxicology. Furthermore, since toxicology is a vast subject and is fast expanding, the book is likely to be useful to those who have become specialized in one or a few areas in toxicology but wish to brush up in other areas.

In preparing this book, attempts were made to have a relatively comprehensive coverage of the subjects as well as to maintain brevity. The latter was achieved by the inclusion of some appendixes and a large number of references to assist readers interested in additional information.

Part One

General Principles of Toxicology

General Considerations

CHAPTER 1 CONTENTS

People are exposed to a great variety of natural and man-made substances. Under certain conditions such exposures cause adverse health effects, ranging in severity from death to subtle biologic changes. Society's ever-increasing desire to identify and prevent these effects has prompted the dramatic evolution of toxicology as a study of poisons to the present-day complex science.

DEFINITION AND PURPOSE OF TOXICOLOGY

To state it simply and concisely, toxicology is the study of the nature and mechanism of toxic effects of substances on living organisms and other biologic systems. It also deals with quantitative assessment of the severity and frequency of these effects in relation to the exposure of the organisms.

The assessment of health hazards of industrial chemicals, environmental pollutants, and other substances represents an important element in the protection of the health of the worker and members of communities. In-depth studies of the nature and mechanism of the effects of toxicants are invaluable in the invention of specific antidotes and other ameliorative measures. Along with other sciences, toxicology contributes to the development of safer chemicals used as drugs, food additives, pesticides, and many useful industrial chemicals. Even the toxic effects per se are exploited in the pursuit of more effective insecticides, anthelmintics, antimicrobials, and agents used in chemical warfare.

3

SCOPE AND SUBDISCIPLINES

Toxicology has a broad scope. It deals with toxicity studies of chemicals used (1) in medicine for diagnostic, preventive, and therapeutic purposes, (2) in the food industry as direct and indirect additives, (3) in agriculture as pesticides, growth regulators, artificial pollinators, and animal feed additives, and (4) in the chemical industry as solvents, components, and intermediates of plastics and many other types of chemicals. It is also concerned with the health effects of metals (as in mines and smelters), petroleum products, paper and pulp, toxic plants, and animal toxins.

Because of its broad scope as well as the need to accomplish different goals, toxicology has a number of subdisciplines. For example, a person may be exposed, accidentally or otherwise, to very large amounts of a toxicant, and become grossly intoxicated. If the identity of the toxicant is not known, *analytical toxicology* will be called upon to identify the toxicant through analysis of body fluids, stomach contents, suspected containers, etc. Those engaged in *clinical toxicology* will administer antidotes, if available, to counter the specific toxicity, and take other measures to ameliorate the symptoms and signs and hasten the elimination of the toxicant from the body. There may also be legal implications, and that will be the task of *forensic toxicology*.

Intoxication may occur as a result of occupational exposure to toxicants. This may result in acute or chronic adverse effects. In either case, the problem is in the domain of *occupational toxicology*. The general public is exposed to a variety of toxicants, via air and water as well as from food as additives, pesticides, and contaminants, often at low levels that may be harmless acutely but may have long-term adverse effects. The sources of these substances, their transport, degradation, and bioconcentration in the environment, and their effects on humans are dealt with in *environmental toxicology*. *Regulatory toxicology* attempts to protect the public by setting laws, regulations, and standards to limit or suspend the use of very toxic chemicals and define use conditions for others. Some of the relevant laws in the United States are listed in Appendix 1-1.

To set meaningful regulations and standards, extensive profiles of the toxic effects are essential. Such profiles can only be established with a great variety of relevant toxicological studies, which form the foundation of regulatory toxicology. The basic part of such studies is referred to as *conventional toxicology*. In addition, knowledge of the mechanism of action, provided by *mechanistic toxicology*, enhances the toxicological evaluation and provides a basis for other branches of toxicology.

EARLY DEVELOPMENTS

The earliest human was well aware of the toxic effects of a number of substances, such as venoms of snakes, the poisonous plants hemlock and aconite, and the toxic mineral substances arsenic, lead, and antimony. Some of these were actually used intentionally for their toxic effects to commit homicide and suicide. For centuries, homicides with toxic substances were not uncommon in Europe. To protect against poisoning, there were continual efforts directed toward the discovery and development of preventive and antidotal measures. However, a more critical evaluation of these measures was only begun by Maimonides (1135–1204) with his famous *Poisons and Their Antidotes*, published in 1198.

More significant contributions to the evolution of toxicology were made in the sixteenth century and later. Paracelsus stated: "No substance is a poison by itself. It is the dose that makes a substance a poison" and "the right dose differentiates a poison and a remedy." These statements laid the foundation of the concept of the "dose-response relation" and the "therapeutic index" developed later. In addition, he described in his book *Bergsucht* (1533–1534) the clinical manifestations of chronic arsenic and mercury poisoning as well as miner's disease. This might be considered the forefather of occupational toxicology. Orfila wrote an important treatise (1814–1815) describing a systematic correlation between the chemical and biologic information on certain poisons. He also devised methods for detecting poisons and pointed to the necessity for chemical analysis for legal proof of lethal intoxication. The introduction of this approach ushered in a specialty area of modern toxicology, namely, forensic toxicology.

RECENT DEVELOPMENTS

In the face of a growing population, modern society demands improvements of health and living conditions, including nutrition, clothing, dwelling, and transportation. To meet this goal, a great variety of chemicals, many of them in large quantities, must be manufactured and used. It has been estimated that tens of thousands of different chemicals are in commercial production in industrialized countries. In one way or another, these chemicals come in contact with various segments of the population: People are engaged in their manufacture, handling, use (e.g., painters, applicators of pesticides), consumption (e.g., drugs, food additives), or misuse (e.g., suicide, accidental poisoning). Furthermore, people may be exposed to the more persistent chemicals via various environmental media and be affected more insidiously. To illustrate the devastating effects of toxicants, some examples of massive acute and long-term poisonings are listed in Appendix 1-2. In some of these episodes, a considerable amount of sophisticated toxicological investigation was done before the etiology was ascertained.

These and other tragic outbreaks of massive chemical poisonings have resulted in intensified testing programs, which have revealed the great diversity of the nature and site of toxic effects. This revelation, in turn, has called for more studies using a greater number of animals, a greater number of indicators of toxicity, etc. There is, therefore, a need to render the task of toxicologically assessing the vast number of chemicals using increasingly more complex testing procedures more manageable. As an attempt to fulfill this need, criteria have been proposed and adopted for the selection of chemicals to be tested according to their priority. In addition, the "tier systems" allow decisions to be made at different stages of toxicologic testing, thus avoiding unnecessary studies. This procedure has been particularly useful in the testing for carcinogenicity, mutagenicity, and immunotoxicity because of the large expenses involved and the great multitude of test systems that are available (chaps. 7, 8, 10, and 22).

Because of the large number of people exposed to these chemicals, society cannot defer appropriate control until serious injuries have appeared. The modern toxicologist, therefore, must attempt to identify, where possible, indicators of exposure and early, reversible signs of health effects. These will permit the formulation of decisions at the right time to safeguard the health of individuals, either as occupational workers or in exposed communities. The achievements in these areas have assisted responsible personnel in instituting appropriate medical surveillance of occupational workers and other exposed populations. Notable examples are the use of cholinesterase inhibition as an indictor of exposure to organophosphorous pesticides and various biochemical parameters to monitor for lead exposure. Such "biological markers" are intended to measure exposure to toxicants or their effects as well as to detect susceptible population groups (NRC Committee on Biological Markers, 1987); they are used for clinical diagnosis, monitoring of occupational workers, and facilitating safety/risk assessment (WHO, 1993). Examples of biomarkers are described in the relevant sections.

Advances made in biochemical and toxicokinetic studies, as well as those in genetic toxicology and immunotoxicology, morphologic studies on a subcellular level, and biochemical studies on a molecular level, have all contributed to a better understanding of the nature, site, and mechanism of action of toxicants. For example, technological breakthroughs enabled in vitro studies to demonstrate that whether the hepatocytes or the nonparenchymal cells are affected by a chemical carcinogen is related to differences in their ability to repair the DNA damage induced by the chemical. Studies using isolated nephrons have provided insight on the site and mode of action of nephrotoxicant (chap. 13). Various other types of in vitro studies have demonstrated the possibility of their use in screening toxicants for specific effects such as mutagenicity and dermal irritancy. Numerous studies have shown that the responses to toxicants are better correlated with the effective dose, that is, the concentration of the toxicant at the site of action, rather than the administered dose. Furthermore, where the effect results mainly or entirely from an active metabolite, the concentration of the metabolite rather than that of the parent chemical is important.

To translate scientific knowledge into basic tools for the health profession, the toxicologist is ever more involved in the determination of safe exposure limits or an assessment of the risks. The former includes the "acceptable daily intakes" (WHO, 1962) and the "threshold limit values" (*Federal Register*, 1971), whereas the latter is used in connection with substances the effects of which are believed to have no threshold or for which the threshold cannot be determined; such as genotoxic carcinogens and mutagens.

These determinations involve comprehensive studies of the toxic properties, demonstration of dosages that produce no observable adverse effects, establishment of dose-effect and dose-response relationships, and toxicokinetic and biotransformation studies.

The greatly increased scope and the multiplicity of subdisciplines as just outlined provide a vivid view of recent progress in toxicology.

SOME CHALLENGES AND SUCCESSES

The so-called aniline tumors were reported by Rehn (1895), a German surgeon, in the urinary bladders of three men who had worked in an aniline factory. The role of aniline and aniline dyes was confirmed only some 40 years later, after much experimental investigation in animals (e.g., Hueper et al., 1938) and extensive epidemiologic studies by Case et al. (1954) had been carried out. This discovery led to improved occupational standards and more stringent controls of food colors derived from coal tar.

In the late 1950s, thalidomide was widely used as a sedative. It has a very low acute toxicity and readily met the toxicity testing protocol prevailing at that time. However, a rare form of congenital malformation, phocomelia (the virtual absence of extremities), was observed among some offspring of mothers who had taken this drug during the first trimester (Lenz and Knapp, 1962). This tragedy led to the explosive development of teratology, an important specialty area of toxicology. The importance of modifying factors has been dramatized by the tragic effect of cobalt among heavy beer drinkers (see chap. 5).

The once prevalent lead poisoning in certain areas of industrialized countries has now largely disappeared. This great accomplishment in the field of public health resulted from the implementation of control measures devised on the basis of the knowledge gained from the numerous toxicologic studies of lead.

Many cases of serious illness that culminate in permanent paralysis and death have been reported in Minamata and Niigata in Japan in the 1950s and 1960s, respectively (Study Group on Minamata Disease, 1968; Tsubaki and Irukayama, 1977). The cause of the illness was eventually traced to methylmercury in the fish caught locally. The fish was contaminated with this chemical, which had been discharged as such into the water by a factory, or the contaminant was derived from elemental mercury discharged by the factory and methylated through microorganisms in the mud. Measures to rehabilitate the surviving patients and legal control of the factories have been instituted.

On the other hand, the cause of another mysterious illness in Japan, known as itai-itai disease, remains unsolved, although cadmium apparently played a role. The patients had resided for many years in areas that were in the vicinity of mines and where the cadmium levels in rice and water were excessive.

A more solid foundation in the assessment of risks of chemical carcinogens resulted from recent advances in epidemiologic studies, long-term animal studies, short-term mutagenesis/carcinogenesis tests, and mechanistic studies, as well as the realization that carcinogens differ in their potency, latency, and mode of action (chaps. 7 and 22).

FUTURE PROSPECTS

The need for new substances will undoubtedly continue. Some of them will treat or prevent a variety of diseases that are currently untreatable or unpreventable. Others will render food more plentiful, tastier, and hopefully more healthful. Still others will improve living conditions in a variety of ways. At the same time, people are more conscious of subtle adverse effects on health, and expect the new substances to be "absolutely safe." Furthermore, the disposal of these substances and their by-products is expected to cause no environmental hazards adversely affecting humans and the ecosystem.

To satisfy these seemingly irreconcilable societal demands, the toxicologist must carry out a series of studies on each substance: Is it readily absorbed, distributed to specific organs, stored, and/or readily excreted? Is it detoxicated or bioactivated? What kind of toxic effects does it induce and what are the host and environmental factors that can alter these effects? How does it produce the effect on a cellular and molecular level? What type of "general toxicity" does it produce? What organs are its targets? What is its predominant mechanism of action? Answers to these and other questions will provide a scientific basis for assessing its safety and risk for the intended use.

It is evident that the multitude of studies involved will place an increasing demand on the limited facilities for toxicologic testing and on the short supply of qualified personnel. It is of utmost importance therefore that toxicity data generated anywhere be accepted internationally. However, to ensure general acceptance, the data must meet certain standards. The "Good Laboratory Practice" promulgated by the U.S. Food and Drug Administration (FDA, 1980) and the Organization of Economic Cooperation and Development (OECD, 1982) must be adopted by all countries involved in toxicological testing.

To streamline the long and costly testing of each chemical separately, there have been schemes that test a representative chemical extensively and verify the results on other members of the group with minimal testing. This practice has been adopted successfully when the substances included in a group are essentially similar. A recent proposal to ban all chlorine compounds, however, appears to have gone too far in ignoring the great diversity of the toxic nature and potency of such a large group of substances (Karol, 1995). It will be a major challenge to determine how diverse a variety of chemicals can be rationally grouped for toxicological testing and assessment purposes.

Other trends designed to simplify and hasten the testing include a reduction in the use of laboratory animals and methods to supplement or supplant such studies with in vitro studies. This is done partly in response to a societal call on humane grounds. Isolated organs, cultured tissues and cells, and lower forms of life will be increasingly used. Furthermore, such test systems will likely be faster and less expensive, and will augment the variety of studies, especially those related to the mechanism of toxicity. Other types of improvements of the testing procedure with respect to simplicity and reliability will continue to be made.

As noted earlier, to provide a scientific basis for proper assessment of the safety/risk of a chemical and for a variety of other purposes, toxicology is increasingly becoming a multifaceted science. To facilitate the acquisition of a broad knowledge of toxicology, this book is divided into four major areas. General topics related to absorption, distribution, and excretion of toxicants, their transformation in the body, the various types of toxic effects they exert, and the host and environmental factors that modify these effects are covered in Part I. Procedures used to discover the general and specific adverse health effects and organs/systems that are the targets of the toxicants are elaborated in Parts II and III within the broad areas of testing procedures and target organs, respectively. A number of important toxic substances are briefly discussed in Part IV to illustrate the diverse nature of toxicity. The last chapter outlines the widely adopted approaches to the assessment of safety/risk of noncarcinogenic and carcinogenic chemicals. In addition, two indexes are appended, listing chemicals and subjects, respectively, to assist the reader in retrieving relevant parts of the text.

REFERENCES

Case, R. A. M., Hosker, M. E., McDonald, D. B., and Pearson, J. T. 1954. Tumours of the urinary bladder in workmen engaged in the manufacture and use of certain dyestuff intermediates in the British chemical industry. *Br. J. Ind. Med.* 11:75–104.

Federal Register. 1971. Threshold Limit Values adopted by the American Conference of Governmental Industrial Hygienists, 1968. Vol. 36, No. 105, May 29. Washington, DC: U.S. Government Printing Office.

Food and Drug Administration. 1980. Code of Federal Regulations, Title 21, Food and Drugs. Part 58. Washington, DC: U.S. Government Printing Office.

Hueper, W. C., et al. 1938. Experimental production of bladder tumors in dogs by administration of beta-naphthylamine. *J. Ind. Hyg. Toxicol.* 20:46.

Karol, M. H. 1995. Toxicologic principles do not support the banning of chlorine: A Society of Toxicology position paper. *Fundam. Appl. Toxicol.* 24:1–2.

Lenz, W., and Knapp, K. 1962. Thalidomide embryopathy. *Arch. Environ. Health* 5:100–105.

NRC Committee on Biological Markers. 1987. Biological markers in environmental health research. *Environ. Health Perspect.* 74:3–9.

Organization of Economic Cooperation and Development. 1982. Good Laboratory Practice in the Testing of Chemicals. Paris Cedex, France: OECD.

Rehn, L. 1895. Blasengeschwulste bei Fuchsin-Arbeiten. *Arch. Klin. Chir.* 50:588.

Study Group on Minamata Disease. 1968. *Minamata disease.* Minamata, Japan: Minamata University.

Tsubaki, T., and Irukayama, K. 1977. *Minamata disease: Methyl mercury poisoning in Minamata and Niigata, Japan.* New York: Elsevier Scientific.

World Health Organization. 1962. Sixth Report of the Joint FAD/WHO Expert Committee on Food Additives. Geneva: WHO.

World Health Organization. 1993. Biomarkers and Risk Assessment: Concepts and Principles. *Environmental Health Criteria* 155. Geneva: WHO.

Appendix 1-1   U.S. Laws That Have a Basis in Toxicology

Responsible agency	Law
Food and Drug Administration (FDA)	Federal Food, Drug, and Cosmetic Act
Environmental Protection Agency (EPA)	Federal Insecticide and Rodenticide Act
	Clean Air Act
	Safe Drinking Water Act
	Toxic Substances Control Act
Consumer Product Safety Commission (CPSC)	Consumer Product Safety Act
	Federal Hazardous Substance Act
Occupational Safety and Health Administration (OSHA)	Occupational Safety and Health Act

Appendix 1-2 Examples of Outbreaks of Mass Poisoning

Location and year	Toxicant	Adverse effect	Number affected
Detroit, MI, 1930	Tri-o-cresyl phosphate in "ginger jake"	Delayed neurotoxicity	16,000
London, UK, 1952	Sulfur dioxide and suspended particulate matter in air	Increased deaths from heart and lung diseases	3,000
Toyama, Japan, 1950s	Cadmium in rice	Severe kidney and bone disease	200[a]
Minamata, Japan, 1950s	Methylmercury in fish	Severe neurological disease ("Minamata disease")	200[a, b]
Southeast Turkey, 1956	Hexachlorobenzene in wheat	Porphyria, neurological diseases	4,000
Morocco, 1959	Tri-o-cresyl phosphate in adulterated oil	Delayed neurotoxicity	10,000
Japan, 1956–1977	Clioquinol	Subacute myelo-opticoneuropathy (SMON)	10,000
Western Europe, late 1950s and early 1960s	Thalidomide	Phocomelia	10,000
Fukuoka, Japan, 1968	Polychlorinated biphenyls (PCB)	Skin disease, general weakness	1,700
Iraq, 1972	Methylmercury in wheat	Deaths from neurological disease	500
		Nonfatal cases	50,000
Madrid, Spain, 1981	Toxic oil in food	Deaths with various symptoms and signs	340
		Nonfatal cases	20,000
Bhopal, India, 1984	Methylisocyanate released into air	Deaths from acute lung disease	6,000
		Nonfatal cases	200,000

[a]Many more cases with mild or moderate symptoms and signs of intoxication.
[b]Hundreds of cases occurred in Niigata, Japan, in 1960s.

11

Absorption, Distribution, and Excretion of Toxicants

CHAPTER 2 CONTENTS

INTRODUCTION

Apart from local effects at the site of contact, a toxicant can cause injury only after it is absorbed by the organism. Absorption can occur through the skin, the gastrointestinal tract, the lungs, and several minor routes. Furthermore, the nature and intensity of the effects of a chemical on an organism depend on its concentration in the target organs. The concentration depends not only on the administered dose but also on other factors, including absorption, distribution, binding, and excretion. For a chemical to be absorbed, distributed, and eventually excreted, a toxicant must pass through a number of cell membranes. A cell membrane generally consists of a biomolecular layer of lipid molecules with proteins scattered throughout the membrane (see Fig. 2-1).

Figure 2-1 Schematic diagram of biologic membrane. Spheres represent head groups (phosphatidylcholine), and zig-zag lines indicate tail ends of lipids. Black, white, and stippled spheres indicate different kinds of lipids. Large bodies represent proteins; some are located on the surface, others within the membrane (modified from Singer and Nicholson, 1972, p. 720, by permission of the author and the American Association for the Advancement of Science, copyright © 1972).

There are four mechanisms by which a toxicant may pass through a cell membrane; the most important of them is passive diffusion through the membrane. The others are filtration through the membrane pores, carrier-mediated transport, and engulfing by the cell. The last two mechanisms are different in that the cell takes an active part in the transfer of a toxicant across its membranes.

Passive Diffusion

Most toxicants cross cell membranes by simple, passive diffusion. The rate of passage is related directly to the concentration gradient across the membrane, and to the lipid solubility. For example, mannitol is hardly absorbed (<2%); acetylsalicylic acid is fairly well absorbed (21%); and thiopental is even more readily absorbed (67%). It is noteworthy that the chloroform : water partition of the nonionized forms of these chemicals are, respectively, <0.002, 2.0, and 100. For references to this and other examples see Hogben et al. (1958).

Many toxicants are ionizable. The ionized form is often unable to penetrate the cell membrane because of its low lipid solubility. On the other hand, the nonionized form is likely lipid-soluble enough to do so, and its rate of penetration is dependent on the lipid solubility. The extent of ionization of weak organic acids and bases depends on the pH of the medium. Thus, for the former, such as benzoic acid, diffusion is facilitated in an acidic environment, where they exist mainly in the nonionized form;

Figure 2-2 Disposition of benzoic acid and aniline in gastric juice and plasma. Figures immediately below the structural formulas represent proportions of ionized and nonionized forms (from Timbrell, 1991, p. 44).

for the latter, such as aniline, diffusion is facilitated in a basic environment (Figs. 2-2 and 2-3).

Filtration

The membranes of the capillaries and the glomeruli have relatively large pores (about 70 nm) and allow molecules smaller than albumin (molecular mass 60,000 Da) to pass through. Bulk flow of water through these pores results from hydrostatic and/or osmotic pressure and can act as carrier of toxicants. The pores in most cells, however, are relatively small (about 4 nm) and allow chemicals only up to a molecular weight of 100–200 to

Figure 2-3 Disposition of benzoic acid and aniline in intestinal juice and plasma (from Timbrell, 1991, p. 45).

pass through. Chemicals of larger molecules, therefore, can filter into and out of the capillaries. They can, therefore, establish equilibrium between the concentrations in the plasma and in the extracellular fluid, but they cannot do so by filtration between the extracellular and intracellular fluids.

Carrier-Mediated Transport

This involves the formation of a complex between the chemical and a macromolecular carrier on one side of the membrane. The complex then diffuses to the other side of the membrane, where the chemical is released. Thereafter the carrier returns to the original surface to repeat the transport process. The carrier has a limited capacity. When it is saturated, the rate of transport is no longer dependent on the concentration of the chemical and assumes zero-order kinetics. Structure, conformation, size, and charge are important in determining the affinity of a chemical for a carrier site, and competitive inhibition can occur among chemicals with similar characteristics.

Active transport involves a carrier that moves molecules across a membrane against a concentration gradient, or, if the molecule is an ion, against an electrochemical gradient. It requires the expenditure of metabolic energy and can be inhibited by poisons that interfere with cell metabolism.

Facilitated diffusion is similar to active transport but does not move molecules against a concentration gradient. Furthermore, it is not energy dependent, and metabolic poisons will not inhibit this process.

Engulfing by the Cell (Endocytosis)

Particles may be engulfed by cells. When the particles are solid the process is called phagocytosis, and when they are liquid it is called pinocytosis. Such special transport systems are important for removal of particulate matter from the alveoli and of certain toxic substances from the blood by the reticuloendothelial system. Absorption of the food additive carrageenan (molecular weight about 40,000) from the gut is also by this process.

ABSORPTION

The main routes by which toxicants are absorbed are the gastrointestinal (GI) tract, lungs, and skin. However, in toxicologic studies, such special routes as intraperitoneal, intramuscular, and subcutaneous injections are also used.

Gastrointestinal Tract

Many toxicants can enter the GI tract along with food and water or alone as drugs or other types of chemicals. With the exception of those that are caustic or very irritating to the mucosa, most toxicants do not exert any toxic effect unless they are absorbed. Absorption can take place along the entire GI tract. For example, certain drugs are administered as sublingual tablets and suppositories to be absorbed in the mouth and the rectum, respectively. However, the mouth and rectum are, in general, insignificant sites of absorption of environmental chemicals.

The stomach is a significant site of absorption, especially for weak acids, which will exist in the diffusible, nonionized, lipid-soluble form. On the other hand, weak bases will be highly ionized in the acidic gastric juice and therefore not readily absorbable. The difference in absorption is further amplified by the circulating plasma. Weak acids will exist mainly in ionized form in plasma and be carried away, whereas weak bases will exist in nonionized form and can diffuse back to the stomach. The influence of these factors, using benzoic acid and aniline as examples, is shown in Fig. 2-2.

In the intestine, weak acids will exist mainly in the ionized form, hence less readily absorbable. However, upon entering the blood, they become ionized and thus will not readily diffuse back. On the other hand, weak bases will exist mainly in the nonionized form, hence more readily absorbable as shown in Fig. 2-3. It should be noted that intestinal absorption is further enhanced by the long contact time and the large surface area provided by the villi and microvilli.

In the intestine, there are special carrier-mediated transport systems that are responsible for the absorption of nutrients, such as monosaccharides, amino acids, and such elements as iron, calcium, and sodium. However, a few toxicants, such as 5-fluorouracil, thallium, and lead, are known to be absorbable from the intestine by active transport systems. In addition, particulate matters such as those of the azo dyes and polystyrene latex can enter the intestinal cell by pinocytosis.

Respiratory Tract

The main site of absorption in the respiratory tract is the alveoli in the lungs. This is especially true for gases such as carbon monoxide, nitrogen oxides, and sulfur dioxide and for vapors of volatile liquids such as benzene and carbon tetrachloride. Their ready absorption is related to the large alveolar area, high blood flow, and proximity of the blood to the alveolar air.

The rate of absorption is dependent on the solubility of the gas in the blood: the more soluble it is, the faster the absorption. However, equilibrium between the air and the blood is reached more slowly for more soluble chemicals, such as chloroform, compared to less soluble chemicals such as ethylene. This is because the more soluble a chemical is, the more of it can be dissolved in the blood. Since the alveolar air can only carry a limited amount of the chemical, more respirations and hence a longer time will be required to attain equilibrium. It will take even longer if the chemical is also deposited in the fat tissue.

In addition to gases and vapors, liquid aerosols and airborne particles may also be absorbed. In general, large particles (>10 μm) do not enter the respiratory tract; when they do, they are deposited in the nose and disposed of by wiping, blowing, and sneezing. Very small particles (<0.01 μm) are likely to be exhaled. Those in the range of $0.01-10$ μm are deposited in various parts of the respiratory tract. The larger ones are likely to be deposited in the nasopharynx and absorbed either through the epithelium of this region or through the gastrointestinal tract epithelium after they are swallowed along with the mucus. Smaller particles are deposited in the trachea, bronchi, and bronchioli and are then either aspirated onto the mucociliary escalator or engulfed by phagocytes. The particles carried up by the escalator will be coughed up or swallowed. The phagocytes with engulfed particles will be absorbed into the lymphatics. Some free particles can also migrate into the lymphatics. Soluble particles may be absorbed through the epithelium into the blood.

A detailed examination of the deposition of particles of various sizes in different parts of the respiratory tract is provided by a Task Group on Lung Dynamics (1966). However, as a rough estimate, 25% of inhaled particles are exhaled, 50% are deposited in the upper respiratory tract, and 25% are deposited in the lower respiratory tract (Morrow et al., 1966).

Skin

In general, the skin is relatively impermeable, and therefore it constitutes a good barrier, separating the organism from its environment. However, some chemicals can be absorbed through the skin in sufficient quantities to produce systemic effects.

A chemical may be absorbed via the hair follicles or through the cells of the sweat glands or those of the sebaceous glands. These are, however, minor routes for absorption since they constitute only a small surface area of the skin. Therefore, the percutaneous absorption of a chemical is essentially through the skin proper, which consists of the epidermis and dermis (see Fig. 14-1).

The first phase of percutaneous absorption is diffusion of the toxicant through the epidermis, which, especially its stratum corneum, is the most important barrier. The stratum corneum consists of several layers of thin, cohesive, dead cells that contain chemically resistant material (protein filament). Small amounts of polar substances appear to diffuse through the outer surface of the protein filaments of the hydrated stratum corneum; nonpolar substances dissolve in and diffuse through the lipid matrix between the protein filaments.

In the human stratum corneum, there are significant differences in structure and chemistry from one region of the body to another, which are reflected in the permeability to chemicals. For example, toxicants cross the scrotum readily, cross the abdominal skin less readily, and cross the sole and palm with great difficulty (Zbinden, 1976).

The second phase of percutaneous absorption is diffusion of the toxicant through the dermis, which contains a porous, nonselective, aqueous diffusion medium. Therefore it is much less effective as a barrier than the stratum corneum, and, as a consequence, abrasion or removal of the latter causes a marked increase in the percutaneous absorption. Acids, alkalis, and mustard gases will also increase the absorption by injuring this barrier. Some solvents, notably dimethyl sulfoxide (DMSO), also increase dermal permeability.

DISTRIBUTION

After a chemical enters the blood, it is distributed rapidly throughout the body. The rate of distribution to each organ is related to the blood flow through the organ, the ease with which the chemical crosses the local capillary wall and the cell membrane, and the affinity of components of the organ for the chemical.

Barriers

The *blood–brain barrier* is located at the capillary wall. The capillary endothelial cells there are tightly joined, leaving few or no pores between these cells (Bradbury, 1984). Thus, the toxicant has to pass through the capillary endothelium itself. A lack of vesicles in these cells further reduces their transport ability. Finally, the protein concentration of the interstitial fluid in the brain is low, in contrast to that in other organs; protein binding therefore does not serve as a mechanism for the transfer of toxicants from the blood to the brain. For these reasons, the penetration of toxicants into the brain is dependent on their lipid solubility. An outstanding example is the toxicant methylmercury, which enters the brain readily and the main toxicity of which is on the central nervous system. In contrast, inorganic mercury compounds are not lipid soluble, do not enter the brain readily, and exert their main adverse effects not on the brain but on the kidney.

The *placental barrier* differs anatomically among various animal species. There are six layers of cells between fetal and maternal blood in some species, whereas in others there is only one layer. Furthermore, the number of layers may change as the gestation progresses. Although the relationship of the number of layers of the placenta to its permeability needs quantitative determination, the placental barrier does impede the transfer of toxicants to the fetus, which is therefore protected to some extent. However, the concentration of a toxicant such as methylmercury may be higher in certain fetal organs, such as the brain, because of the less effective fetal blood–brain barrier. On the other hand, the fetal concentration of the food coloring amaranth is only 0.03–0.06% of that of the mother (Munro and Willes, 1978).

Other barriers are also present in such organs as the eyes and testicles. In addition, the erythrocyte plays an interesting role in the distribution of certain toxicants. For example, its membrane acts as a barrier against the penetration of inorganic mercury compounds but not that of alkylmercury. Furthermore, there is affinity of the erythrocyte cytoplasm for alkylmercury compounds. Because of these factors, the concentration of inorganic mercury compounds in the erythrocytes is only about half that in the plasma, whereas that of methylmercury in the erythrocyte is about ten times that in the plasma (WHO, 1976).

Binding and Storage

As noted earlier, binding of a chemical in a tissue can result in a higher concentration in that tissue. There are two major types of binding. The covalent type of binding is irreversible and is, in general, associated with significant toxic effects. The noncovalent binding usually accounts for a major portion of the dose and is reversible. Therefore, this process plays an important role in the distribution of toxicants in various organs and tissues. There are several types of noncovalent binding as outlined by Riviere (1994).

Plasma proteins can bind normal physiologic constituents in the body as well as many foreign compounds. Most of the latter are bound to the albumin and are therefore not immediately available for distribution to the extravascular space. However, since the binding is reversible, it permits the bound chemical to dissociate from the protein, thereby replenishing the level of unbound chemical, which may then cross the capillary endothelium. The toxicologic significance of the binding can be illustrated by the possible induction of coma by the administration of sulfonamide drugs to patients who are taking antidiabetic drugs. The antidiabetic drugs are bound to the plasma proteins but can be replaced by the sulfonamide drugs, which have a greater affinity for the plasma protein. The antidiabetic drugs thus released may precipitate a hypoglycemic coma.

The *liver* and *kidney* have a higher capacity for binding chemicals. This characteristic may be related to their metabolic and excretory functions. Certain proteins have been identified in these organs for their specific binding property, such as metallothionein, which is important for the binding of cadmium in the liver and kidney and possibly also for the transfer of the metal from the liver to the kidney. Binding of a substance can increase its concentration in an organ rapidly. For example, 30 min after a single administration of lead, its concentration in the liver is 50 times higher than that in the plasma.

The *adipose tissue* is an important storage depot for lipid-soluble substances such as DDT, dieldrin, and polychlorinated biphenyls (PCB). They appear to be stored in the adipose tissue by simple dissolution in the neutral fats. There exists the potential that the plasma concentration of the substances stored in the fat may rise sharply as a result of rapid mobilization of fat following starvation. Conjugation of fatty acid to toxicants such as DDT may also be a mechanism by which these chemicals are retained in the lipid-containing tissues and cells of the body (Leighty et al., 1980).

Bone is a major site for storage for such toxicants as fluoride, lead, and strontium. The storage takes place by an exchange adsorption reaction between the toxicants in the interstitial fluid and the hydroxyapatite crystals of bone mineral. By virtue of similarities in size and charge, F^- may readily replace OH^-, and calcium may be replaced by lead or strontium. These stored substances can be released by ionic exchange and by dissolution of bone crystals through osteoclastic activity.

EXCRETION

After absorption and distribution in the organism, toxicants are excreted, rapidly or slowly. A generally accepted indicator of the rate of elimination of a toxicant is its "half-life" ($t_{1/2}$), which is the time required for 50% of it to be removed from the bloodstream.

The toxicants are excreted as the parent chemicals, as their metabolites, and/or as conjugates of them. The principal route of excretion is the urine, but the liver and lungs are also important excretory organs for certain types of chemicals. In addition, there are a number of minor routes of excretion.

Urinary Excretion

The kidney removes toxicants from the body by the same mechanisms as those used in the removal of end products of normal metabolism, namely, glomerular filtration, tubular diffusion, and tubular secretion.

The glomerular capillaries have large pores (70 nm); therefore, most toxicants will be filtered at the glomerulus, except those that are very large (greater than 60,000 Da) or are tightly bound to plasma protein. Once a toxicant enters the glomerular filtrate, it will either be passively reabsorbed across the tubular cells if it has a high lipid/water partition coefficient or remain in the tubular lumen and be excreted if it is a polar compound.

A toxicant can also be excreted through the tubules into the urine by passive diffusion. Since urine is normally acidic, this process plays a role in the excretion of organic bases. On the other hand, organic acids are unlikely to be excreted by passive diffusion through the tubular cells. However, weak acids are often metabolized to stronger acids, thereby increasing the percentage of the ionic forms that are not reabsorbed through the tubular cells and are thus excreted.

Certain toxicants can be secreted by the cells of the proximal tubules into the urine. There are two distinct secretory mechanisms, one for organic acids (e.g., glucuronide and sulfate conjugates) and the other for organic bases. Protein-bound toxicants can also be secreted, provided the binding is reversible. Furthermore, chemicals of similar characteristics compete for the same transport system. For example, probenecid can increase the serum level of penicillin and prolong its activity by blocking its tubular excretion.

Biliary Excretion

The liver is also an important organ for the excretion of toxicants, especially for compounds with high polarity (anionic and cationic), conjugates of compounds bound to plasma proteins, and compounds with molecular weights greater than 300. In general, once these compounds are in the bile, they are not reabsorbed into the blood and are excreted via the feces. However, there are exceptions, such as the glucuronide conjugates, which can be hydrolyzed by intestinal flora, enabling the reabsorption of the free toxicants.

The importance of the biliary route of excretion for some chemicals has been well demonstrated in experiments that showed a severalfold increase of the acute toxicity in animals with ligated bile ducts. Such chemicals include digoxin, indocyanine green, ouabain, and, most dramatically, diethylstilbestrol (DES). The toxicity of DES is increased by a factor of 130 in rats with ligated bile ducts (Klaassen, 1973).

Lungs

Substances that exist in the gaseous phase at body temperature are excreted mainly by the lungs. Volatile liquids are also readily excreted via the expired air. Highly soluble liquids such as chloroform and halothane are excreted slowly because of their storage in the adipose tissue and the limited ventilation volume. Excretion of toxicants from the lung is accomplished by simple diffusion through cell membranes.

Other Routes

The gastrointestinal tract is not a major route of excretion of toxicants. However, because the human stomach and intestine each secretes about 3 L of fluid per day, some toxicants are excreted along with the fluid. The excretion is mainly by diffusion and thus the rate depends on the pK_a of the toxicant and the pH of the stomach and intestine.

The excretion of toxicants in mother's milk is not important as far as the host organism is concerned. However, the presence of toxic substances in milk may be toxicologically significant because they can be passed in the milk from the mother to the nursing child and from cows to humans. The excretion is also via simple diffusion. Since milk is slightly acidic, basic compounds will reach a higher level in milk than in plasma, while the opposite is true with acidic compounds. Lipophilic compounds such as DDT and PCB also reach a higher level in milk because of its higher fat content.

Sweat and saliva are also minor routes of excretion of toxicants. The excretion is also by diffusion; thus it is confined to the nonionized, lipid-soluble forms of the toxicants. Substances excreted in the saliva are usually swallowed and then become available for absorption in the GI tract.

LEVELS OF TOXICANTS IN THE BODY

As noted earlier, the nature and intensity of the effects of a chemical depend on its concentration at the site of action, namely, the effective dose rather than the administered dose. The level in the target organ is, in general, a function of the blood level. However, binding of a toxicant in a tissue will increase its level, whereas tissue barriers tend to reduce the level. Since the blood level is more readily determined, especially over a time period, it is the parameter often used in toxicokinetic studies.

While the toxicant is being absorbed, its blood level rises. In the meantime, the rates of its excretion, biotransformation (see chap. 3), and the distribution to other organs and tissues also increase. The curve depicting the blood level against time and the area under that curve (AUC) are useful tools in toxicokinetics. In a series of experimental studies, Smyth and Hottendorf (1980) demonstrated that the AUC for a solution of a chemical is, in general, greater than that for its suspension, and it is greater for acidic than basic chemicals. They also illustrated the effects of the route of administration, dose level, and dosing vehicle on the AUC.

The influence of the rate of excretion on the blood level is vividly shown in Fig. 2-4. Saccharin is rapidly excreted; hence its blood level drops rapidly, even after repeated administration. On the other hand, methylmercury is excreted very slowly; its gradual accumulation culminates in a near plateau only after 270 d (Munro and Willes, 1978).

Figure 2-4 Comparative chemobiokinetics of saccharin and methylmercury chloride (adapted from Munro and Willes, 1978, p. 138).

Methods for determining the rate and extent of absorption, distribution, binding, storage, and excretion at various organs and tissues are readily found in the literature. A summary of some of them is given in a World Health Organization publication (WHO, 1986).

REFERENCES

Bradbury, M. W. B. 1984. The structure and function of the blood-brain barrier. *Fed. Proc.* 43:186–190.

Hogben, C. A. M., Tocco, D. J., Brodie, B. B., and Schanker, L. S. 1958. On the mechanism of intestinal absorption of drugs. *J. Pharmacol. Exp. Ther.* 125:275–282.

Klaassen, C. D. 1973. Comparison of the toxicity of chemicals in newborn rats to bile duct-ligated and sham-operated rats and mice. *Toxicol. Appl. Pharmacol.* 24:37–44.

Leighty, E. G., Fentiman, A. F., Jr., and Thompson, R. M. 1980. Conjugation of fatty acids to DDT in the rat: Possible mechanism for retention. *Toxicology* 15:77–82.

Morrow, P. E., Hodge, H. C., Newman, W. F., Maynard, E. A., Blanchet, H. J., Jr., Fassett, D. W., Birk, R. E., and Mavrodt, S. 1966. Deposition and retention models for internal dosimetry of the human respiratory tract. *Health Phys.* 12:173–207.

Munro, I. O., and Willes, A. F. 1978. Reproductive toxicity and the problems of in vitro exposure. In *Chemical toxicology of food*, eds. A. Galli, R. Paoletti, and G. Veterazzi, pp. 133–145. Amsterdam: Elsevier/North Holland.

Riviere, J. E. 1994. Absorption and distribution. In *Introduction to biochemical toxicology*, eds. E. Hodgson and P. E. Levi. Norwalk, CT: Appleton & Lange.

Singer, S. J., and Nicolson, G. C. 1972. The fluid mosaic model of the structure of cell membranes. *Science* 175:720–731.

Smyth, A. D., and Hottendorf, G. H. 1980. Application of pharmacokinetics and biopharmaceutics in the design of toxicological studies. *Toxicol. Appl. Pharmacol.* 53:179–195.

Task Group on Lung Dynamics 1966. Deposition and retention models for internal dosimetry of the human respiratory tract. *Health Phys.* 12:173–207.

Timbrell, J. A. 1991. *Principles of biochemical toxicology.* London: Taylor & Francis.

World Health Organization. 1976. Mercury. Environmental Health Criteria 1, p. 70. Geneva: WHO.

World Health Organization. 1986. Principles of Toxicokinetic Studies. Environmental Health Criteria 57. Geneva: WHO.

Zbinden, G. 1976. Percutaneous drug permeation. In *Progress in toxicology*, Vol. 2, pp. 50–57. New York: Springer-Verlag.

ADDITIONAL READING

Klaassen, C. D., and Rozman, K. 1993. Absorption, distribution and excretion of toxicants. In *Casarett and Doull's toxicology*, eds. M. O. Amdur, J. Doull, and C. D. Klaassen, pp. 50–87. New York: McGraw-Hill.

Matthews, H. B. 1980. Elimination of toxicants and their metabolites. In *Introduction to biochemical toxicology*, eds. E. Hodgson and F. E. Guthrie. New York: Elsevier.

Biotransformation of Toxicants

CHAPTER 3 CONTENTS

GENERAL CONSIDERATIONS

As noted in the previous chapter, a toxicant can be absorbed into an organism via different routes. After absorption it is distributed to various parts of the body, including the excretory organs, and is thus available for excretion. Many chemicals are known to undergo biotransformation (metabolic transformation) while in the organs and tissues. The most important site of such reactions is the liver, the others being the lungs, stomach, intestine, skin, and kidneys.

There are two types of biotransformation:

1 Phase I, involving oxidation, reduction, and hydrolysis, may be considered degradation reactions;

2   Phase II, involving the production of a compound (a conjugate) that is biosynthesized from the toxicant, or its metabolite, plus an endogenous metabolite, may be considered conjugation reactions.

Biotransformation is, therefore, a process that, in general, converts the parent compounds into metabolites and then forms conjugates, but it may involve only one of these reactions. For example, benzene undergoes oxidation, a phase I reaction, to form phenol, which conjugates with sulfate, a phase II reaction. However, when the administered chemical is phenol, it will conjugate with sulfate without a phase I reaction. The metabolites and conjugates are usually more water soluble and more polar, hence more readily excretable. Biotransformation can therefore be considered a mechanism of detoxication by the host organism.

However, it must be noted that in certain cases the metabolites are more toxic than the parent compounds. Such reactions are known as "bioactivation."

The rate of biotransformation and the type of biotransformation of a toxicant differ from one species of animal to another and even from one strain to another, a fact that often accounts for the difference of toxicity in these animals (see chap. 5). The age and sex of the animal and exposures to other chemicals may also alter the biotransformation. Knowledge of such factors is important in the design of toxicologic studies and in the interpretation of health hazards of toxicants to humans.

PHASE I (DEGRADATION) REACTIONS

The three types of phase I reactions, namely, oxidation, reduction, and hydrolysis, are briefly described:

Oxidation

The biotransformation of a great variety of chemicals involves oxidative processes. The most important enzyme systems catalyzing the processes involve cytochrome P-450 and NADPH cytochrome P-450 reductase. In these reactions, one atom of molecular oxygen is reduced to water and the other is incorporated into the substrate.

The cytochrome-linked monooxygenases (oxidases) are located in the endoplasmic reticulum. When a cell is homogenized, the endoplasmic reticulum breaks down to small vesicles known as microsomes. Because of the location of these enzymes and the great variety of chemicals that they may catalyze, they are also known as microsomal, mixed-function oxidases (MFO). In addition, oxidation of a number of toxicants is catalyzed by nonmicrosomal oxidoreductases that are located in the mitochondrial fraction or in the 100,000-g supernatant of tissue homogenates.

Oxidation may take place in a variety of reactions, and often more than one metabolite is formed. The following are some examples:

A   Microsomal oxidation
1   Aliphatic oxidation involves oxidation of the aliphatic side chains of aromatic chemicals: e.g., *n*-propylbenzene → 3-phenylpropan-1-ol, 3-phenylpropan-2-ol, and 3-phenylpropan-3-ol, as well as aliphatic compounds such as *n*-hexane.
2   Aromatic hydroxylation generally proceeds through an epoxide intermediate: e.g., naphthalene → naphthalene-1,2-epoxide → 1-naphthol + 2-naphthol.
3   Epoxidation: e.g., aldrin → dieldrin.
4   Oxidative deamination: e.g., amphetamine → phenylacetone.
5   *N*-Dealkylation: e.g., *N,N*-dimethyl-*p*-nitrophenyl carbamate → *N*-methyl-*p*-nitrophenyl carbamate.
6   *O*-Dealkylation: e.g., *p*-nitroanisole → *p*-nitrophenol.
7   *S*-Dealkylation: e.g., 6-methylthiopurine → 6-mercaptothiopurine.
8   *N*-Oxidation: e.g., trimethylamine → trimethylamine oxide.
9   *N*-Hydroxylation: e.g., aniline → phenylhydroxylamine.
10   *P*-Oxidation: e.g., diphenylmethylphosphine → diphenylmethylphosphine oxide.
11   Sulfoxidation: e.g., methiocarb → methiocarb sulfone.
12   Desulfuration involves the replacement of S by O: e.g., parathion → paraoxon.

B   Nonmicrosomal oxidations
1   Amine oxidation: Monoamine oxidase is located in mitochondria and diamine oxidase is a cytosolic enzyme. Both are involved in the oxidation of the primary, secondary, and tertiary amines, such as 5-hydroxytryptamine and putrescine, into corresponding aldehydes.
2   Alcohol and aldehyde dehydrogenations are catalyzed, respectively, by alcohol dehydrogenase and aldehyde dehydrogenase: e.g., ethanol → acetaldehyde → acetic acid.

Reduction

Toxicants may undergo reductions through the function of reductases. These reactions are less active in mammalian tissues but more so in intestinal bacteria. A notable example is the reduction of prontosil to sulfanilamide.

A   Microsomal reduction

1   Nitro reduction: e.g., nitrobenzene → nitrosobenzene → phenylhydroxylamine → aniline.

2 Azo reduction: e.g., azobenzene → aniline.

B Nonmicrosomal reductions occur via the reverse reaction of alcohol dehydrogenases (see Oxidation, B-2 earlier).

Hydrolysis

Many toxicants contain ester-type bonds and are subject to hydrolysis. These are essentially esters, amides, and compounds of phosphate. Mammalian tissues, including the plasma, contain a large number of nonspecific esterases and amidases, which are involved in hydrolysis. The esterases, usually located in the soluble fraction of the cell, may be broadly categorized into four classes (Testa and Jenner, 1976):

1 Arylesterases, which hydrolyze aromatic esters.
2 Carboxylesterases, which hydrolyze aliphatic esters.
3 Cholinesterases, which hydrolyze esters in which the alcohol moiety is choline.
4 Acetylesterases, which hydrolyze esters in which the acid moiety is acetic acid.

In contrast to esterases, amidases cannot be classified according to substrate specificity. Furthermore, enzymatic hydrolysis of amides proceeds much more slowly than that of esters, probably a result of the lack of substrate specificity.

PHASE II (CONJUGATION) REACTIONS

Phase II reactions involve several types of endogenous metabolites that, as noted earlier, may form conjugates with the toxicants per se or their metabolites. These conjugates are generally more water soluble and more readily excretable. This is because the physiological transport mechanisms for the endogenous metabolites also recognize the conjugates and hence facilitate their excretion.

Glucuronide Formation

This is the most common and most important type of conjugation. The enzyme catalyzing this reaction is UDP-glucuronyl transferase (uridine disphosphate glucuronyl transferase) and the coenzyme is UDPGA (uridine-5'-diphospho-α-D-glucuronic acid). This enzyme is also located in the endoplasmic reticulum. There are four classes of chemical compounds that are capable of forming conjugates with glucuronic acid: (1) aliphatic or aromatic alcohols, (2) carboxylic acids, (3) sulfhydryl compounds, and (4) amines.

Sulfate Conjugation

This reaction is catalyzed by sulfotransferases. These enzymes are found in the cytosolic fraction of liver, kidney, and intestine. The coenzyme is PAPS (3'-phosphoadenosine 5'-phosphosulfate). The functional groups of the foreign compounds for sulfate transfer are phenols and aliphatic alcohols as well as aromatic amines.

Methylation

This reaction is catalyzed by methyl transferases. The coenzyme is SAM (S-adenosylmethionine). Methylation is not a major route of biotransformation of toxicants because of the broader availability of UDPGA, which leads to the formation of glucuronides. Furthermore, it does not always increase the water solubility of the methylated products.

Acetylation

Acetylation involves transfer of acetyl groups to primary aromatic amines, hydrazines, hydrazides, sulfonamides, and certain primary aliphatic amines. The enzyme and coenzyme involved are respectively N-acetyl transferases and acetyl coenzyme A. In certain cases, such as isoniazid, acetylation results in a decrease in water solubility of an amine and an increase in toxicity.

Amino Acid Conjugation

This conjugation is catalyzed by amino acid conjugates and coenzyme A. Aromatic carboxylic acids, arylacetic acids, and aryl-substituted acrylic acids can form conjugates with α-amino acids, mainly glycine, but also glutamine in humans and certain monkeys and ornithine in birds.

Glutathione Conjugation

This important reaction is effected by glutathione S-transferases and the cofactor glutathione. Glutathione conjugates subsequently undergo enzymatic cleavage and acetylation, forming N-acetylcysteine (mercapturic acid) derivatives of the toxicants, which are readily excreted. Examples of chemicals such as epoxides and aromatic halogens that conjugate with glutathione are shown in Fig. 3-1. In addition, glutathione can conjugate unsaturated aliphatic compounds and displace nitro groups in chemicals.

In the process of biotransformation of toxicants, a number of highly reactive electrophilic metabolites are formed. Some of these metabolites can react with cellular constituents and cause cell death, induce tumor

Figure 3-1 Conjugation of epoxide and dehalogenation catalyzed by glutathione (GSH) transferase (from Timbrell, 1991).

formation, or affect immune function. The role of glutathione is to react with the electrophilic metabolites and thus prevent their harmful effects on the cells. However, exposure to very large amounts of such reactive substances can deplete the glutathione, thereby resulting in marked toxic effects. An example of the depletion of glutathione by acetaminophen and the concomitant increase in covalent binding to macromolecules is shown in Fig. 3-2. Similarly, 3-methylindole is bioactivated mainly in lungs and, after depleting the glutathione, will induce lung damages (Adams et al., 1988). Furthermore, certain glutathione conjugates may become toxic (Anders et al., 1988).

For additional information on the biological functions of glutathione in the conjugation of electrophiles and as antioxidant, see DeLeve and Kaplowitz (1991).

BIOACTIVATION

Certain chemically stable compounds can be converted to chemically reactive metabolites. The reactions are generally catalyzed by cytochrome P-450-dependent monooxygenase systems, but other enzymes, including those of the intestinal flora, are involved in certain cases. Furthermore, additional phase I or phase II reactions may be required. The reactive metabolites, such as epoxides, can become covalently bound to cellular macromolecules and cause necrosis and/or cancer. Others, such as free radicals, can cause lipid peroxidation resulting in tissue damage. Descriptions of the bioactivation of various classes of chemicals are available in

Figure 3-2 Protective effect of gluta-thione against covalent binding of acet-aminophen to liver proteins (from Wills, 1981).

the literature, such as the chapter by Levi (1994). The following are some notable examples. Appendix 3-1 lists a number of chemicals that are known to be bioactivated.

Epoxide Formation

Many aromatic compounds are converted to epoxides by microsomal mixed-function oxygenase systems. The biotransformation of bromoben-zene to its epoxide and subsequent reactions serve as an interesting ex-ample of bioactivation and its consequences. These are depicted in Fig. 3-3.

Although bromobenzene epoxide may become covalently bound to tis-sue macromolecules and cause injury, the alternative routes of metabolism

Figure 3-3 The bromobenzene epoxide formed from the parent chemical may covalently bind to macromolecules, but such binding may be minimal when the other metabolic routes are predominant (from Gillette and Mitchell, 1975).

may prevent or reduce the injury. The most important of these routes is the conjugation with glutathione. This reaction is important in that it serves as a protective mechanism. Only after the hepatic levels of reduced glutathione have been greatly depleted will the bromobenzene epoxide significantly bind to macromolecules and result in hepatic necrosis. Depletion of glutathione occurs when a huge dose of bromobenzene is present or when there has been an induction of microsomal enzymes; both conditions increase the amount of bromobenzene epoxide. Other reactions include a nonenzymatic arrangement to form p-bromophenol and the formation of 3,4-dihydro-3,4-dihydroxybromobenzene catalyzed by hydrase.

Other chemicals that undergo epoxidation include aflatoxin B_1, benzene, benzo[a]pyrene, furosemide, olefins, polychlorinated and polybrominated biphenyls, trichloroethylene, and vinyl chloride. The bioactivation takes place mainly in the liver, and the resulting reactive metabolites induce toxicity through covalent binding with macromolecules in the tissue, resulting in necrosis or cancer formation.

N-Hydroxylation

Microsomal enzymes from many tissues can N-hydroxylate a variety of chemicals. Some of the N-hydroxy metabolites, such as those of acetaminophen, 2-acetylaminofluorene (2-AAF), urethane, and certain aminoazo dyes, can cause cancer or tissue necrosis through covalent binding, whereas others, such as certain aromatic amines, can induce hemolysis or methemoglobinemia.

N-Hydroxy metabolites are also subject to conjugation reactions. Their conjugates with glucuronic acid are readily excreted; those formed with sulfuric or acetic acid, however, may be unstable and thus can be mutagenic, carcinogenic, and highly toxic (Weisburger and Weisburger, 1973).

Free Radical and Superoxide Formation

Certain halogen-containing compounds undergo metabolism to form free radicals. For example, carbon tetrachloride forms trichloromethyl radical, which causes peroxidation of polyunsaturated lipid as well as covalently binds to protein and unsaturated lipid. These initial reactions are followed by disturbances of various cellular components, as described in chap. 12. Halothane and bromotrichloromethane are other examples of chemicals that may form free radicals. The herbicide paraquat is known to produce superoxide radicals (Halliwell et al., 1992).

Other Pathways

Ethanol can be oxidized by a dehydrogenase to acetaldehyde, which has been implicated in some of the manifestations of alcohol toxicity. Pyrrolizidine alkaloids are dehydrogenated to reactive pyrrole derivatives, which are carcinogenic. There is evidence confirming that the acute toxicity of aliphatic nitriles is attributable to the cyanide released through hepatic microsomal enzyme activities (Willhite and Smith, 1981).

Activation in the GI Tract

Nitrites and certain amines can react in the acidic environment of the stomach to form nitrosamines, many of which have been shown to be potent carcinogens, and nitrates, which, under certain conditions, can be converted to nitrites that may induce methemoglobinemia. The artificial sweetener cyclamate is converted by intestinal bacteria to cyclohexylamine, which can induce testicular atrophy. Cycasin is converted to its aglycone, methylazoxymethanol, which is hepatotoxic and can induce tumors.

COMPLEX NATURE OF BIOTRANSFORMATION

Toxicants generally undergo several types of biotransformation, resulting in a variety of metabolites and conjugates. Some of the various metabolites and conjugates of bromobenzene are shown in Fig. 3-3. Organophosphorous insecticides, such as fenithrothion, chlorofenvinphos, and omethoate, can be metabolized through dealkylation, oxidation, desulfuration, or hydrolysis, yielding ten or more different metabolites.

Parathion, an organophosphorous pesticide, is bioactivated in the liver to paraoxon, which is a much more potent cholinesterase inhibitor. Infusion of parathion by way of the vena cava, bypassing the liver, therefore produced little cholinesterase inhibition, but a moderate effect was induced following infusion by way of the portal vein. On the other hand, infusion of paraoxon via the vena cava nearly completely blocked the cholinesterase activity, whereas it had negligible effect after an infusion via the portal vein, since it is detoxicated in the liver (Westermann, 1961).

A reactive metabolite formed in a phase I reaction can be further metabolized, such as carbon tetrachloride and halothane. Such a metabolite may also be followed by a phase II reaction to produce another reactive metabolite. 2-Acetylaminofluorene, for example, after N-hydroxylation can undergo acetylation or form sulfate or glutathione conjugates, all of which are highly reactive.

The relative importance of various types of biotransformation of a toxicant depends on many host, environmental, and chemical factors as well as the dose of the toxicant. Since the metabolites resulting from different biotransformations are often markedly different in their effects, the toxicity of a chemical can be greatly altered by these factors, as discussed in chap. 5.

Some of the metabolic reactions take place in sequence; hence interference with the normal metabolic pathway may have considerable influ-

Figure 3-4 Typical routes of foreign compound metabolism in humans (from Reeves, 1981).

ence on the toxic effects. For example, ethanol is normally metabolized through the intermediary product acetaldehyde. In normal humans the acetaldehyde formed is rapidly further metabolized to acetate, which in turn is converted to carbon dioxide and water. However, if the aldehyde dehydrogenase is inhibited, such as after the administration of disulfiram, the level of acetaldehyde rises and results in distress symptoms such as nausea, vomiting, headache, and palpitations.

A toxicant may be transformed in one organ to a stable proximate metabolite, which is transported to another organ and metabolizes to the ultimate toxic metabolite (Cohen, 1986).

Reeves (1981) provides a number of examples of biotransformations of "typical" chemicals, as well as a limited generalization of the typical routes of foreign compound metabolism in humans (Fig. 3-4).

REFERENCES

Adams, J. D., Jr., Laegreid, W. W., Huijzer, J. C., Hayman, C., and Yost, G. S. 1988. Pathology and glutathione status in 3-methylindole-treated rodents. *Res. Commun. Chem. Pathol. Pharmacol.* 60:323–336.

Anders, M. W., Lash, L., Dekant, W., Elfarra, A. E., and Dohn, D. R. 1988. Biosynthesis and biotransformation of glutathione *S*-conjugates to toxic metabolites. *CRC Crit. Rev. Toxicol.* 18:311.

Cohen, G. M. 1986. Basic principles of target organ toxicity. In *Target organ toxicity*, ed. G. M. Cohen, pp. 1–16. Boca Raton, FL: CRC Press.

DeLeve, L. D. and Kaplowitz, N. 1991. Glutathione metabolism and its role in hepatotoxicity. *Pharmacol. Ther.* 52:287–305.

Gillette, J. R., and Mitchell, J. R. 1975. Drug actions and interactions: Theoretical considerations. In: *Handbook of experimental pharmacology. New series*, eds. O. Eichler, A. Farah, H. Herken, and A. D. Welch, vol. 28, pp. 359–382. New York: Springer-Verlag.

Halliwell, B., Gutteridge, J. M. C., and Cross, C. E. 1992. Free radicals, antioxidants and human diseases--Where are we now? *J. Lab Clin. Med.* 119:598–620.

Levi, P. E. 1994. Reactive metabolites and toxicity. In *Introduction to biochemical toxicology*, eds. P. E. Hodgson and P. E. Levi, pp. 219–239. Norwalk, CT: Appleton & Lange.

Mazel, P., and Pessayre, D. 1976. Significance of metabolite-mediated toxicities in the safety evaluation of drugs and chemicals. In *New concepts in safety evaluation*, vol. 1, part 1, eds. M. A. Mehlmen, R. E. Shapiro, and H. Blumenthal. Washington, DC: Hemisphere.

Reeves, A. L. 1981. The metabolism of foreign compounds. In *Toxicology: Principles and practices*, vol. 1, ed. A. L. Reeves, pp. 1–28. New York: John Wiley.

Testa, B., and Jenner, P. 1976. *Drug metabolism: Chemical and biochemical aspects*. New York: Marcel Dekker.

Timbrell, J. A. 1991. *Principles of biochemical toxicology*. London: Taylor & Francis.

Weisburger, J. H., and Weisburger, E. K. 1973. Biochemical formation and pharmacological, toxicological and pathological properties of hydroxylamines and hydroxamic acids. *Pharmacol. Rev.* 25:166.

Westerman, E. O. 1976. *Introduction to general toxicology*, eds. E. J. Ariens, A. M. Simonis, and J. Offermeier, p. 147. New York: Academic Press.

Willhite, C. C., and Smith, R. P. 1981. The role of cyanide liberation in the acute toxicity of aliphatic nitriles. *Toxicol. Appl. Pharmacol.* 59:589–602.

Wills, E. D. 1981. The role of glutathione in drug metabolism and the protection of the liver against toxic metabolites. In *Testing for toxicity*, ed. J. W. Gorrod, p. 108. London: Taylor & Francis.

GENERAL PRINCIPLES

Appendix 3-1 Examples of Bioactivation

Parent compound	Toxic metabolite	Mechanism of toxicity	Toxic effect
Acetaminophen	N-Hydroxy derivative	Covalent binding	Hepatic necrosis
2-Acetylaminoflu- orene (AAF)	N-Hydroxy-AAF, sul- fate ester	Covalent binding	Cancers
Aflatoxin B₁	Aflatoxin 8,9-epoxide	Covalent binding	Hepatic cancer
Allyl formate	Acrolein	Covalent binding	Hepatic necrosis
Amygdalin	Mandelonitrile, gut flora	Cyanide formation	Cytotoxic hypoxia
Benzene	Benzene epoxide	Covalent binding	Bone-marrow depression
Benzo[a]pyrene (BaP)	BaP 7,8-epoxide → BaP 7,8-diol 9, 10- epoxide	Covalent binding	Cancers
Bromobenzene	Bromobenzene epoxide	Covalent binding	Hepatic, renal, bronchiolar necrosis
Carbon tetrachloride	Trichloromethane free radical	Covalent binding	Hepatic necrosis, hepatic cancer
Carcinogenic alkylnitrosami- nes	α-Hydroxylation	Alkylation	Hepatic cancer
Carcinogenic ami- noazo dyes	N-Hydroxy derivatives	Covalent binding	Hepatic cancer
Carcinogenic pol- ycyclic hydrocarbons	Epoxides, many organs	Covalent binding	Cancers, cytotoxicity
Chloroform	Phosgene	Covalent binding	Hepatic, renal necrosis
Cycasin	Methylazoxymethanol, gut flora	Alyklation	Cancers, hepatic necrosis
Cyclophospha- mide	Many proposed	Alkylation	Cytotoxicity
Fluoroacetate	Fluorocitrate	Enzyme inhibition	Lethal synthesis
Furosemide	Epoxide?	Covalent binding	Hepatic, renal necrosis
Parent compound	Toxic metabolite	Mechanism of toxicity	Toxic effect
Halothane	Free radical	Covalent binding	Hepatic necrosis
Isoniazid	Acetylhydrazine (me- tabolite of)	Covalent binding	Hepatic necrosis
Methemoglobin- producing aro- matic amines and nitro compounds	N-Hydroxy metabolites	Cyclic oxidoreduction	Methemoglobine- mia
Methoxyflurane	Inorganic fluoride	Enzyme inhibition	Renal failure
Naphthylamine	N-Hydroxy naphthylamine	Covalent binding	Bladder cancer
Nitrates	Nitrites, gut flora	Hemoglobin oxidation	Methemoglobin
Nitrites plus sec- ondary or terti- ary amines	Nitrosamines	Alkylation	Hepatic, pulmonary cancers

Appendix 3-1   (Continued)

Parent compound	Toxic metabolite	Mechanism of toxicity	Toxic effect
Parathion	Paraoxon	Covalent binding to cholinesterase	Neuromuscular paralysis
Purine and pyrimidine base analogues	Mononucleotides, nucleotide triphosphates	Lethal synthesis, lethal incorporation	Cytotoxicity
Safrole	1'-Hydroxysafrole (metabolite of)	Covalent binding	Cancers
Urethane	N-Hydroxyurethane	Alkylation	Cancers, cytotoxicity
Vinyl chloride	Eposide	Covalent binding	Liver cancer

Source: Adapted from Mazel and Pessayre (1976).
Note: Site of bioactivation is the liver except as otherwise noted.

Toxic Effects

CHAPTER 4 CONTENTS

GENERAL CONSIDERATIONS

Toxic effects are greatly variable in nature, potency, target organ, and mechanism of action. A better understanding of their characteristics can improve assessment of the associated health hazards. It can also facilitate the development of rational preventive and therapeutic measures.

All toxic effects result from biochemical interactions between the toxicants (and/or their metabolites) and certain structures of the organism. The structure may be nonspecific, such as any tissue in direct contact with corrosive chemicals. More often it is specific, involving a particular subcellular structure. A variety of structures may be affected.

The nature of effects may vary from organ to organ. The organ-specific effects are discussed in some detail in the chapters in Part III. In some cases, the reason why a particular organ is affected is known. This knowledge is useful in many ways. A few examples are described in this chapter.

SPECTRUM OF TOXIC EFFECTS

The great variety of toxic effects can be grouped according to the target organ, mechanism of action, or other characteristics such as those discussed next.

Local and Systemic Effects

Certain chemicals can cause injuries at the site of first contact with an organism. These local effects can be induced by caustic substances on the gastrointestinal tract, by corrosive materials on the skin, and by irritant gases and vapors on the respiratory tract.

Systemic effects result only after the toxicant has been absorbed and distributed to other parts of the body. Most toxicants exert their main effects on one or a few organs. These organs are referred to as the "target organs" of these toxicants. A target organ does not necessarily have the highest concentration of the toxicants in the organism. For example, the target organ of DDT is the central nervous system, but it is concentrated in adipose tissues.

Reversible and Irreversible Effects

Reversible effects of toxicants are those that will disappear following cessation of exposure to them. Irreversible effects, in contrast, will persist or even progress after exposure is discontinued. Certain effects are obviously irreversible. These include carcinomas, mutations, damages to the neurons, and liver cirrhosis.

Certain effects are considered irreversible even though they disappear some time after cessation of exposure. For example, the "irreversible" cholinesterase-inhibiting insecticides inhibit the activity of this enzyme for a period of time that approximates that required for the synthesis and replacement of the enzyme.

The effect produced by a toxicant may be reversible if the organism is exposed at a low concentration and/or for a short duration, whereas irreversible effects may be produced at higher concentrations and/or for longer durations of exposure.

Immediate and Delayed Effects

Many toxicants produce immediate toxic effects, which develop shortly after a single exposure, a notable example being cyanide poisoning. Delayed effects occur after a lapse of some time. Carcinogenic effects generally become manifest 10–20 yr after the initial exposure in humans; even in rodents a lapse of many months is required. To determine these and other delayed effects of toxicants, long-term studies are essential.

Morphologic, Functional, and Biochemical Effects

Morphologic effects refer to gross and microscopic changes in the morphology of the tissues. Many of these effects, such as necrosis and neoplasia, are irreversible and serious. Functional effects usually represent reversible changes in the functions of target organs. Functions of the liver and kidney (e.g., rate of excretion of dyes) are commonly tested in toxicologic studies.

Functional effects are in general reversible, whereas morphologic effects are not, and functional changes are generally detected earlier or in animals exposed to lower doses than those with morphologic changes. In addition, functional tests are valuable in following the progress of effects on target organs in long-term studies in animals and in humans. However, the results are often more variable.

Although all toxic effects are associated with biochemical alterations, in routine toxicity testing, "biochemical effects" usually refer to those without apparent morphologic changes. An example of such effects is the cholinesterase inhibition following exposure to organophosphate and carbamate insecticides. δ-Aminolevulinic acid dehydratase (ALAD) inhibition in lead poisoning is another example (see chaps. 19 and 20).

Allergic and Idiosyncratic Reactions

Allergic reaction (also known as hypersensitivity and sensitization reaction) to a toxicant results from previous sensitization to that toxicant or a chemically similar one. The chemical acts as a hapten and combines with an endogenous protein to form an antigen, which in turn elicits the formation of antibodies. A subsequent exposure to the chemical will result in an antigen–antibody interaction, which provokes the typical manifestations of allergy. Thus this reaction is different from the usual toxic effects, first because a previous exposure is required, and second because a typical sigmoid dose-response curve is usually not demonstrable with allergic reactions. Nevertheless, threshold doses were demonstrable for the induction as well as the challenge in dermal sensitization (Koschier et al., 1983).

Generally an idiosyncratic reaction is a genetically determined abnormal reactivity to a chemical. Some patients exhibit prolonged muscular reaction and apnea following a standard dose of succinylcholine. These patients have a deficiency of serum cholinesterase, which normally degrades the muscle relaxant rapidly. Similarly, people with a deficiency in NADH methemoglobinemia reductase are abnormally sensitive to nitrites and other chemicals that produce methemoglobinemia.

Graded and Quantal Responses

Effects on body weight, food consumption, and enzyme inhibition are examples of graded responses. On the other hand, mortality and tumor formation are examples of quantal (all-or-none) responses. Both types of responses can be statistically analyzed as illustrated in chap. 6.

The relationship between dose and response usually follows an S-shaped curve. Figure 4-1 is a schematic representation of most chemicals (B) and that of certain essential nutrients (A). The latter is exemplified by

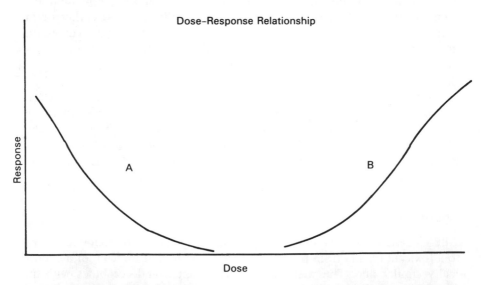

Figure 4-1 Schematic representation of dose-response relationship. Curve A: Most essential nutrients, with which the response (deficiency syndrome) increases along with decreased intake. Curve B: Most chemicals, with which the response (toxic effects) increases along with increased instake. Certain substances, such as selenium, exhibit both types of responses.

thiamine and ascorbic acid. Insufficient intake of these vitamins will induce deficiency syndromes, but larger intakes will be readily eliminated in the urine. Selenium is an essential element but excessive intake will be toxic (see chap. 20); therefore its dose-response relationship is represented by curves A and B.

As the dose of a toxicant increases so does the response, either in terms of the proportion of the population responding or in terms of the severity of graded responses. Furthermore, additional toxic effects may also appear along with increased doses. For example, methylmercury induces paresthesia at low doses, but it also induces ataxia, dysarthria, deafness, and death at higher doses, as shown in Fig. 20-2, which depicts both dose-response and dose-effect relationships.

TARGET ORGANS

Toxicants do not affect all organs to the same extent. An understanding of the mechanisms that determine organ specificity will assist in the advancement of various aspects of toxicology. While the reason is not always clear, the probable mechanisms by which many toxicants act specifically on certain organs are known. In general, the underlying mechanism is either a greater susceptibility of the target organ or a higher concentration of the chemical and/or its metabolite at the site of action. The higher concentration may arise under a variety of conditions.

Sensitivity of the Organ

Neurons and myocardium depend primarily on adenosine triphosphate (ATP) generated by mitochondrial oxidation with little capacity for anaerobic metabolism, and there are rapid ionic shifts through the cell membrane. They are, therefore, especially sensitive to lack of oxygen resulting from disorders of the vascular system or of the hemoglobin (e.g., carbon monoxide poisoning).

Rapidly dividing cells, such as those in the bone marrow and the intestinal mucosa, are more susceptible to mitotic poisons (e.g., methotrexate).

Distribution

The respiratory tract and the skin are target organs of industrial and environmental toxicants because these are the sites of absorption. An example is provided by bischloromethyl ether. It produces skin tumors in humans when applied topically, but will induce tumors in the respiratory tract after exposure by inhalation.

On a unit weight basis, the liver and kidney have a higher volume of blood flow, and thus they are in general exposed to toxicants to a greater extent. In addition, these organs have greater metabolic and excretory functions, which also render them more susceptible to toxicants. Being lipophilic, methylmercury can cross the blood–brain barrier and exert its toxic effects on the nervous system. Inorganic mercury compounds, in contrast, are not able to cross the blood–brain barrier and are not neurotoxic.

Radiation may damage DNA and induce tumors. Ultraviolet light has little penetrating power and therefore will only produce skin tumors, whereas ionizing radiation may penetrate tissues and cause leukemia and other types of cancer.

Selective Uptake

Certain cells have a high affinity for selected chemicals. For example, in the respiratory tract, the type I and type II alveolar epithelial cells, which have an active uptake system for endogenous polyamines, will take up paraquat, a structurally similar chemical. This process can result in local tissue damage even when paraquat is administered orally.

Melanin is present in the eye, inner ear, etc. Drugs such as chloroquine and kanamycin that have an affinity for melanin may accumulate, after prolonged administration, in these organs and cause damage. Strontium-90 is selectively deposited in the bone and can induce tumors of the bone.

Biotransformation

As a result of *bioactivation*, reactive metabolites are formed. Liver, being a major site of biotransformation, is susceptible to the action of many toxicants. However, there are exceptions. For example, certain metabolites are sufficiently stable; they may affect other organs after being transported there. Thus bromobenzene, though bioactivated in the liver, can affect the kidney.

With some toxicants, the bioactivation at certain sites predominates their effects. For example, the organophosphorothioate insecticides, such as parathion, are bioactivated mainly in the liver, but the abundance of detoxifying enzymes and of reactive but noncritical binding sites there prevents any overt signs of toxicity. On the other hand, brain tissue has much fewer bioactivating enzymes, but because the bioactivation takes place near the critical target sites, that is, the synapses, the main toxic manifestations of this group of toxicants arise from the nervous system.

The bioactivating enzymes are not necessarily evenly distributed in an organ or tissue. For example, the Clara cells (nonciliated bronchiolar epithelial cells) constitute only 1% of the cells in the lung, yet they contain a major portion of the pulmonary cytochrome P-450. They are therefore more susceptible to damage by such toxicants as 4-ipomeanol and CCl_4. A similar situation exists in the kidney. The proximal tubules, especially the S3 cells, which are located in the pars recta portion of these tubules, have the highest concentrations of this enzyme system; hence the most susceptible parts of the kidney are the proximal tubules, especially its pars recta portion.

Repair Mechanism

A toxicant may affect a specific organ because of a lack of the required repair mechanism. For example, N-methyl-N-nitrosourea (MNU) produces tumors in the rat mainly in the brain, occasionally in the kidney, but not in the liver. Kleihues and Cooper (1976) demonstrated that the liver is capable of enzymatically excising the O^6-alkyl-guanine induced by MNU from the DNA, whereas the brain is deficient in this respect. The capacity of the kidney falls between those of the liver and brain.

MECHANISMS OF ACTION

While the mechanisms of action of all toxicants are not fully understood, a number of biochemical reactions are likely involved. The underlying processes/subcellular sites are listed, along with some exemplary toxicants, in Table 4-1. The table clearly shows the diverse nature of the mechanisms as well as the multiple processes/sites that are involved in the action of a number of toxicants. For many of the toxicants listed in Table 4-1, the mechanisms are described, along with their toxic manifestations, in the relevant chapters.

Of the various mechanisms of action, disturbance of calcium homeostasis merits special mention because of its importance and complexity. The extracellular level of Ca^{2+} is more than ten times higher than that in the cytosol.

The differential is maintained by a variety of mechanisms including the Ca^{2+}-transporting ATPase at the plasma membrane, the store in the endoplasmic reticulum, mitochondria, and nucleus, as well as the binding with intracellular calmodulin. Increases of cytosolic Ca^{2+} may be caused via different mechanisms. For example, CCl_4 and bromobenzene act through inhibition of Ca_{2+}-ATPase, acetaminophen and CCl_4 through damages of plasma membrane, and cadmium by release of Ca^{2+} from mitochondria. The rise in cytosolic Ca^{2+} may affect the cytoskeleton and thereby damage cellular integrity either directly or through Ca^{2+}-activated proteases. In addition, TCDD may promote "apoptosis" (programmed cell death) by combining with Ah receptor, increasing intracellular Ca^{2+} activating endonuclease and causing DNA breakdown (Timbrell, 1992; Halliwell and Cross, 1994).

Table 4-1 Some Mechanisms of Toxic Action

Mechanism of action	Process / subcellular site	Examples of toxicants
Interference with normal receptor-ligand interaction	Neurotransmitters Hormone receptors Enzymes Transport proteins	Botulinum toxin, organophosphate pesticides Amitrole, DES, retinoic acid, TCDD Fluoroacetate, cyanide, organophosphate pesticides CO, nitrites
Interference with membrane function	Excitable membrane ion influx Membrane fluidity Lysosomal membranes Mitochondrial membranes	DDT, saxitoxin, tetrodotoxin Organic solvents (e.g., CCl_4, chloroform), ethanol CCl_4, phosphorus, phalloidin CCl_4, organotins, phosphorus
Interference with cellular energy production	Hemoglobin Oxidative phosphorylation uncoupling Electron transport inhibition Carbohydrate metabolism inhibition	CO, nitrites Dinitrophenol, organotins Cyanide, rotenone Fluoroacetate
Covalent binding to biomolecules	Lipids peroxidation Glutathione depletion Protein thiols oxidation Nucleic acids	CCl_4, ozone, paraquat, phenytoin Acetaminophen Acetaminophen, phenytoin Carcinogens, mutagens, teratogens
Perturbation of calcium homeostasis	Cytoskeleton, etc. Apoptosis	Arsenic, cobalt, doxorubicin, paraquat, phalloidin TCDD

Source: Adapted from Klaassen and Eaton (1993).

Note: The toxic effects of a number of the toxicants are described in other sections. For the relevant pages, refer to the Chemical Index.

Most of the reactions take place at various subcellular sites. Table 12-1 lists a number of hepatotoxicants along with the organelles that they affect.

MOLECULAR TARGETS: CHEMICAL NATURE

Proteins

Receptors   Receptors are located across plasma membrane, or in cytosol or nucleus, and serve to transmit physical or chemical signals to the cell. There are many types of receptors serving a variety of functions. Some of them are known to be affected by toxicants (see next section).

Enzymes   Enzymes are common targets of toxicants. The enzyme effects may be specific, such as the inhibition of acetylcholinesterase. They may be reversible, as is the case with a number of carbamate insecticides on cholinesterase. Irreversible enzyme inhibition is exemplified by DFP (diisopropyl fluorophosphate), which covalently binds with the enzymes.

The effects may be nonspecific. For example, lead and mercury are inhibitors of a great variety of enzymes. However, some enzymes are more susceptible. For example, δ-aminolevulinic acid dehydrase is especially sensitive to lead, and its activity in erythrocytes is used as an early indicator of lead poisoning.

The last step of the oxidation of many chemicals is catalyzed by the cytochrome oxidase chain. Hydrocyanic acid (HCN) can bind with the iron in these enzymes and block their redox function. The aerobic respiration of cells is then arrested and biochemical asphyxia ensues.

An enzyme can also be inhibited by a chemical derived by synthesis from the toxicant, such as fluoroacetic acid and its derivatives. The process is known as *lethal synthesis*. Fluoroacetic acid is metabolized as acetic acid in the citric acid cycle, and fluorocitric acid is synthesized, instead of citric acid. Since fluorocitric acid is an inhibitor of aconitase, further metabolism, and consequently the energy production, is blocked.

In a somewhat similar manner, amino acid antagonists (e.g., azaserine and fluorophenylalanine) can interfere with the utilization of specific amino acids in the synthesis of proteins.

The energy that is liberated by biochemical oxidation is normally stored in the form of high-energy phosphates. Uncoupling agents such as dinitrophenol interfere with the synthesis of energy-rich phosphates, and thus the energy is liberated as heat instead of being stored.

Carriers   Carriers such as hemoglobin can be affected by a toxicant through preferential binding. For example, carbon monoxide can bind hemoglobin at the site where oxygen is normally bound. Because of its greater affinity for hemoglobin, it can inactivate hemoglobin and cause manifestations of oxygen deficiency in tissues.

Oxygen transport can also be impaired by an accumulation of methemoglobin, which is an oxidation product of hemoglobin with no oxygen-binding ability. In normal individuals the trace amount of methemoglobin is readily reduced to hemoglobin. Certain toxicants, such as nitrites and aromatic amines, can enhance the formation of methemoglobin and overwhelm the normal process of its reduction to hemoglobin. People with glucose-6-phosphatase dehydrogenase deficiency have a lower capacity to regenerate hemoglobin from methemoglobin and are thus prone to have methemoglobinemia.

Structural Proteins   Extracellular structural proteins such as collagen are unlikely to be affected by toxicants. However, toxicants such as ozone and asbestos may cause an increase in fibroblasts and deposition of collagen in the lung (chap. 11). Intracellular structural proteins, such as cytoskeleton, may be damaged by toxicants, such as arsenic and paraquat (Li and Chou, 1992; Li et al, 1987).

Coenzymes

Coenzymes are essential for the normal function of enzymes. Their levels in the body can be diminished by toxicants that inhibit their synthesis. For example, pyrithiamine can inhibit thiamine kinase, which is responsible for the formation of the coenzyme thiamine pyrophosphate. NADPH can be destroyed in the presence of free radicals, which can be produced by such toxicants as carbon tetrachloride.

Metal-dependent enzymes can be inhibited by chelating agents (e.g., cyanides and dithiocarbamates) through removal of metal coenzymes such as copper and zinc.

Lipids

Peroxidation of polyenoic fatty acids has been suggested as a mechanism of the necrotizing action of a number of toxicants, such as carbon tetrachloride.

Cell membrane derangement may result after exposure to various types of toxicants. The general anesthetics ether and halothane, as well as many other lipophilic substances, can accumulate in the cell membranes and thereby interfere with transport of oxygen and glucose into the cell. The cells of the central nervous system are especially susceptible to a lowering of oxygen tension and glucose level and are therefore among the first to be deleteriously affected by these substances. Membrane dissolution can follow contact with organic solvents and amphoteric detergents. The ions of mercury and cadmium can complex with phospholipid bases and expand the surface area of the membrane, thereby altering its function. Lead ion can increase the fragility of erythrocytes and result in hemolysis. The oxygen-carrying function of hemoglobin is lost after it escapes from the hemolyzed erythrocytes.

Nucleic Acids

Covalent binding between a toxicant (such as alkylating agents) and replicating DNA and RNA can cause cancer, mutation, and teratogenesis. Such toxicants may also exert immunosuppressive effects.

Antimetabolites such as aminopterin and methotrexate may be incorporated into DNA and RNA and then interfere with their replication.

Others

Hypersensitivity reactions result from repeated exposure to a particular substance or to its chemically related substances. The latter phenomenon is referred to as cross-sensitization. The substance, if it is a large polypeptide, acts as an antigen and stimulates the body to form antibodies. Otherwise, the substance acts as a hapten and combines with proteins in the body to form antigens. The reaction between an antigen from a later exposure and the corresponding antibodies results in the release of histamine, bradykinin, and others. The reaction has a typical pattern irrespective of the nature of the antigen. Photosensitization reaction is somewhat similar except sunlight is also required for its induction (see chaps. 10, 11, and 14).

Corrosive agents such as strong acids and bases can destroy local tissues by precipitating cellular proteins. Irritation of the underlying tissues occurs as a consequence.

Blockade of renal and biliary tubules may follow the precipitation of relatively insoluble toxicants or their metabolites. For example, acetylsulfapyridine, a metabolite of sulfapyridine, may block renal tubules, and harmol glucuronide from harmol may cause cholestasis.

RECEPTORS

Historical Notes

It has long been observed that a number of poisons and toxins exert certain specific biologic effects. John N. Langley proposed in 1905 the concept of a "receptive substance." That the receptors are protein in nature was first suggested by Welsh and Taub (1951).

To demonstrate the protein nature of acetylcholine receptors, Lu (1952) showed that the stimulant effect of acetylcholine on isolated rabbit ileum was lost after the ileum was treated with the proteolytic enzyme trypsin (10 mg/100 ml, for 30 min). That the effect was on the receptor rather than the muscle was demonstrated by the fact that the treated ileum still responded to barium chloride, a direct-acting muscle stimulant. In 1971, Cuatrecasas observed that trypsin, at the same concentration as that used by Lu, eliminated the activity of insulin receptor.

In the 1970s cholinergic receptors (ChR) were solubilized, isolated, and characterized by several groups of investigators. The amino acid composition of ChR was reported by Heilbronn et al. (1975). They also found that ChR contained about 6% carbohydrates. While it has been generally agreed that the ligand–receptor complex would initiate responses in the cells, it was Rodbell et al. (1971) who proposed a "transducer" was required to act between the receptor and the effector. This "transducer" was later confirmed as the G-proteins (see Gilman, 1987).

Functional Categories

There are many types of receptors, located either in the cell membrane, the cytosol, or the nucleus. They serve a variety of functions such as metabolism, secretion, muscular contraction, neural activity, and proliferation. In general they are placed in the following categories:

Neurotransmitter receptors include the cholinergic (nicotinic, located in ganglia and skeletal muscles, and muscarinic in smooth muscles and brain), α- and β-adrenergic, dopamine, serotonin, opiates (e.g., endorphin), and histamine (H_1 and H_2) receptors.

Hormone receptors are for insulin, cortisone, adrenocorticotropin (ACTH), thyrotropin, estrogen, progesterone, angiotensin, glucagon, prostaglandin, and others.

Certain chemicals such as antidepressants and antitumor agents bind with specific macromolecules that may be considered *drug receptors*. These receptors may well have endogenous messengers (such as endorphins and enkephalins for opiates), but these are as yet undiscovered. Another example of such agents is benzodiazepine, for which receptors, and possible endogenous effectors, have been discovered. Furthermore, antagonists have been synthesized (Lal et al., 1988).

Other receptors are located on *enzymes* and *carrier proteins*. They may also be affected by toxicants as listed in Table 4-1.

Structure and Signal Transduction

The various functional categories of receptors just described exert their biological effects upon binding with an appropriate ligand, which may be an endogenous or exogenous substance. These effects are preceded by a series of biochemical activities, the signaling, which vary according to the structural characteristics of the receptor. Structurally they may be placed in four classes of receptors. These are (1) G-protein coupled receptors, (2) ligand-gated ion channels, (3) voltage-gated channels, and (4) intracellular receptors.

    1   With the G-protein coupled receptors (Fig. 4-2:1), binding with a ligand results in the activation of the G-protein, converting GTP (guanosine triphosphate) to GDP (guanosine diphosphate), which activates or inhibits a specific enzyme (adenylate cyclase or phospholipase C), followed by the formation of a "second messenger," such as cAMP (from ATP), diacylglycerol, or phosphoinositol. The second messenger then initiates the cellular response: the biologic effect. Typical ligands for this class of receptors are adrenergic, muscarinic, cholinergic, and dopaminergic neurotransmitters and their analogs (e.g., ephedrine), as well as others such as diphtheria toxin.

    2   The second class of receptors is transmembrane proteins with an ion channel (Fig. 4-2:2). Upon binding with a ligand, the receptor undergoes conformational changes resulting in the opening of the channel. This process allows changes of Na^+, K^+, Cl^-, or Ca^{2+} concentrations across the

Figure 4-2 Schematic representation of the four classes of receptors: (1) G-protein coupled receptor, (2) ligand-gated ion channel, (3) voltage-gated ion channel, and (4) intracellular receptor (adapted from Mailman and Lawler, 1994).

plasma membrane. Nicotinic cholinergic and gamma-aminobutyric acid$_A$ (GABA$_A$) receptors belong to this class. In addition, glutamate and chemicals such as kainate, diazepam, barbiturates, and picrotoxin also act on this type of ion-channel receptors.

3 The voltage-gated conductance channels (Fig. 4-2:3) are located across plasma membranes of excitable cells such as neurons and their axons. At present, no endogenous ligands are known. However, the neurotoxins tetrodotoxin and saxitoxin (see chap. 16) bind to a site near the extracellular opening of the Na$^+$ channel and block the entry of Na$^+$ through the channel, thereby interfering with the conduction of nerve impulse.

4 Intracellular receptors are located in the cytosol or nucleus (Fig. 4-2:4). The main endogenous ligands are estrogens, androgens, progestins, glucocorticoids, and mineralocorticoids. A representative toxicant that binds with this type of receptor is 2,3,7,8-tetrachlorodibenzo-p-dioxin (TCDD). It binds with the Ah receptor in the cytosol, but moves to the nucleus after the binding (see next section). For additional details see Mitchell (1992) and Mailman and Lawler (1994).

The ligand that binds with the receptor may be an "agonist" or an "antagonist." An agonist induces the "physiologic" function of the receptor, whereas an antagonist blocks its functions. For example, methacholine is an agonist interacting with certain cholinergic receptors, mimicking the effects of acetylcholine, whereas atropine, an antagonist, blocks these effects. Both types of effects may be adverse to health. In addition, an agonist may cause a toxic effect by failing to dissociate from the receptor readily enough, thereby preventing further action of the endogenous messenger, and an antagonist can compete with the messenger for the site on the receptor and block the action of the latter. In addition, a toxicant may induce tolerance to its toxicity by reducing the number of receptors, as shown by Costa et al. (1981) with chronic treatment with an organophosphate acetylcholinesterase inhibitor.

Receptors in Toxicology

The receptor concept has been valuable in advancing our understanding of certain biochemical, physiologic, and pharmacologic effects, as well as facilitating the development of drugs. Its role in toxicology is evidenced by an increasing number of receptors being recognized as mediators of effects of toxicants.

Poland and Knutson (1982) reviewed the extensive literature on TCDD (2,3,7,8-tetrachlorodibenzo-p-dioxin) and related halogenated aromatic hydrocarbons with respect to their toxicity, their ability to induce AHH (aryl hydrocarbon hydroxylase), and their affinity for a cytosol receptor. It was suggested that TCDD binds with the Ah (aromatic hydrocarbon) receptor.

The TCDD–receptor complex translocates to the nucleus and there interacts with specific genomic recognition sites. This initiates the transcription and translation of the specific genes that code for AHH. A preponderance of evidence suggests that most of the TCDD toxicities are receptor mediated. It was also noted that the concentration of this cytosol receptor is much higher in the liver of C57BL/6 mice than in that of DBA/2 mice and that the former strain of mice was much more susceptible than the latter with respect to TCDD-induced thymus involution, teratogenesis, and hepatic porphyria. Furthermore, the genetic evidence indicated that the *Ah* locus in mice was the structural gene for the cytosol receptor (see also Whitlock, 1990; Okey et al., 1994).

Many neurotoxicants act through receptors on central nervous system (CNS), peripheral nervous system (PNS), and autonomic nervous systems. Other examples are receptors for TPA (12-*O*-tetradecanoyl phorbol 13-acetate) and retinoic acid. TPA, a tumor promoter, binds with a receptor that initiates a chain of events leading to selected replication of initiated cells (Blumberg et al., 1983). Retinoic acid, as TCDD, acts on an estrogen receptor to exert teratogenic and other effects (see Lu et al., 1994). A few examples of toxicants that act through receptors are mentioned in the previous section. Furthermore, many immunotoxicants act through specific receptors on T cells, B cells, cytokines, polymorphic nuclear cells, and monocytes (Lad et al., 1995), and certain organophosphorous (OP) compounds act not only through acetylcholinesterase (AChE) but also on muscarine receptors (Huff and Abou-Donia, 1995).

REFERENCES

Blumberg, P. M., Delcos, B. K., Dunn, J. A., Jaken, S., Leach, K. L., and Yeh, E. 1983. Phorbol ester receptors and the in vitro effects of tumor promoters. *Ann. NY Acad. Sci.* 407:303–315.

Costa, L. G., Schwab, B. W., Hand, H., and Murphy, S. D. 1981. Reduced [H^3] quinuclidinyl benzilate binding to muscarinic receptors in disulfoton-tolerant mice. *Toxicol. Appl. Pharmacol.* 60:441–450.

Cuatrecasas, P. 1971. Perturbation of the insulin receptor of isolated fat cells with proteolytic enzymes. *J. Biol. Chem.* 246:6522–6531.

Gilman, A. G. 1987. G-proteins: Transducers of receptor-generated signals. *Annu. Rev. Biochem.* 56:615–649.

Halliwell, B., and Cross, C. E. 1994. Oxygen-derived species: Their relation to human disease and environmental stress. *Environ. Health Perspect.* 102 (suppl. 10):5–12.

Heilbronn, E., Mattsson, C., and Elfman, L. 1975. Biochemical and physical properties of the nicotinic ACh receptor from *Torpedo marmorata*. In *Properties of purified cholinergic and adrenergic receptors*, vol. 37, ed. M. Wollemann, pp. 27–37. New York: Elsevier.

Huff, R. A., and About-Donia, M. B. 1995. In vitro effect of chloropyrifos oxon on muscarinic receptors and adenylate cyclase. *Neurotoxicology.* 16:281–290.

Klaassen, C. D., and Eaton, D. L. 1993. Principals of toxicology. In *Casarett and Doull's toxicology*, eds. M. O. Amdur, J. Doull, and C. D. Klaassen, 4th ed, pp. 12–49. New York: McGraw-Hill.

Kleihues, P., and Cooper, H. K. 1976. Repair excision of alkylated bases from DNA *in vivo*. *Oncology* 33:86–88.

Koschier, F. J., Burden, E. J., Brunkhorst, C. S., and Friedman, M. A. 1983. Concentration-dependent elicitation of dermal sensitization in guinea pigs treated with 2,4-toluene diisocyanate. *Toxicol. Appl. Pharmacol.* 67:401–407.

Lad, P. M., Kapstein, J. S. and Lin, C. E., eds. 1995. *Signal traduction in leukocytes. G-protein-related and other pathways.* Boca Raton, FL: CRC Press.

Lal, H., Kumer, B., and Forster, M. J. 1988. Enhancement of learning and memory in mice by a benzodiazepine antagonist. *FASEB J.* 2:2707–2711.

Li, W., and Chou, I.-N. 1992. Effects of sodium arsenite on the cytoskeleton and cellular glutathione levels in cultured cells. *Toxicol. Appl. Pharmacol.* 114:132–139.

Li, W., Zhao, Y., and Chou, I.-N. 1987. Paraquat-induced cytoskeletal injury in cultured cells. *Toxicol. Appl. Pharmacol.* 91:96–106.

Lu, F. C. 1952. The effects of proteolytic enzymes on the isolated rabbit intestine. *Br. J. Pharmacol.* 7:624–640.

Lu, Y., Wang, X., and Safe, S. 1994. Interaction of 2,3,7,8-tetrachlorodibenzo-*p*-dioxin and retinoic acid in MCF-7 human breast cancer cells. *Toxicol. Appl. Pharmacol.* 127:1–8.

Mailman, R. B. and Lawler, C. P. 1994. Toxicant-receptor interactions: Fundamental principles. In *Introduction to biochemical toxicology*, eds. E. Hodgson and P. E. Levi, pp. 319–344. Norwalk, CT: Appleton & Lange.

Mitchell, R. H. 1992. Inositol lipids in cellular signalling mechanisms. *Trends Biochem. Sci.* 17:274–276.

Okey, A. B., Riddick, D. S., and Harper, P. A. (1994) The Ah receptor: Mediator of the toxicity of 2,3,7,8-tetrachlorodibenzo-*p*-dioxin (TCDD) and related compounds. *Toxicol. Lett.* 70: 1–22.

Poland, A., and Knutson, J. C. 1982. 2,3,7,8-Tetrachlorodibenzo-*p*-dioxin and related halogenated aromatic hydrocarbons: Examination of the mechanism of toxicity. *Annu. Rev. Pharmacol. Toxicol.* 22:517–554.

Rodbell, M., Birnbaumer, L., Pohl, S. L., and Kraus, H. M. J. 1971. The glycagon sensitive adenyl cyclase system in plasma membranes of rat liver. V. An obligatory role of guanyl nucleotides in glucagon action. *J. Biol. Chem.* 246:1877–1887.

Timbrell, J. A. 1992. *Principles of biochemical toxicology.* London: Taylor & Francis.

Welsh, J. H., and Taub, R. 1951. The significance of the carbonyl group and ether oxygen in the reaction of acetylcholine with receptor substance. *J. Pharmacol. Exp. Ther.* 103: 62–73.

Whitlock, J. P., Jr. 1990. Genetic and molecular aspects of 2,3,7,8-tetrachlorodibenzo-*p*-dioxin action. *Annu. Rev. Pharmacol. Toxicol* 30:251–277.

ADDITIONAL READING

Jackson, T. 1991. Structure and function of G protein coupled receptors. *Pharmacol. Ther.* 50: 425–442.

Modifying Factors of Toxic Effects

GENERAL CONSIDERATIONS

While toxicity is an inherent property of a substance, the nature and extent of the toxic manifestations in an organism that is exposed to the substance depend on a variety of factors. The obvious ones are the dose and duration of exposure.

They also include such less obvious host factors as the species and strain of the animal, its sex and age, and its nutritional and hormonal status. Various environmental (physical and social) factors also play a part. In addition, the toxic effect of a chemical may be influenced by simultaneous and consecutive exposure to other chemicals.

The toxic effects may be modified in a number of ways: alterations of the absorption, distribution, and excretion of a chemical; an increase or decrease of its biotransformation; and changes of the sensitivity of the receptor at the target organ.

A clear understanding of the existence of these factors and of their mode of action is important in designing the protocols of toxicologic investigation. It is equally important in evaluating the significance of the toxicologic data and in assessing the safety/risk to humans under specified conditions of exposure.

The most common mechanism underlying various modifying factors is differences in the rate of detoxication. However, differences in bioactivation, and toxicokinetic, toxicodynamic, physiologic, and anatomic characteristics are responsible for a number of modifying factors. Examples are listed in Appendix 5-1.

HOST FACTORS

Species, Strain, and Individual

Differences of toxic effect from one species to another have long been recognized. Knowledge in this field has been used to develop, for example, pesticides, which are more toxic to pests than to humans and other mammals. Among various species of mammals, most effects of toxicants are somewhat more similar. This fact forms the basis of predicting the toxicity to humans from results obtained in toxicologic studies conducted in other mammals, such as the rat, mouse, dog, rabbit, and monkey. There are, however, notable differences in toxicity even among mammals (Williams, 1974).

Some of these differences can be attributed to variations in detoxication mechanisms. For example, the sleeping time induced in several species of laboratory animals by hexobarbital shows marked differences, which are obviously attributable to the activity of the detoxication enzyme, as shown in Table 5-1.

Differences in response to hexobarbital, although less marked, also exist among various strains of mice (Jay, 1955). Other examples include

Table 5-1   Species Differences in Duration of Action and Metabolism of Hexobarbital

Species	Duration of action (min)	Plasma half-life (min)	Relative enzyme activity (μg/g/h)	Plasma level on awakening (μg/ml)
Mouse	12	19	598	89
Rabbit	49	60	196	57
Rat	90	140	135	64
Dog	315	260	36	19

Source: Reprinted with permission from Quinn et al. (1958). Copyright © 1958, Elsevier Science Inc.
Note: Dose of barbiturate 50 mg/kg in dogs, 100 mg/kg in the other animals.

ethylene glycol and aniline. Ethylene glycol is metabolized to oxalic acid, which is responsible for the toxicity, or to carbon dioxide. The magnitude of the toxicity of ethylene glycol in animals is in the following order: cat > rat > rabbit, and this is the same for the extent of oxalic acid production. Aniline is metabolized in the cat and dog mainly to o-aminophenol, which is more toxic, but it is metabolized mainly to p-aminophenol in the rat and hamster, which are less susceptible to aniline.

Differences in bioactivation also account for many dissimilarities of toxicity. A notable example is 2-naphthylamine, which produced bladder tumors in the dog and human but not in the rat, rabbit, or guinea pig. Dogs and humans, but not the others, excrete the carcinogenic metabolite 2-naphthyl hydroxylamine (Miller et al., 1964). Acetylaminofluorene (AAF) is carcinogenic to many species of animals but not to the guinea pig. However, the N-hydroxy metabolite of AAF is carcinogenic to all animals including the guinea pig, demonstrating that the difference between the guinea pig and the other animals is not in their response to the toxicant but in the bioactivation (Weisburger and Weisburger, 1973).

Although differences in biotransformation, including bioactivation, account for species variation in susceptibility to a great majority of chemicals, other factors such as absorption, distribution, and excretion also play a part. In addition, variations in physiologic functions are important in toxic manifestations in response to such toxicants as squill. This toxic chemical is a good rodenticide because rats cannot vomit, whereas humans and many other mammals can eliminate this poison by vomiting (Doull, 1980). Anatomic differences may also be responsible, such as with butylated hydroxyanisole (BHA) (see chap. 18).

Apart from the differences in susceptibility that exist from one species to another and from one strain to another, there are also variables among individuals of the same species and same strain. While the magnitude of such individual variations is usually relatively small, there are exceptions. This phenomenon has been widely studied among humans. For example, there are "slow inactivators," who are deficient in acetyltransferase. Such individuals acetylate isoniazid only slowly and are thus likely to suffer from peripheral neuropathy resulting from an accumulation of isoniazid. On the other hand, people with more efficient acetyltransferase require larger doses of isoniazid to obtain its therapeutic effect and are thus more likely to suffer from hepatic damage.

Differences in response to succinylcholine provide another example. Individuals with an atypical or a low level of plasma cholinesterase may exhibit prolonged muscular relaxation and apnea following an injection of a standard dose of this muscle relaxant. Glucose-6-phosphate dehydrogenase deficiency and altered stability of reduced glutathione are responsible for hemolytic anemia in subjects exposed to primaquine, antipyrine, and similar agents. A more extensive list of potentially hemolytic chemicals and drugs has been compiled by Calabrese et al. (1979).

Less dramatic but more consistently greater susceptibility to many drugs have been reported to exist among Indonesians and perhaps also other Asians (Darmansjah and Muchtar, 1992).

Sex, Hormonal Status, and Pregnancy

Male and female animals of the same strain and species usually react to toxicants similarly. There are, however, notable quantitative differences in their susceptibility, especially in the rat. For example, many barbiturates induce more prolonged sleep in female rats than in males. The shorter duration of action of hexobarbital in male rats is related to the higher activity of the liver microsomal enzymes to hydroxylate this chemical. This higher activity can be reduced by castration or pretreatment with estrogen. Similarly, male rats demethylate aminopyrine and acetylate sulfanilamide faster than females, and the males are thus less susceptible.

Female rats are also more susceptible than the males to such organophosphorus insecticides as azinphosmethyl and parathion. Castration and hormone treatment reverse this difference. Furthermore, weanling rats of both sexes are equally susceptible to these toxicants. However, unlike hexobarbital, parathion is metabolized more rapidly in the female rat than in the male. This faster metabolism of parathion results in a higher concentration of its metabolite, paraoxon, which is more toxic than the parent compound. This higher toxicity resulting from greater bioactivation in female rats, compared to males, is also true with aldrin and heptachlor, which undergo epoxidation. The female rat is also more susceptible to warfarin and strychnine. On the other hand, male rats are more susceptible than females to ergot and lead.

Differences in susceptibility between the sexes are also seen with other chemicals. For example, chloroform is acutely nephrotoxic in the male mouse but not in the females. Castration or the administration of estrogens reduces this effect in the males, and treatment with androgens enhances susceptibility to chloroform in the females. The greater susceptibility of male mice was explained on the basis of a much higher concentration of cytochrome P-450 (Smith et al., 1983). Nicotine is also more toxic to the male mouse, and digoxin is more toxic to the male dog. However, the female cat is more susceptible to dinitrophenol and the female rabbit is more so to benzene.

Imbalances of non-sex hormones can also alter the susceptibility of animals to toxicants. Hyperthyroidism, hyperinsulinism, adrenalectomy, and stimulation of the pituitary–adrenal axis have all been shown to be capable of modifying the effects of certain toxicants (Doull, 1980; Hodgson, 1987).

Age

It has long been recognized that neonates and very young animals in general are more susceptible to toxicants such as morphine. For a great majority of toxicants, the young are 1.5–10 times more susceptible than adults (Goldenthal, 1971).

The available information indicates that the greater susceptibility of the young animals to many toxicants can be attributed to deficiencies of various detoxication enzyme systems. Both phase I and phase II reactions may be responsible. For example, hexobarbital at a dose of 10 mg/kg induced a sleeping time of longer than 360 min in 1-d-old mice compared to 27 min in the 21-d-old. The proportion of hexobarbital metabolized by oxidation in 3 h in these animals was 0% and 21–33%, respectively (Jondorf et al., 1959). On the other hand, chloramphenicol is excreted mainly as a glucuronide conjugate. When a dose of 50 mg/kg was given to 1- or 2-d-old infants, the blood levels were 15 g/ml or higher over a period of 48 h. In contrast, children aged 1–11 yr maintained such blood levels for only 12 h (Weiss et al., 1960).

However, not all chemicals are more toxic to the young. Certain substances, notably central nervous system (CNS) stimulants, are much less toxic to neonates. Lu et al. (1965) reported that the LD_{50} of DDT was more than 20 times greater in newborn rats than in adults, in sharp contrast to the effect of age on malathion (Table 5-2). This insensitivity to the toxicity of DDT may be reassuring in assessing the potential risk of this pesticide, because of the very much larger intake in young babies via breast feeding and cow's milk, especially on the unit body weight basis.

The effect of age on the susceptibility to other CNS stimulants, including other organochlorine insecticides (e.g., dieldrin), appears less marked (generally in the range of 2–10 times). Most organophosphorous

Table 5-2 Effect of Age on Acute Toxicity of Malathion, DDT, and Dieldrin in Rats

Pesticide	Age	LD_{50} (mg/kg) with 95% confidence limits
Malathion	Newborn	134.4 (94.0–190.8)
	Preweaning	925.5 (679.01–261.0)
	Adult	3697.0 (3179.0–4251.0)
DDT	Newborn	>4000.0
	Preweaning	437.8 (346.3–553.9)
	Adult	194.5 (158.7–238.3)
Dieldrin	Newborn	167.8 (140.8–200.0)
	Preweaning	24.9 (19.7–31.5)
	Adult	37.0 (27.4–50.1)

Source: From Lu et al. (1965). Copyright © 1965, Elsevier Science Inc.

pesticides such as malathion are more toxic to the young; Schradan (oc-tamethyl pyrophosphoramide) and phenylthiourea are notable exceptions (Brodeur and DuBois, 1963).

Apart from differences in biotransformation, other factors also play a role. For example, a lower susceptibility at the receptor has been found to be the reason for the relative insensitivity of young rats to DDT (Henderson and Woolley, 1969).

Certain toxicants are absorbed to a greater extent by the young than by the adult. For example, young children absorb 4–5 times more lead than adults (McCabe, 1979) and 20 times more cadmium (Sasser and Jarbor, 1977). The greater susceptibility of the young to morphine is attributable to a less efficient blood–brain barrier, as is vividly illustrated in Fig. 5-1 (Kupferberg and Way, 1963). Penicillin and tetracycline are excreted more slowly and hence are more toxic in the young (Lu, 1970). Ouabain is about 40 times more toxic in the newborn than in the adult rat because the adult rat's liver is much more efficient in removing this cardiac glycoside from the plasma. The higher incidence of methemoglobinemia in young infants has been explained on the basis that their lower gastric acidity allows upward migration of intestinal microbial flora and the reduction of nitrates to a greater extent. Furthermore, they have a higher proportion of fetal hemoglobin, which is more readily oxidized to methemoglobin (WHO, 1977).

Figure 5-1 Brain and blood levels of free morphine at specific time intervals after intra-peritoneal injections of morphine. Bracketed vertical lines show the standard error, using four animals per point (from Kupferberg and Way, 1963).

There is evidence that the newborn is more susceptible to such carcinogens as aflatoxin B_1. Furthermore, the fetuses, but not the embryos, of rodents are much more susceptible. For example, there was a 50-fold increase in the potency of ethylnitrosourea. This is also true with nonhuman primates, except the maximal effects occur during the first third of gestation. If this is true with human fetuses, then they may be exposed to carcinogens before the mothers are aware of their pregnancies (Rice, 1979).

Old animals and humans are also more susceptible to certain chemicals. This problem has not been studied as extensively as in the young. However, the available evidence indicates that the aged patients are generally more sensitive to many drugs. The possible mechanisms include reduced detoxication and an impaired renal excretion (Goldstein, 1990). In addition, the distribution of chemicals in the body may also be altered because of increased body fat and decreased body water (Jarvik et al., 1981). A number of drugs have been found to be likely to induce more severe signs of toxicity. These include most CNS depressants, certain antibiotics, cardiac glycosides, and hypotensive agents (WHO, 1981).

Nutritional Status

The principal biotransformation of toxicants, as noted in chap. 3, is catalyzed by the microsomal mixed-function oxidase system (MFO). A deficiency of essential fatty acids generally depresses MFO activities. This is also true with protein deficiency. The decreased MFO has different effects on the toxicity of chemicals. For example, hexobarbital and aminopyrine are detoxicated by these enzymes and are thus more toxic to rats and mice with these nutrient deficiencies. On the other hand, the toxicities of aflatoxin, carbon tetrachloride, and heptachlor are lower in such animals because of their depressed bioactivation of these toxicants. Rats fed low-protein diets were 2–26 times more sensitive to a variety of pesticides (Boyd, 1972). MFO activities are decreased in animals fed high levels of sugar.

A number of carcinogenesis studies have demonstrated that restriction of food intake decreases tumor yield. Deficiency of protein generally lowers tumorigenicity of carcinogens, such as aflatoxin B_1 and dimethylnitrosamine. The importance of diet on carcinogenesis is further demonstrated by the fact that rats and mice fed diets rich in fats have higher tumor incidences compared to those that are given a restricted diet.

Vitamin A deficiency depresses the MFO. In general, this is also true with deficiencies of vitamins C and E. But thiamine deficiency has the opposite effect. Vitamin A deficiency, in addition, increases the susceptibility of the respiratory tract to carcinogens (Nettesheim et al., 1979).

Some foods contain appreciable amounts of chemicals that are strong inducers of the MFO, such as safrole, flavones, xanthines, and indoles. In addition, potent inducers such as DDT and polychlorinated biphenyls (PCB) are present as contaminants in many foods.

Diseases

The liver is the main organ wherein biotransformation of chemicals takes place. Such diseases as acute and chronic hepatitis, cirrhosis of the liver, and hepatic necrosis often decrease the biotransformation. The microsomal and nonmicrosomal enzyme systems as well as the phase II reactions may be affected.

Renal diseases may also affect the toxic manifestations of chemicals. This effect stems from disturbances of the excretory and metabolic functions of the kidney. Heart diseases, when severe, can increase the toxicity of chemicals by impairing the hepatic and renal circulation, thus affecting the metabolic and excretory functions of these organs. Respiratory tract disorders such as asthma render the subjects much more susceptible to air pollutants such as SO_2.

ENVIRONMENTAL FACTORS

Physical Factors

Changes in temperature may alter the toxicity. For example, colchicine and digitalis are more toxic to the rat than to the frog. But their toxicity to the frog can be increased by raising the environmental temperature. The duration of the response, however, is shorter when the temperature is higher. The effect of environmental temperature on the magnitude and duration of the response is apparently related to the temperature-dependent biochemical reactions responsible for the effect and for the biotransformation of the chemical.

Interest in the effect of barometric pressure on the toxicity of chemicals stems from human exposure to them in space and in saturation diving vehicles. At high altitudes, the toxicity of digitalis and strychnine is decreased whereas that of amphetamine is increased. The influence of changes in barometric pressure on the toxicity of chemicals seems attributable mainly, if not entirely, to the altered oxygen tension rather than to a direct pressure effect.

Whole-body irradiation increases the toxicity of CNS stimulants but decreases that of CNS depressants. However, it has no effect on analgesics such as morphine. More details and literature citations have been provided by Doull (1980).

The effects of toxicants often show a diurnal pattern that is mainly related to the light cycle. In the rat and the mouse, the activities of cytochrome P-450 are the greatest at the beginning of the dark phase.

Social Factors

It is well known that animal husbandry and a variety of social factors can modify the toxicities of chemicals: the handling of the animals, the housing (singly or in groups), the types of cage, and bedding materials are all important factors. Some examples of the influence of environmental factors on toxicity are given in chap. 6.

CHEMICAL INTERACTION

Types of Interaction

The toxicity of a chemical in an organism may be increased or decreased by a simultaneous or consecutive exposure to another chemical (Table 6-1). If the combined effect is equal to the sum of the effect of each substance given alone, the interaction is considered to be *additive*, for example, combinations of most organophosphorous pesticides on cholinesterase activity. If the combined effect is greater than the sum, the interaction is considered to be *synergistic*, for example, carbon tetrachloride and ethanol on the liver, and asbestos exposure and cigarette smoking on the lung. In the latter example, Selikoff et al. (1968) reported that there was a 5-fold increase in lung cancer incidence among asbestos workers, an 11-fold increase among cigarette smokers, and a 55-fold increase among asbestos workers who were cigarette smokers. The term *potentiation* is used to describe the situation in which the toxicity of a substance on an organ is markedly increased by another substance that alone has no toxic effect on that organ. For example, isopropanol has no effect on the liver, but it can increase considerably the hepatotoxicity of carbon tetrachloride.

Similarly, trichloroethylene, which has little effect on the liver, increases the hepatotoxicity of carbon tetrachloride, as measured by the release of liver enzymes alanine aminotransferase, sorbitol dehydrogenase, and aspartate aminotransferase (Borzelleca et al., 1990).

The exposure of an organism to a chemical may reduce the toxicity of another. *Chemical antagonism* denotes the situation wherein a reaction between the two chemicals produces a less toxic product, for example, chelation of heavy metals by dimercaprol. *Functional antagonism* exists when two chemicals produce opposite effects on the same physiologic parameters, such as the counteraction between CNS stimulants and depressants. *Competitive antagonism* exists when the agonist and antagonist act on the same receptor, such as the blockade of the effects of nicotine on ganglia by ganglionic blocking agents. *Noncompetitive antagonism* exists when the toxic effect of a chemical is blocked by another not acting on the same receptor. For example, atropine reduces the toxicity of acetylcholinesterase (AChE) inhibitors not by blocking the receptors on the AChE, but by blocking the receptors for the acetylcholine (ACh) accumulated.

Mechanisms of Action

Chemical interactions are achieved through a variety of mechanisms. For instance, nitrites and certain amines can react in the stomach to form nitrosamines, the majority of which are potent carcinogens, and thus greatly increase the toxicity. On the other hand, the action of many antidotes is based on their interaction with the toxicants; for example, thiosulfate is used in cases of cyanide poisoning. Furthermore, a chemical may displace another from its binding site on plasma protein and thereby increase its effective concentration. A chemical may modify the renal excretion of weak acids and weak bases by altering the pH of urine. Competition for the same renal transport system by one chemical can hinder the excretion of another. A notable example is the administration of probenecid along with penicillin to reduce the renal excretion of the antibiotic, thereby prolonging its duration of action.

One important type of interaction involves the binding of chemicals with their specific receptors. An antagonist blocks the action of an agonist, such as a neurotransmitter or a hormone, by preventing the binding of the agonist to the receptor.

Another important type of interaction results from alterations of the biotransformation of a chemical by another. Some chemicals are *inducers* of xenobiotic-metabolizing enzymes. They augment the activities of these enzymes, perhaps mainly by de novo synthesis. The common inducers include phenobarbital, 3-methylcholanthrene (3-MC), PCB, DDT, and benzo[a]pyrene (BaP). The inducers may lower the toxicity of other chemicals by accelerating their detoxication. For example, pretreatment with phenobarbital shortens the sleeping time induced by hexobarbital and the paralysis induced by zoxazolamine. Such pretreatment also reduces the plasma level of aflatoxins (Wong et al., 1981). In addition, 3-MC pretreatment greatly reduces the liver necrosis produced by bromobenzene, probably by increasing the activity of the epoxide hydrase (see Fig. 3-3). On the other hand, pretreatment with phenobarbital augments the toxicity of acetaminophen and bromobenzene, apparently by increasing the toxic metabolites formed. Repeated administration of a chemical may induce its metabolizing enzymes, as has been shown with vinyl chloride.

Piperonyl butoxide, isoniazid, and SKF 525A and related chemicals are *inhibitors* of various xenobiotic-metabolizing enzymes. For instance, piperonyl butoxide increases the toxicity of pyrethrum in insects by inhibiting their MFO that detoxifies this insecticide. Isoniazid, when taken along with diphenylhydantoin, lengthens the plasma half-life of the antiepileptic drug and increases its toxicity. Iproniazid inhibits monoamine oxidase and increases the cardiovascular effects of tyramine, which is found in cheese and which is normally readily metabolized by the oxidase.

Characteristics of Enzyme Induction

Because of the importance of the effect of enzyme induction, much work has been done on certain inducers, notably phenobarbital and polycyclic aromatic hydrocarbons (PAHs). These two types of inducers differ in several respects. For example, phenobarbital markedly increases the liver weight and the smooth endoplasmic reticulum, but PAHs such as 3-MC and BaP have little effect on these parameters. Phenobarbital augments mainly the amounts of cytochrome P-450 and NADPH-cytochrome c reductase. PAHs have little effect on these enzymes, but they increase the amount of cytochrome P-448, which is also known as P_1-450, and aryl hydrocarbon hydroxylase (AHH), as discussed in chap. 4. These isozymes have different substrate specificity and hence alter the effects of toxicants differently (see Sipes and Gandolfi, 1993).

Interaction as Toxicologic Tools

Studies on chemical interaction are conducted not only to determine the effects of combinations of chemicals, but the data thereof are useful in assessing health hazards associated with exposures to such combinations. These studies are also done to elucidate the nature and the mode of action of the toxicity of a chemical by the administration of another as well as to bring out weak or latent effects of chemicals. For example, a number of studies have been done to demonstrate the carcinogenic effects of saccharin by administering it along with potent carcinogens.

REFERENCES

Borzelleca, J. F., O'Hara, T. M., Gennings, C., Granger, R. H., Sheppard, M. A., and Condie, L. W. 1990. Interactions of water contaminants. *Fundam. Appl. Toxicol* 14:477–490.

Boyd, E. M. 1972. *Protein deficiency and pesticide toxicity.* Springfield, IL: Charles C Thomas.

Brodeur, J., and DuBois, K. P. 1963. Comparison of acute toxicity of anticholinesterase insecticides to weanling and adult male rats. *Proc. Soc. Exp. Biol. Med.* 114:509–511.

Calabrese, E. J., Moore, G., and Brown, R. 1979. Effects of environmental oxidant stressors on individuals with a G-6-PD deficiency with particular reference to an animal model. *Environ. Health Perspect.* 29:49–55.

Darmansjah, I., and Muchtar, A. 1992. Dose-response variation among different populations. *Clin. Pharmacol. Ther.* 52:449–452.

Doull, J. 1980. Factors influencing toxicology. In *Casarett and Doull's toxicology*, eds. J. Doull, C. D. Klaasen, and M. O. Amdur, p. 75. New York: Macmillan.

Goldenthal, E. I. 1971. A compilation of LD_{50} values in newborn and adult animals. *Toxicol. Appl. Pharmacol.* 18:185–207.

Goldstein, R. S. 1990. Drug-induced nephrotoxicity in middle-aged and senescent rats. *Proc. V Int. Congress of Toxicology*, pp. 412–421. London: Taylor & Francis.

Henderson, G. L., and Woolley, D. A. 1969. Studies on the relative insensitivity of the immature rat to the neurotoxic effects of DDT. *J. Pharmacol. Exp. Ther.* 170:173–180.

Hodgson, E. 1987. Modification of metabolism. In *Modern toxicology*, eds. E. Hodgson and P. E. Levi, pp. 85–121. New York: Elsevier.

Jarvik, L. F., Greenblatt, D. J., and Harman, D. 1981. *Clinical pharmacology and the aged patient.* New York: Raven Press.

Jay, G. E., Jr. 1955. Variation in response of various mouse strains to hexobarbital (Evipal). *Proc. Soc. Exp. Biol. Med.* 90:378–380.

Jondorf, W. R., Maickel, R. P., and Brodie, B. B. 1959. Inability of newborn mice and guinea pigs to metabolize drugs. *Biochem. Pharmacol.* 1:352–354.

Kupferberg, H. J., and Way, E. L. 1963. Pharmacologic basis for the increased sensitivity of the newborn rat to morphine. *J. Pharmacol. Exp. Ther.* 141:105–112.

Lu, F. C., Jessup, D. C., and Lavellee, A. 1965. Toxicity of pesticides in young versus adult rats. *Food Cosmet. Toxicol.* 3:591–596.

Lu, F. C. 1970. Significance of age of test animals in food additive evaluation. In *Metabolic aspects of food safety*, ed. F. J. C. Roe, pp. 285–308. Oxford: Blackwell.

McCabe, E. B. 1979. Age and sensitivity to lead toxicity: A review. *Environ. Health Perspect.* 29:29–33.

Miller, E. C., Miller, J. H., and Enomotor, M. 1964. The comparative carcinogenetics of 2-acetylaminofluorene and its *N*-hydroxy metabolite in mice, hamsters and guinea pigs. *Cancer Res.* 24:2018–2032.

Nettesheim, P., Snyder, C., and Kim, J. C. S. 1979. Vitamin A and the susceptibility of respiratory tract tissues to carcinogenic insult. *Environ. Health Perspect.* 29:89–93.

Quinn, G. P., Axelrod, J., and Brodie, B. B. 1958. Species, strain and sex differences in metabolism of hexobarbitone, amidopyrine, antipyrine and aniline. *Biochem. Pharmacol.* 1:152–159.

Rice, J. M. 1979. Perinatal period and pregnancy: Intervals of high risk for chemical carcinogens. *Environ. Health Perspect.* 29:23–27.

Sasser, L. B., and Jarbor, G. E. 1977. Intestinal absorption and retention of cadmium in neonatal rat. *Toxicol. Appl. Pharmacol.* 41:423–431.

Selikoff, I. J., Hammond, E. C., and Churg, J. 1968. Asbestos exposure, smoking, and neoplasia. *J. Am. Med. Assoc.* 204:106–112.

Sipes, I. G., and Gandolfi, A. J. 1993. Biotransformation of toxicants. In *Casarett and Doull's toxicology*, eds. M. O. Amdur, J. Doull, and C. D. Klaassen, pp. 88–126. New York: McGraw-Hill.

Smith, J. H., Maita, K., Adler, V., Schacht, T., Sleight, S. D., and Hook, J. B. 1983. Effect of sex hormone status on chloroform nephrotoxicity and renal drug metabolizing enzymes. *Toxicol. Lett.* 28(suppl. 1):23.

Weisburger, J. H., and Weisburger, E. K. 1973. Biochemical formation and pharmacological, toxicological and pathological properties of hydroxylamines and hydroxamic acids. *Pharmacol. Rev.* 25:166.

Weiss, c. G., Glazko, A. J., and Weston, A. 1960. Chloramphenicol in the newborn infant. A physicologic explanation of its toxicity when given in excessive doses. *N. Engl. J. Med.* 262:787–794.

Williams, R. T. 1974. Inter-species variations in the metabolism of xenobiotics. *Biochem. Soc. Trans.* 2:359–377.

Wong, Z. A., Wei, Chiang-I, Rice, D. W., and Hsieh, D. P. H. 1981. Effects of phenobarbital pretreatment on the metabolism and toxicokinetics of aflatoxin B_1 in the rhesus monkey. *Toxicol. Appl. Pharmacol.* 60:387–397.

World Health Organization. 1977. Nitrates, nitrites and *N*-nitroso compounds. Environmental Health Criteria 5. Geneva: WHO.

World Health Organization. 1981. Health care in the elderly: Report of the technical group on use of medicaments by the elderly. *Drugs* 22:279–294.

ADDITIONAL READING

Birnbaum, L. S. 1991. Pharmacokinetic basis of age-related changes in sensitivity to toxicants. *Annu. Rev. Pharmacol.* 31:101–128.

Appendix 5-1   Mechanisms[a] Underlying Certain Modifying Factors

Toxicant	Responsible mechanism	Toxic response
1. Bioactivation differences		
2-Naphthylamine	2-Naphthyl hydroxylamine	Bladder tumor in dog, human, but not rat, mouse
Acetylaminofluorene	N-Hydroxy metabolite	Carcinogenic in rat, mouse and hamster, but not in guinea pigs
2. Toxicokinetic characteristics		
Lead, cadmium	Greater absorption in the young	Greater toxic effects
Penicillin, tetracycline	Slower excretion in the young	Longer half-life
Morphine	Blood–brain barrier inefficient in the young	Greater CNS effect
3. Toxicodynamic characteristics		
DDT	Susceptibility of receptor	Less susceptible in the young
4. Anatomic characteristics		
BHA, BHT	Presence of forestomach in rat	Hyperplasia of forestomach
5. Physiologic characteristics		
Squill	Vomiting reflex	Absence in rat leading to toxic effect

[a]Other than detoxication.

Appendix 5-2 Strain-Related Differences in Drug-Induced Responses

Parameter	Tissue	Strain/stock	
		Resistant[a]	Susceptible
Ciprofibrate-induced peroxisomal proliferation	Liver	Sprague-Dawley	Long-Evans
Acetaminophen-induced necrosis	Kidney	Sprague-Dawley	F344
Streptozotocin-induced autoimmune reactivity	Popliteal lymph node	F344	Sprague-Dawley or Wistar
Amiodarone-induced phospholipidosis	Lung	Sprague-Dawley	F344
Diethylstilbesterol-induced carcinoma	Mammary tissue	COP	F344
Saccharin-induced histopathologic changes	Urinary bladder	Sprague-Dawley	Wistar
Mepirizole-induced ulceration	Duodenum	DONYRU	Sprague-Dawley or F344
Azaserine-induced carcinoma	Pancreas	F344	Wistar
β-Adrenoceptor suppression of lipolysis	Adipocyte	Wistar	Sprague-Dawley
Diethylstilbesterol-induced prolactin section	Pituitary	Sprague-Dawley	F344

Note. Adapted from S. Kacew and M. F. W. Festing, "Role of rat strain in the differential sensitivity to pharmaceutical agents and naturally occurring substances," *Journal of Toxicology and Environmental Health*, 47:1–30.
[a]Resistant does not imply a lack of effect but a significantly lower responsiveness than susceptible.

Part Two

Testing Procedures for Conventional and Nontarget Organ Toxicities

Conventional Toxicity Studies

CHAPTER 6 CONTENTS

INTRODUCTION

Usefulness

As noted in prior chapters, toxicants vary greatly in their potency, target organ, and mode of action. To provide proper orientation for additional in-depth targeted studies, conventional toxicity studies are generally carried out first. These studies are designed to provide indications of the appropriate dosage range, the probable adverse effect, and the target organ (e.g., liver), system (e.g., respiratory), or special toxicity (e.g., carcinogenicity).

In addition to providing preliminary information for proper orientation of additional investigations, however, the conventional toxicity studies per se yield data that can be used to assess the nature of the adverse effects and the "no-observed-adverse-effect level" (NOAEL) of the toxicant, which are required in the safety assessment described in chap. 22. For example, approximately half of the pesticides evaluated by the WHO Expert Committee on Pesticide Residues in the past thirty years have been based on conventional toxicity studies, in spite of the extensive database that is also available (Lu, 1995).

Categories

In order to examine the different effects associated with various lengths of exposure, the conventional studies are generally divided into three categories: (1) *Acute toxicity studies* involve either a single administration of the chemical under test or several administrations within a 24-h period. (2) *Short-term* (also known as subacute and subchronic) toxicity studies involve repeated administrations, usually on a daily or 5 times per week basis, over a period of about 10% of the life span, namely 3 mo in rats and 1 or 2 yr in dogs. However, shorter durations such as 14- and 28-d treatments have also been used by some investigators. (3) *Long-term* toxicity studies involve repeated administrations over the entire life span of the test animals or at least a major fraction of it, for example, 18 mo in mice, 24 mo in rats, and 7–10 yr in dogs and monkeys.

ACUTE TOXICITY STUDIES

These studies are designed either to determine the median lethal dose (LD_{50}) of the toxicant or a rough estimate of it. The LD_{50} has been defined as "a statistically derived expression of a single dose of a material that can be expected to kill 50% of the animals." In addition, such studies may also indicate the probable target organ of the chemical and its specific toxic effect and provide guidance on the doses to be used in the more prolonged studies.

In certain cases, especially those with low acute toxicities, it may not be necessary to determine precise LD_{50}s. Simple lethality data can serve useful purposes. For example, synergistic and antagonistic effects can be demonstrated using a few animals as shown by the data presented in Table 6-1. Furthermore, even the information that a sufficiently large dose causes few or no deaths may suffice. This *limit test* has been applied. For example, a number of food colors were given to rats at a dose of 2 g/kg. Since none of the rats died, it was considered sufficient to rule out any serious acute toxicity and no LD_{50} was determined (Lu and Lavallée, 1965). This view was accepted by the Joint FAO/WHO Expert Committee on Food Additives (WHO, 1966). The U.S. Environmental Protection Agency (EPA, 1994) recommends the use of 5 g/kg for a limit test.

When the route of exposure is inhalation, the end point is then either the median lethal concentration (LC_{50}) with a given duration of exposure or the median lethal time (LT_{50}) with a given concentration of the chemical in the air.

Experimental Design

Selection of Species of Animal In general, the rat, and sometimes the mouse, are selected for use in determining the LD_{50}. Their preference stems from the fact that they are economical, readily available, and easy to handle. Further, there are more toxicologic data on these species of animals, a fact that facilitates comparisons of toxicities of other chemicals.

Sometimes a nonrodent species is desirable. This is true especially when the LD_{50} values in rats and mice are markedly different or when the pattern or rate of biotransformation in humans is known to be significantly different from rats and mice.

The LD_{50} determination is preferably done in animals of both sexes, and also in adult and young animals, because of their differences in susceptibility.

Table 6-1   Using Lethality in Demonstrating Chemical Interaction

KBrO$_3$ (mg/kg)	Lethality (number of deaths/number on test)		
	Control (saline)	Cysteine[a] (400 mg/kg)	Diethyl maleate[b] (0.7 ml/kg)
169	5/5	0/5	
130	5/5	0/5	
49	0/5		4/5
29	0/5		4/5

Source: Adapted from Kurakawa et al. (1987).
Note: With five animals per dose group, the interactions between KBrO$_3$ and an "antagonist" (cysteine) and a "synergist" (diethyl maleate) are evident.
[a]Antagonistic.
[b]Synergistic.

Route of Administration Generally, the toxicant is administered by the route by which humans would be exposed. The oral route is most commonly used. The dermal and inhalation routes are used increasingly, not only for chemicals that are intended for human use by such routes but also for chemicals whose health hazards to personnel handling these chemicals are to be assessed (see chaps. 11 and 14). Parenteral routes are mainly used in assessing the acute toxicity of parenteral drugs. In addition, immediate or very prompt and complete or nearly complete absorption generally follow intravenous and intraperitoneal injection.

Dosage and Number of Animals To properly ascertain an LD_{50}, it is necessary to try to select a dose that would kill about half of the animals, another that would kill more than half (preferably less than 90%), and a third dose that would kill less than half (preferably more than 10%) of the animals. The Organization of Economic Cooperation and Development (OECD, 1992), among others, recommends a "sighting" study to aid in the selection of the doses, which can be accomplished with no more than five animals. Dosing of the animals is done sequentially, with at least a 24-h interval to allow adjustment of the dose the next animal is to receive.

In general, the precision of the LD_{50} is improved by increasing the number of animals per dose and by decreasing the ratio between successive doses. Some investigators use 40–50 animals per LD_{50} test and select ratios of 1.2–1.5. However, others (e.g., Weil, 1952) proposed the use of four animals per dose and a ratio of 2.0 between successive doses. Another simple test procedure has been described (Bruce, 1985) involving the use of only six to nine animals per test.

On the other hand, there are occasions when a more precise determination of the LD_{50} is desired. A more precise LD_{50} can be obtained with a smaller ratio between successive doses. For example, a ratio of 1.2 has been used (Lu et al., 1965) in demonstrating a lack of appreciable diurnal variation and a 4-fold difference in toxicity between batches. On the same batches of malathion, but using a ratio of 2 between successive doses, no conclusions could be drawn from the one hundred LD50 determinations with respect to the differences between batches because of the wide confidence limits (C. B. Shaffer, unpublished data).

In determining the LD_{50} in large animals, such as dogs, generally a much smaller number of them is used.

Observations and Examinations

After administering the toxicant to the animals, they should be examined for the number and time of death in order to estimate the LD_{50}. More importantly, their signs of toxicity should be recorded. Table 6-2 provides a list of body organs and systems that might be affected, along with the

Table 6-2 Relationship Between Toxic Signs and Body Organs or Systems

System	Toxic signs
Autonomic	Relaxed nictitating membrane, exophthalmos, nasal discharge, salivation, diarrhea, urination, piloerection
Behavioral	Sedation, restlessness, sitting position–head up, staring straight ahead, drooping head, severe depression, excessive preening, gnawing paws, panting, irritability, aggressive and defensive hostility, fear, confusion, bizarre activity
Sensory	Sensitivity to pain; righting, corneal, labyrinth, placing, and hindlimb reflex; sensitivity to sound and touch; nystagmus, phonation
Neuromuscular	Decreased and increased activity, fasciculation, tremors, convulsions, ataxia, prostration, straub tail, hindlimb weakness, pain and hindlimb reflexes (absent or diminished), opisthotonos, muscle tone, death
Cardiovascular	Increased and decreased heart rate, cyanosis, vasoconstriction, vasodilation, hemorrhage
Respiratory	Hypopnea, dyspnea, gasping, apnea
Ocular	Mydriasis, miosis, lacrimation, ptosis, nystagmus, cycloplegia, pupillary light reflex
Gastrointestinal, gastrourinary	Salivation, retching, diarrhea, bloody stool and urine, constipation, rhinorrhea, emesis, involuntary urination and defecation
Cutaneous	Piloerection, wet dog shakes, erythema, edema, necrosis, swelling

Source: McNamara (1976).

specific signs of toxicity. The observation period should be sufficiently long so that delayed effects, including death, would not be missed. The period is usually 7–14 d but may be much longer.

Gross autopsies should be performed on all animals that have died as well as at least some of the survivors, especially those that are morbid at the termination of the experiment. Autopsy can provide useful information on the target organ, especially when death does not occur shortly after the dosing. Histopathologic examination of selected organs and tissues may also be indicated.

Evaluation of the Data

Dose-Response Relationship When the mortality, or the frequency of other effects expressed in percentages, is plotted against the dose on a logarithmic scale, an S-shaped curve is obtained (Fig. 4-1, curve B) . The central portion of the curve (between 16% and 84% response) is sufficiently straight for estimating the LD_{50} or ED_{50}. However, a much wider range of the curve can be straightened by converting the percentages to probit units. This procedure is especially useful in estimating, for example, the LD_{01} or LD_{99}, when the extreme ends of this curve have to be used.

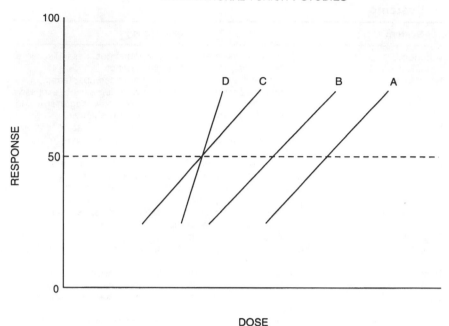

Figure 6-1 Median lethal doses and slopes of the dose-response (death) relationships of four chemicals. Chemical A is less toxic than the others. Chemical C is as toxic as D at the median lethal dose level but is more toxic at lower dose levels. Chemical B is less toxic than D at the median lethal dose level, but it may be more or less so at lower doses.

The probit units correspond to normal equivalent deviations around the mean, for example, +1, +2, +3 ... and −1, −2, −3 ... deviations, whereas the mean value itself has a zero deviation. However, to avoid negative numbers, the probit units are obtained by adding five to these deviations. The corresponding figures in these systems are as follows:

Deviations	Probit	% Response
−3	2	0.1
−2	3	2.3
−1	4	15.9
0	5	50.0
1	6	84.1
2	7	97.7
3	8	99.9

Detailed methods for estimating the LD_{50} and its standard errors are given in many papers and books on statistics, including those of Bliss (1957), Finney (1971), and Weil (1952).

Table 6-3 Acute LD_{50} Values for a Variety of Chemical Agents

Agent	Species	LD_{50} (mg/kg body weight)
Ethanol	Mouse	10,000
Sodium chloride	Mouse	4,000
Ferrous sulfate	Rat	1,500
Morphine sulfate	Rat	900
Phenobarbital, sodium	Rat	150
DDT	Rat	100
Picrotoxin	Rat	5
Strychnine sulfate	Rat	5
Nicotine	Rat	1
d-Tubocurarine	Rat	0.5
Hemicholinium-3	Rat	0.2
Tetrodotoxin	Rat	0.1
Dioxin (TCDD)	Guinea pig	0.001
Botulinum toxin	Rat	0.00001

Source: Loomis (1978).

Relative Potency The potency of a toxicant varies significantly. Table 6-3 illustrates the range of LD_{50} values.

To render the LD_{50} values more meaningful, it is advisable to determine also their standard errors (or the confidence limits) and the slopes of the dose-response curves. The importance of the slope can be readily appreciated when comparing two substances with similar LD_{50}s. The one with a flatter slope will likely cause more deaths than the other at doses smaller than the LD_{50}s (Fig. 6-1, chemicals C and D). The examples in Table 6-4 illustrate the marked differences in slopes.

Table 6-4 Dose-Response Relationships

Aflatoxin B_1[a]		Botulinum toxin[b]			
Dose (ppb)	Response (tumor)	Dose (pg)	Response (death)	Dose (pg)	Response (death)
0	0/18	1	0/10	34	11/30
1	2/22	5	0/10	37	10/30
5	1/22	10	0/30	40	16/30
15	4/21	15	0/30	45	26/30
50	20/25	20	0/30	50	26/30
100	28/28	24	0/30	55	17/30
		27	0/30	60	22/30
		30	4/30	65	20/30

Note: Relatively shallow dose-response relationship exists with aflatoxin B_1, wherein a 100-fold increase existed between the minimal and maximal effective doses, in contrast to the steep slope of botulinus toxin, wherein there was a mere 50% increase.

[a]Data quoted from Food Safety Council (1980).

[b]Data supplied by E. J. Schantz (Food Research Institute, University of Wisconsin, Madison, WI 53706). Part of the data also appears in the Report of Food Safety Council (1980).

Uses of LD$_{50}$ Values and Signs of Toxicity

These values are useful in a number of ways. Primary is classification of chemicals according to relative toxicity. A common classification is as follows:

Category	LD$_{50}$
Supertoxic	5 mg/kg or less
Extremely toxic	5–50 mg/kg
Highly toxic	50–500 mg/kg
Moderately toxic	0.5–5 g/kg
Slightly toxic	5–15 g/kg
Practically nontoxic	>15 g/kg

Others include evaluation of the hazard from accidental overdosage; planning subacute and chronic toxicity studies in animals; providing information about (a) the mechanism of toxicity, (b) the influence of age, sex, and other host and environmental factors, and (c) the variations in response among different animal species and strains; providing information about the susceptibility of a particular animal population; contributing to the overall information required in planning therapeutic trials of drugs in humans; and quality control of chemicals, to detect toxic impurities and physical changes affecting bioavailability.

For toxicants with important health implications (e.g., TCDD), LD$_{50}$s are determined in several species of animals. The extent of variation of these values indicates the range of differences in the toxicokinetics and/or toxicodynamics among these species.

Guidelines for acute oral, dermal, and inhalation toxicity studies have been published by various national and international agencies (e.g. U.S. EPA, 1994). However, the prevailing advice is to estimate approximate LD$_{50}$s unless otherwise indicated.

Multiple End-Point Evaluation

To derive additional information concerning the chemical on test, the toxic signs, such as those listed in Table 6-2, should be critically observed and recorded for evaluating nonlethal end points. These end points may assist in characterizing the nature of the toxicant.

SHORT-TERM AND LONG-TERM TOXICITY STUDIES

Humans are more often exposed to chemicals at levels much lower than those that are acutely fatal, but they are exposed over longer periods of time. To assess the nature of the toxic effects under these more realistic situations, short-term and long-term toxicity studies are conducted. These studies are also known as subacute (or subchronic) and chronic toxicity studies. The procedures involved in these two types are very similar except for their duration.

Experimental Design

Species and Number   Generally, two or more species of animals are used. Ideally, the animals chosen should biotransform the chemical in a manner essentially identical to humans. Since this is often unattainable, the rat and the dog are usually selected. This preference is based on their appropriate size, ready availability, and the great preponderance of toxicologic information on chemicals in these animals. The value of using more than one species is demonstrated, inter alia, by Contrera et al. (1993).

Equal numbers of male and female animals should be used. Generally, 10–50 rats are used in each dose group as well as in the control group. As a rule, this procedure will provide data that are statistically analyzable. Smaller numbers of dogs (48 per group) are used because of the greater number of examinations that can be made on each animal and because of their size and the expense involved.

Route of Administration   The chemical should be administered by the route of the intended use or exposure in humans. For most chemicals, the common route is oral. The preferred procedure is to incorporate the chemical in the diet, although the drinking water is sometimes used as the vehicle. The latter method is advisable when the chemical may react with a component in the diet. The chemical, especially if it is reactive, volatile, or unpalatable, is often administered by gavage or in gelatin capsules, a procedure more often used in dogs. The daily dose of the chemical may also be incorporated in a bolus of canned dog food.

Dermal application, exposure by inhalation, and parenteral routes are used for special purposes, such as industrial and agricultural products and drugs.

Dosage and Duration   Since the aim of these studies is to determine the nature and site of the toxic effects as well as the "no-observed-adverse-effect level," it is advisable to select three doses: a dose that is high enough to elicit definite signs of toxicity but not high enough to kill many of the animals, a low dose that is expected to induce no toxic effect, and an intermediate dose. Sometimes, one or more additional doses are included to ensure that these objectives are achieved. As noted earlier, a control group should be included. These animals will not receive the chemical under test but must be given any vehicle used.

The doses are generally selected on the basis of the information obtained in the acute toxicity studies, using both the LD_{50} and the slope of the dose-response curve. Any information on related chemicals and on their metabolism, especially the presence or absence of bioaccumulation, is also taken into account. A range-finding study is sometimes done. It consists of dosing five rats of each sex at each of three or four dose levels for 7 d. The criteria for toxic effects are mortality, body weight gain, relative liver and kidney weights, and feed consumption. The results from 7-d tests are generally better than the LD_{50} values in predicting the dose levels for the longer term toxicity study.

In studies in rats, the dose levels may be constant concentrations and expressed in milligrams per kilogram diet (ppm) or constant dosage and expressed in milligrams per kilogram body weight of the animals. As the animal grows, there are changes in the body weight as well as in the food consumption. For the constant dose regimen, the concentration of the chemical must therefore be adjusted periodically to maintain a relatively constant dose in mg/kg body weight. This is usually done at weekly intervals during the period of rapid growth and biweekly thereafter.

In the short-term studies, the duration in rats is generally 90 d. In the dog, the duration is often extended to 6 mo or even 1 yr. The duration of long-term studies in rats is generally 24 mo, and 7 yr or more in dogs.

Observations and Examinations

Body Weight and Food Consumption   These should be determined weekly. Decreased body weight gain is a simple yet sensitive index of toxic effects. Food consumption is also a useful indicator. In addition, a marked decrease in food consumption can induce effects that mimic or aggravate the toxic manifestations of the chemical. In such cases, paired feeding or parenteral feeding may have to be instituted. Where the animals receiving the toxicant are affected more than those maintained on a reduced feed alone, the toxicant, apart from the undernutrition, is responsible for the effect.

General Observations   These should include appearance, behavior, and any abnormality. Dead and moribund animals should be removed from the cages for gross and possibly microscopic examination. Frequent observation is necessary to minimize cannibalism.

Laboratory Tests   *Hematologic* examinations usually include hematocrit, hemoglobin, erythrocyte count, total leukocyte count, and differential leukocyte count. All dogs should be sampled before the initiation of treatment and at one week, one month, and at the end. Tests at other intervals may be warranted. Because of the small blood volume of rats, only half of them are sampled at various intervals, while the others are sampled only at the end. Special tests such as reticulocyte count, platelet count, methemoglobin, and glucose-6-phosphate dehydrogenase (G-6-PD) may be indicated.

Clinical laboratory tests usually include fasting blood glucose, serum aspartate aminotransferase (AST or SGOT), alanine aminotransferase (ALT or SGPT), alkaline phosphatase (AP), total protein, albumin, globulin, blood urea nitrogen (BUN), and such elements as sodium, potassium, calcium, and chloride. Other tests may be done where indicated. For example, cholinesterase activity is assessed when testing organophorus and carbamate pesticides.

Urinalysis usually includes color, specific gravity, pH, protein, glucose, ketones, formed elements (red blood cells, etc.), and crystalline and amorphous materials.

Postmortem Examination   Whenever possible, all animals that are found dead or dying should be subjected to a gross pathologic examination. If the state of the tissue permits, histologic examinations should also be done. In addition, the weights of a number of organs, either in absolute values or in terms of the body weights, should be determined as they serve as useful indicators of toxicity.

The organs that are usually weighed are liver, kidneys, adrenals, heart, brain, thyroid, and testes or ovaries. Those that are histologically examined are the following: all gross lesions, brain (three levels), spinal cord, eye and optic nerve, a major salivary gland, thymus, thyroid, heart, aorta, lung with a bronchus, stomach, small intestine (three levels), large intestine (two levels), adrenal gland, pancreas, liver, gallbladder (if present), spleen, kidney, urinary bladder, skeletal muscle, and bone and its marrow.

A list indicating the correlation between general observations, clinical laboratory tests, and postmortem examinations is produced as Appendix 6-1.

Guidelines for short-term and long-term studies have been published by the World Health Organization (WHO, 1978, 1990), and the U.S. Environmental Protection Agency (U.S. EPA, 1994), among others.

Evaluation

Comprehensive short-term and long-term toxicity studies, using the various parameters of observations and examinations just described, usually yield information on the toxicity of the chemical under test with respect to the target organs, the effects on these organs, and the dose-effect and dose-response relationships. Such information often provides an indication of the additional specific types of studies that should be conducted. The quantitative data from the short-term and other studies have been suggested for use in the determination of the "no-observed-adverse-effect level" (NOAEL). This suggestion, however, has not been widely accepted because it is considered more prudent to use the data from long-term studies. This is especially true for chemicals (e.g., food additives, pesticides, environmental pollutants) to which humans may be subjected to lifetime exposure. On the other hand, short-term studies may suffice in testing such chemicals as most pharmaceuticals, which are used for short durations.

The NOAEL from the long-term studies, along with data on their acute toxicity and metabolism as well as information from genetic, reproductive, and any other studies, is used in determining their "acceptable daily intakes" (ADI) for humans. For further discussion on the procedure used for this purpose, see chap. 22.

GOOD LABORATORY PRACTICE

In 1975 and 1976, the U.S. Food and Drug Administration (FDA) raised questions about the integrity of toxicologic data received from certain laboratories. On inspecting these facilities, FDA discovered a number of unacceptable laboratory practices, such as selective reporting, underreporting, lack of adherence to a specified protocol, poor animal care procedures, poor recordkeeping, and inadequate supervision of personnel. In an attempt to improve the validity of the data, FDA proposed a set of regulations for good laboratory practice in 1978. These were later included in the Regulation for the Enforcement of the Federal Food, Drug, and Cosmetic Act.

These regulations (FDA, 1987) contain detailed guidance on provisions for the following:

1 Personnel, stipulating the responsibilities of the study director, testing facility management, and quality assurance unit.
2 Facilities for animal care, animal supply, and handling test and control chemicals.
3 Equipment, regarding its design, maintenance, and calibration.
4 Testing facilities operation, including standard operating procedures, reagents and solutions, and animal care.
5 Test and control chemicals, such as their characterization and handling.
6 The protocol and conduct of a laboratory study.
7 Records, their storage, retrieval, and retention, as well as the preparation and contents of reports.
8 Disqualifications of testing facilities.

The U.S. Environmental Protection Agency also proposed a set of good laboratory practice standards. They contain provisions similar to those of the FDA regulation regarding health effects testing. However, the U.S. EPA standards also contain provisions for environmental effects testing (U.S.

EPA, 1994). At an international level, the OECD (1982) has also produced a set of similar guidelines.

REFERENCES

Bliss, C. L. 1957. Some principles of bioassay. *Am. Sci.* 45:449–466.

Bruce, R. D. 1985. An up-and-down procedure for acute toxicity testing. *Fundam. Appl. Toxicol.* 5:151–157.

Contrera, J. F., Aub, D., Barbehann, E., et al. 1993. A retrospective comparison of the results of 6 and 12 month nonrodent toxicity studies. *Adverse Drug React. Toxicol. Rev.* 12: 63–76.

Finney, D. J. 1971. *Probit analysis.* Cambridge: Cambridge University Press.

Food and Drug Administration. 1987. Good laboratory practice regulations; Final rule. *Fed. Reg.* 52:33768–33782.

Food Safety Council. 1980. Proposed system for food safety assessment. *Food Cosmet. Toxicol.* 16, suppl. 2.

Kurakawa, Y., Takamura, N., et al. 1987. Comparative studies on lipid peroxidation in the kidney of rats, mice and hamsters and the effect of cysteine, glutathione and diethyl maleate treatment on mortality and nephrotoxicity after administration of potassium bromate. *J. Am. Coll. Toxicol.* 6:487–501.

Loomis, T. 1978. *Essentials of toxicology*, 3d ed. Philadelphia: Lea & Febiger.

Lu, F. C. 1995. A review of the acceptable daily intakes of pesticides assessed by WHO. *Regul. Toxicol. Pharmacol.* 21:352-364.

Lu, F. C., Jessup, D. C., and Lavallée, A. 1965. Toxicity of pesticides in young versus adult rats. *Food Cosmet. Toxicol.* 3:591–596.

Lu, F. C. and Lavallée, A. 1965. The acute toxicity of some synthetic colors used in drugs and foods. *Can. Pharm. J.* 97:30.

McNamara, B. P. 1976. Concepts in health evaluation of commercial and industrial chemicals. In *New concepts in safety evaluation*, eds. M. A. Mehlman, R. E. Shapiro, and H. Blumenthal, pp. 61–140. Washington, DC: Hemisphere.

Organization of Economic Cooperation and Development. 1982. Good Laboratory Practice in the Testing of Chemicals. Paris: OECD.

Organization of Economic Cooperation and Development. 1992. OECD Guidelines for Testing Chemicals. Acute Oral Toxicity. Paris: OECD.

U.S. Environmental Protection Agency. 1994. Health Effects Test Guidelines. Hazard Evaluation. Code of Federal Regulations, Title 40, Part 792 and 798.

Weil, C. S. 1952. Tables for convenient calculation of median effective dose (LD_{50} or ED_{50}) and instructions for their use. *Biometrics* 8:249–263.

Workshop on Subchronic Toxicity Testing. 1980. Proceedings of the Workshop, EPA-560/11-80-028, eds. N. Page, D. Sawbney, and M. G. Ryon. Springfield, VA: National Technical Information Service.

World Health Organization. 1966. Specifications for Identity and Purity and Toxicological Evaluation of Food Colors. WHO/Food Add./66.25. Geneva: WHO.

World Health Organization. 1978. Principles and Methods for Evaluating the Toxicity of Chemicals. Part I. Environmental Health Criteria 6. Geneva: WHO.

World Health Organization. 1990. Principles for Toxicological Assessment of Pesticide Residues in Food. Environ. Health Criteria. 104: Geneva: WHO.

ADDITIONAL READING

Ecobichon, D. J. 1992. *The basis of toxicity testing.* Boca Raton, FL: CRC Press.

Appendix 6-1 General Observations, Clinical Laboratory Tests, and Pathology Examinations That May be Used in Short- and Long-Term Toxicity Studies

Organ or organ system	General observations	Clinical laboratory tests on blood	Pathology examination[a]
Liver	Discoloration of mucus membranes, edema, ascites	ALT (SGPT), AP, AST (SGOT), cholesterol, total protein, albumin, globulin	Liver[b]
Urinary system	Urine volume, consistency, color	BUN, total protein, albumin, globulin	Kidney and urinary bladder[b]
Gastrointestinal (GI) system	Diarrhea, vomit, stool, appetite	Total protein, albumin, globulin, sodium, potassium	Stomach, GI tract, gallbladder (if present), salivary gland, pancreas
Nervous system	Posture, movements, responses, behavior		Brain, spinal cord, and sciatic nerve
Eye	Appearance, discharge, ophthalmologic examination		Eye and optic nerves
Respiratory system	Rate, coughing, nasal discharge	Total protein, albumin, globulin	One lung with a major bronchus
Hematopoietic system	Discoloration of mucous membranes, lethargy, weakness	Packed red cell volume, hemoglobin, erythrocyte count, total and differential leukocyte count, platelet count, prothrombin time, activated partial thromboplastin time	Spleen, thymus, mesenteric lymph nodes, bone marrow smear and section
Reproductive system	Appearance and palpation of external reproductive organs		Testes and epididymis or ovaries; uterus or prostate and seminal vesicles[b]
Endocrine system	Skin, hair coat, body weight, urine and stool characteristics	Glucose, Na, K, AP (dog), cholesterol	Thyroid, adrenal, pancreas
Skeletal system	Growth, deformation, lameness	Calcium, phosphorus, AP	Bone and breakage strength
Cardiovascular system	Rate and characteristic of pulse, rhythm, edema, ascites	AST	Heart, aorta, small arteries in other tissues
Skin	Color, appearance, odor, hair coat	Total protein, albumin, globulin	Only in dermal studies
Muscle	Size, weakness, wasting, decreased activity	AST, creatine phosphokinase	Only if indicated by observations, clinical chemistry, or gross lesions

Source: Adapted from Workshop on Subchronic Toxicity Testing (1980).

[a]All animals should undergo thorough gross examination; organs or tissues listed should be examined microscopically.

[b]These organs should also be weighed.

Carcinogenesis

CHAPTER 7 CONTENTS

INTRODUCTION

In many countries, cancer is one of the leading causes of death. It is induced by a variety of agents, the most important being certain life-styles, such as smoking cigarettes, drinking alcoholic beverages, or chewing betel. However, chemicals in the community and workplace and some therapeutic agents also play a role. Attempts at reducing cancer incidence are therefore aimed at reducing these hazardous life-styles as well as at identifying these chemical carcinogens, in the hope that human exposure to them can be eliminated or minimized. Chemicals that are considered definite human carcinogens and those considered probable human carcinogens are listed in Appendix 7-1 (IARC, 1987).

Another type of research in carcinogenesis is aimed at improving existing methods and devising new methods for prompt and reliable identification of carcinogenic chemicals. Presently available methods either are too costly and time-consuming or are not sufficiently reliable. This problem stems mainly from the fact that cancer only occurs in response to a chemical long after its first entry into an organism. Often the chemical is no longer detectable in the body by the time the tumor develops.

In addition, the health hazards of carcinogens vary, depending not only on their potency, but also on their mode of action. In this chapter are therefore briefly described various categories of carcinogens based on the weight of evidence and their mode of action; the potency aspect is dealt with in chap. 22.

While human data provide an important role in establishing a substance as a human carcinogen, animal data are often required to substantiate the preliminary human data or to provide a lead to additional investigations in humans; in many cases, the special groups of population are exposed to a variety of possible carcinogens. The different categories of required information and animal tests are also discussed in this chapter.

Definition

The term *chemical carcinogenesis* is generally defined to indicate the induction or enhancement of neoplasia by chemicals. Although in the strict etymologic sense this term means the induction of carcinomas, it is widely used to indicate tumorigenesis. In other words, it includes not only epithelial malignancies (carcinomas) but also mesenchymal malignant tumors (sarcomas) and benign tumors. The extension to benign tumor is justified because no carcinogen that produces only benign tumors has been discovered.

It is generally agreed (e.g., WHO, 1969) that the response of an organism to a carcinogen may be in one or more of these forms:

1 An increase in the frequency of one or several types of tumors that also occur in the controls.
2 The development of tumors not seen in the controls.
3 The occurrence of tumors earlier than in the controls.
4 An increase in the number of tumors in individual animals, compared to the controls.

Classification / Weight of Evidence

Evidence of carcinogenicity consists of human and animal data. However, because of interspecies difference in response to chemicals, sound human data are given much greater weight. In fact, the earliest discoveries of chemical carcinogens were made in humans. Thus, in 1761 Hill found users of tobacco snuff had a high rate of nasal cancer, and Pott observed in 1775 that exposure to soot by chimney sweeps induced cancer of the scrotum. Twenty years later, Sömmering noted that cancer of the lip was often associated with pipe smoking. Rehn discovered in 1895 that bladder tumors occurred among workers in aniline dye factories.

Human evidence of carcinogenesis usually comes from *occupational* settings. For example, 2-naphthylamine was found to produce bladder cancers among some occupational workers. This finding was confirmed in the mouse, rat, rabbit, hamster, dog, and rhesus monkey. Similarly, asbestos induced tumors in the lung and pleural cavity, and these tumors were produced in several species of animals.

In addition, certain *medications* have been found to cause cancers in humans. Examples are cyclophosphamide, which induced bladder cancers among patients, and DES (diethylstilbestrol), which when given to pregnant women in very large doses resulted in vaginal and uterine tumors in their offspring. There is evidence that aflatoxins and arsenic compounds from *environmental sources* have increased the incidence of liver and skin cancers, respectively.

In view of the seriousness of cancer, however, it would be grossly imprudent to wait for relevant results to be generated from long-term human studies to assess each chemical for its carcinogenicity. Consequently, appropriate studies need be carried out in animals. The significance of the results, however, varies greatly among different studies. For example, aflatoxin B_1 induced tumors in a variety of animals, with small doses (ppb), and with a relatively short latent period. On the other hand, saccharin yielded positive results inconsistently, with very large doses (in tens of thousands of parts per million), and only after very long periods of treatment. Furthermore, the experimental design and conduct of the studies also differ in their adequacy (see Evaluation, p. 104).

To facilitate the evaluation of such diverse findings, a *weight of evidence* scheme has been adopted. The findings may be considered *sufficient* when there exists one of the following conditions:

1 Presence of benign and malignant tumors in multiple species or strains or in multiple experiments.
2 Occurrence of tumors at a high rate, or at an unusual site, or of a special type.

Limited evidence means positive results in only one species, strain, or experiment, or when the experimental design or conduct is inadequate. *Inadequate* evidence applies to results that are difficult to interpret. Using these or similar criteria, the U.S. Environmental Protection Agency (U.S. EPA, 1986) and IARC (1987) classified chemical carcinogens in five categories (Table 7-1).

In addition to extensive testing programs being carried out in animals, toxicologists and scientists in relevant disciplines have been vigilant in collecting carcinogenesis data in humans.

MODE OF ACTION

Chemical carcinogenesis, as shown in Fig. 7-1, is a multistage process. Carcinogenic chemicals act by initiating certain genetic changes in a cell, promoting the formation of a neoplasm, converting the neoplasm to a cancer, or enhancing the activity of another chemical.

Bioactivation

Most carcinogenic chemicals per se are inactive. However, they undergo bioactivation in the body to yield reactive metabolites. A common type

Table 7-1 Classification of Carcinogens Based on "Weight of Evidence"

Categories	IARC	EPA	Human data	Animal data
Human carcinogen	1	A	Sufficient	Sufficient or limited
Probable human carcinogen	2A	B1, B2[a]	Limited or inadequate[b]	Sufficient
Possible human carcinogen	2B	C	Absent or inadequate	Sufficient or limited[b]
Not classifiable	3	D	Absent or inadequate	Inadequate or absent
Not carcinogenic	4	E	Absent	Negative evidence in at least two species

[a]EPA classifies carcinogens with sufficient animal data as "probable human carcinogen" and places them in category B1 or B2 depending on the weight of the human data.
[b]IARC accepts positive genotoxicity in lieu of human data.

reactive metabolite is epoxide. For example, aflatoxin B_1 is converted to aflatoxin 8,9-epoxide. Benzene, vinyl chloride, and a number of polycyclic hydrocarbons also form epoxides. Other carcinogens, such as acetylaminofluorene (AAF) and certain aminoazo dyes, form N-hydroxy derivatives (see Appendix 3-1). Certain chemicals are bioactivated to ultimate carcinogens via an intermediary step. An example of this is benzo[a]pyrene (BaP), which forms BaP 7,8-epoxide, the intermediary carcinogen. The latter then transforms to BaP 7,8-diol 9,10-epoxide, the ultimate carcinogen.

Interaction with Macromolecules

The reactive metabolites bind with macromolecules. Some of them, such as proteins, may not play a critical role in carcinogenesis. However, when DNA is the target, the reaction may lead to point mutation, frame-shift mutation, and others. These changes may not persist; they may be reversed by an error-free DNA repair or disappear when the cell dies.

Initiation

If the cell with an altered DNA undergoes mitosis, the alteration will be retained. The cell with the altered DNA is termed an *initiated* cell. Depending on the site of the alteration, the cell may be partially or fully neoplastic. The process generally involves the conversion of proto-oncogene to oncogene.

Proto-oncogenes may be converted to oncogenes through translocation to a different chromosomal site, or other mechanisms such as genetic am-

Figure 7-1 Schematic diagram depicting fate of a genotoxic carcinogen and its relation with carcinogenesis. Events in left-hand column lead to cancer formation, whereas those in right-hand column are harmless. Asterisk indicates step may be important during other stages of carcinogenesis.

plification, insertions, and gene mutation (Bishop, 1987). In addition, there are onco-suppressor genes; a lack of their expression or an inactivation of their products may also lead to carcinogenesis (Weinberg, 1989). One of them, the p53 supressor gene, is mutated in about half of human cancers (Greenblatt et al., 1994).

Promotion

The initiated tumor cell, with altered genotype and phenotype, may remain dormant for a long period of time before it becomes a tumor through cell proliferation in the presence of *promoters* (Butterworth and Goldworthy, 1991). The dormancy is probably due to the suppressant influence of the surrounding normal cells exerted through certain intercellular communication (Trosko and Chang, 1988). The influence can be reduced by cell killing (e.g., from cytotoxic chemicals), cell removal (e.g., partial hepatectomy), growth factors (e.g., hormones), and other factors.

While initiation is generally considered to be a permanent process, promotion is not. Furthermore, it is reversible. Therefore, for an initiated cell to continue to replicate, it must be exposed to a promoter more or less continuously.

Conversion and Progression

These are characterized by biochemical and/or morphological changes in the activity or structures of the genome. The mechanism of action is not fully understood, but may involve activation of the initiated cells by exposure to clastogenic agents or complete carcinogens (Pitot et al., 1988). During this period, the neoplasm may convert from benign to malignant tumor which is invasive and metastatic.

Similar to initiation, progression is an irreversible process. Table 7-2 provides a list of the characteristics of initiation, promotion, and progression. For additional information and references, see Williams and Weisburger (1993).

CATEGORIES OF CARCINOGENS

Carcinogens may also be classified according to their mode of action into genotoxic and epigenetic (nongenotoxic) carcinogens.

Genotoxic (DNA-Reactive) Carcinogens

Genotoxic carcinogens initiate tumors by producing DNA damage (Fig. 7-1). There are two types.

Table 7-2 Morphologic and Biologic Characteristics of the Stages of Initiation, Promotion, and Progression in Hepatocarcinogenesis in the Rat

Initiation	Promotion	Progression
Irreversible with constant "stem cell" potential; initiated "stem cell" not morphologically identifiable	Reversible	Irreversible Measurable and/or morphologically discernible alteration in cell genome's structure
Efficacy sensitive to xenobiotic and other chemical factors	Promoted cell population existence dependent on continued administration of the promoting agent	
Spontaneous (fortuitous) occurrence of initiated cells can be quantitated	Efficiency sensitive to dietary and hormonal factors	Growth of altered cells sensitive to environmental factors during early phase
Requires cell division for "fixation"		
Dose response does not exhibit a readily measurable threshold	Dose response exhibits measurable threshold and maximal effect dependent on dose of initiating agent	Benign and/or malignant neoplasms characteristically seen
Relative effect of initiators depends on quantitation of focal lesions following defined period of promotion	Relative effectiveness of promoters depends on time and dose rate to reach maximal effect and dose rate	"Progressor" agents act to advance promoted cells into this stage but may not be initiating agents

Source: Pitot et al. (1988).

Direct-Acting Carcinogens   These chemicals are also known as ultimate carcinogens. They are electrophilic and can bind to DNA and other macromolecules. Examples are alkyl and aryl epoxides, lactones, sulfate esters, nitrosamides, nitrosoureas, and platinum amine chelates. Because of their high reactivity, these direct-acting carcinogens are often more active in vitro but less so in vivo.

Precarcinogens   These are also known as procarcinogens. They require conversion through bioactivation to become ultimate carcinogens, either directly or via an intermediary stage, the proximate carcinogens. Most of the presently known chemical carcinogens fall into this class. These include the polycyclic aromatic hydrocarbons (PAH), aromatic amines, halogenated hydrocarbons, nitrosamines, cycasin, aflatoxin B, pyrrolizidine alkaloids, safrole, and thioamides. Different types of bioactivations (such as formation of epoxides, N-hydroxy derivatives) are involved in their conversion to the direct-acting agents, as discussed in chap. 3.

These chemicals may also activate proto-oncogene to oncogene, and in-activate onco-suppressor genes.

There are pure initiators, such as *trans*-4-acetyl-aminostilbene, which can convert normal cells but cannot, in the absence of promoters, produce tumors. Complete genotoxic carcinogens, such as 2-AAF, act as initiator as well as promoter (Neumann, 1983).

As noted earlier, timely and error-free DNA repair plays an important part in the prevention of neoplastic transformation. An interesting example is dimethylnitrosamine. Its damage to hepatocyte DNA is rapidly repaired in the rat but only slowly in the hamster, and the latter is thus more sus-ceptible than the rat to this carcinogen. Furthermore, in the rat it induces tumor in the brain where the repair mechanism is deficient (see p. 47).

Epigenetic (Nongenotoxic) Carcinogens

These substances do not damage DNA but enhance the growth of tumors induced by genotoxic carcinogens or induce tumors through other mech-anisms. These are briefly described as follows.

Cocarcinogens These substances enhance the effects of genotoxic carcinogens when given simultaneously. They may act by effecting an in-crease in the concentration of the initiator, the genotoxic carcinogen itself, or that of the reactive metabolite. This can be achieved either by an in-crease of the absorption of the carcinogen, via the gastrointestinal tract or the skin, or by an increase of the bioactivation. The same result can also be achieved through a decrease of the elimination of the initiator either by inhibiting the detoxification enzymes or by depleting the endogenous sub-strates involved in phase II reactions, such as glutathione.

Apart from increasing the concentration of the reactive species at the site of action, cocarcinogens may inhibit the rate or fidelity of DNA repair, or they may enhance conversion of DNA lesions to permanent alterations.

Tobacco smoke contains relatively small amount of genotoxic carcin-ogens, such as PAH and nitrosamines; its marked carcinogenic effects are perhaps attributed to its catechols, which act as cocarcinogens (van Duuren, 1982).

Promoters These chemicals increase the effects of initiators when given subsequently. The classic example of this phenomenon was provided by studies demonstrating that an initial application on mouse skin of a carcinogenic PAH did not induce skin cancer until after applying, at the same site, phorbol esters from croton oil (Berenblum and Shubik, 1947, 1949). The application of the promoters could be delayed for months or even a year without losing the effect. These studies clearly demonstrate the *two-stage* process of carcinogenesis as well as the persistence of the effect of the initiator. Incidentally, croton oil is also cocarcinogenic since it is effective when applied at the same time as the initiator.

The possible mechanisms of action of promoters include (1) stimulation of cell proliferation through cytotoxicity or hormonal effects; (2) inhibition of intercellular communication, thereby releasing the initiated cells from the restraint exercised by the surrounding normal cells; and (3) immunosuppression.

Cytotoxicants such as nitrilotriacetic acid (NTA), a noneutrophying replacement for phosphate in household detergent, produce tumors through cell proliferation resulting from cell injury and death (Anderson et al., 1985). Unleaded gasoline and a number of other chemicals have been shown to induce renal tubular necrosis resulting from deposition of $\alpha_{2\mu}$-globulin. The cell death and subsequent regeneration are believed to cause kidney tumors (Swenberg et al., 1989).

Hormones such as estradiol and diethylstilbestrol have been shown to cause an increase in tumors in animals (e.g., breast cancer in mice) and in humans (e.g., endometrial cancer in menopausal females maintained on estrogen). These substances are not genotoxic but act as promoters. The actual initiators are not known. Androgens have little, if any, carcinogenic effect. The herbicide aminotriazole and certain fungicides induce thyroid tumor also through a hormonal mechanism (McClain, 1989).

Gap junction intercellular communication is an important mechanism in regulating cell growth. A number of chemicals interfere with this mechanism, thereby inducing hyperplasia and acting as promoters in carcinogenesis (Trosko and Chang, 1988). Klaunig (1991) listed, among others, a number of pesticides (e.g. chlordane, DDT, dieldrin, endosulfan, lindane) and pharmaceuticals (phenobarbital and diazepam) as being able to inhibit hepatic gap junctional intercellular communication.

Immunosuppresive drugs such as cyclosporrin A and azathioprine are increasingly being used in conjunction with organ transplantation. They have been shown to cause leukemias and sarcomas in some of these patients and in mice and rats. The genotoxic agents are likely to be viruses, and the immunosuppressive drugs promote the development of the tumors through epigenetic mechanisms (Ryffel, 1992).

Proxisome proliferators consist of a variety of chemicals that have the common property of inducing rodent liver tumors and increasing peroxisomes in liver cells. These chemicals have therefore been considered as a special class of carcinogen (Reddy and Lalwani, 1983). Examples are hypolipidemic drugs such as clofibrate and fenofibrate, certain phthalate plasticizers such as di(2-ethylhexyl) phthalate, and the solvent 1,1,2-trichloroethylene. These chemicals are not genotoxic, but by increasing the number of peroxisomes, they may increase the formation of H_2O_2, leading to the formation of reactive oxygen species and thereby enhancing cell replication (Lake, 1995).

Solid state carcinogens are exemplified by asbestos and implanted materials such as plastics, metal, and glass. These substances show no genotoxicity, and they produce tumors of mesenchymal origin. While the precise mode of action is not known, the tumors they induce are preceded by an exuberant foreign-body reaction including hyperplastic fibrosis with a high frequency of chromosomal changes in the preneoplastic cells (Rashko and Brand, 1983).

Others

Metals and Metalloids Arsenic, chromium, nickel, and their compounds are carcinogenic in animals; some of them are considered to be carcinogens in humans also (IARC, 1987). Arsenic was thought to be an exception in that it is carcinogenic in humans but not in animals. Recent data, however, show that intratracheal instillation of As_2O_3 in Syrian hamsters resulted in an increase in pulmonary adenomas, and after intrauterine exposure, it apparently caused lung tumors in mice.

The mechanisms of metal carcinogenesis are not fully understood but may involve genotoxic and/or epigenetic activities. Sunderman (1984) has listed a number of promising avenues for research. Among them are the formation of cross-links between DNA and proteins or between adjacent DNA strands, and impairment of the fidelity of DNA replication by altering the conformation of DNA polymerases. These substances may be classified as genotoxic carcinogens since they alter the gene expression in one way or another. In addition, damage of the cytoskeleton by certain metals may contribute to their carcinogenicity (Chou, 1989).

Secondary Carcinogens This term has been used to refer to substances that are not directly carcinogenic but can induce cancer following a distinctly noncarcinogenic effect. For example, polyoxyethylene monostearate (Myrj 45), at very high doses, elicited bladder stones that in turn caused bladder tumors. No tumors were observed in any of the animals that had no bladder stones. On the other hand, this term has also been used in connection with those genotoxic carcinogens that require bioactivation.

LONG-TERM CARCINOGENICITY STUDIES

These studies are designed to provide definitive information on the carcinogenic effects of chemicals on the test animals. Because of the great expense and time required, they are undertaken usually after a review of other data, such as the chemical structure and results from short-term mutagenesis tests and long-term chronic toxicity studies, which are described, respectively, in a following section and in chap. 6.

Guidelines on the long-term carcinogenicity studies are outlined in this section. More detailed descriptions and references to some comments are provided in a number of papers (WHO, 1969; OECD, 1981; U.S. ISGC, 1986).

Animals: Species, Strain, Sex, and Number

Rats and mice are generally preferred because of their small size, short life span, ready availability, and an abundance of information on their response to other carcinogens. Hamsters are also used, especially in studies on cancers of the bladder, breast, gastrointestinal tract, and respiratory tract. Dogs and nonhuman primates are occasionally used for their positive response to 2-naphthylamine, and the latter also for their higher phylogenetic order. However, their use is limited because of their large size and relatively long life span, thereby requiring a 7- to 10-yr exposure to the chemical on test.

The characteristics of a preferred strain are (1) known sensitivity to substances of similar chemical structure, (2) low incidence of spontaneous tumors, and (3) similarity of its rate and pattern of biotransformation to those of humans, if known.

Highly inbred strains should not be used, to avoid possible insensitivity. Hybrid mice of two known inbred strains are preferable because they lack the possible insensitivity of inbred strains and they are generally more robust.

Both sexes should be included in these studies; differences in response to the carcinogenic activity of chemicals are well documented. To provide a sufficient number of animals surviving until the appearance of tumors for statistical analysis, it is a common practice to start the tests with 50 animals of each sex per dose group, including the controls.

Inception and Duration

The studies are generally started shortly after weaning the animals to allow maximum duration of exposure. The duration of the studies is generally 24 mo in rats and 18 mo in mice. If the animals are in good condition, the duration may be extended to 30 and 24 mo, respectively.

Route of Administration

The chemical under test should be given to the animals by the route of human exposure and the usual route is oral. This principle readily applies to food additives and contaminants as well as most drugs. For industrial and environmental chemicals, the main route of entry is inhalation. Alternatively, the test chemical may be instilled intratracheally.

When the test substance is to be given orally, it can be mixed with the diet, either in constant concentration (in milligrams of the chemical per kilogram diet, ppm) or in constant dosage (in milligrams of the chemical per kilogram of body weight). In the latter case, it is necessary to adjust the concentration of the chemical in the diet according to the food consumption and the body weight at appropriate intervals. The chemical may also be incorporated in the drinking water instead of the diet, or it may be given by gavage. Commercial animal feed may contain small amounts of carcinogens (e.g., aflatoxins) or enzyme inducers (e.g., DDT), which can modify the effects of the test chemical.

Dermal application is used for industrial chemicals and drugs intended for topical use. This route is mainly intended for detecting local carcinogenicity. However, in some cases, appreciable amounts may be absorbed to induce systemic effects. The choice of vehicle is important: It ought to have little or no toxicity per se and should not react with the chemical under test. Dimethyl sulfoxide is often used.

Doses

Usually two or three dose levels are included in such studies. In addition, control groups are also included for comparison. The doses are selected on the basis of the short-term studies and metabolism data, with the aim that the high dose would produce some minor signs of toxicity but not significantly reduce the life-span of the animals. The two lower doses are generally some fractions of the high dose (e.g., one-half and one-fourth) and are expected to permit the animals to survive in good health or until tumor develops.

The "maximally tolerated dose" (MTD) is generally used as the high dose. It is estimated from 90-d studies and defined as one that would (1) not produce morphologic evidence of toxicity of a severity that interferes with the interpretation of the long-term study, and (2) not comprise so large a fraction of the animal's diet that it might lead to nutritional imbalance (U.S. ISGC, 1986). However, the use of the MTD has been criticized, especially when it is much higher than the expected human exposure; there is the possibility of alteration of metabolic pattern by "overloading" the animals (Mermelstein et al., 1994).

Controls and Combined Treatment

An untreated group consisting of the same number, or a larger number, of animals as each dose group is included. In addition to these negative controls, another group of animals is often incorporated that is given a known carcinogen at a dose level that had shown to be carcinogenic. The positive controls provide more confidence in the results on the test chemical by serving as a check on the sensitivity of the particular lot of animals used as well as the adequacy of the facilities and procedures in the specific laboratory. It will also provide some indication of the relative potency of the test chemical. If a vehicle, such as acetone or dimethyl sulfoxide, is to be used, its possible effect should also be tested in a group of animals.

Observations and Examinations

General Observations   The animals should be examined daily for mortality and morbidity. Dead and moribund animals should be removed from the cage for gross and microscopic examinations whenever the condition of the tissues permits.

Sick animals should be placed in single cages to prevent cannibalism and for quarantine. If indicated, they may be treated with drugs, but any therapy must be recorded. Prolonged drug treatment should be avoided to preclude possible interference with the effect of the chemical under test.

The onset, location, size, and growth of any unusual tissue masses should be carefully examined and recorded. Signs of toxicity and pharmacologic effects should also be noted.

Body weight and food consumption figures allow the calculation of the intake of the chemical on a milligram per kilogram body weight basis. Furthermore, the body weight is a sensitive index of the health status of the animal and should be determined at weekly intervals during the first 3 mo, when the animals are growing, and biweekly afterward.

Postmortem Examinations   All animals found dead or dying should be subjected to gross autopsy. The survivals at the end of the study should be sacrificed and examined. In addition, a number of organs should be weighed, including the liver, kidneys, heart, testes, and brain.

Samples of all tissues should be preserved for histologic examination. Microscopic examinations should be done on all tumor growths and all tissues showing gross abnormalities. Usually the following tissues are also examined: mandibular lymph node, salivary gland, mammary gland, sternebrae, femor or vertebrae (including marrow), thymus, thyroid, parathyroid, trachea, lungs and main bronchi, heart, esophagus, stomach, small intestine, colon, liver, gallbladder, pancreas, spleen, adrenals, kidneys, urinary bladder, prostate, testes, uterus, ovaries, brain (three sections), pituitary, eyes (if grossly abnormal), and spinal cord (if neurologic signs).

Reporting of Tumors   As carcinogenesis can manifest in a variety of forms (see Definition), it is necessary to record the following:

1   The number of various types of tumors (both benign and malignant), and any unusual tumors.
2   The number of tumor-bearing animals.
3   The number of tumors in each animal.
4   The onset of tumors whenever determinable.

RAPID SCREENING TESTS

Short-Term Tests for Mutagenesis/Carcinogenesis

In recent years, a number of relatively simple and much shorter tests have been devised and employed to detect the mutagenic activity of chemicals. These tests utilize a variety of systems, including microbes, insects, and mammalian cells, as well as a battery of parameters such as gene mutation, chromosomal effects, and DNA repair. These mutagenesis tests and tests using cell transformation as end point are described and discussed in the next chapter.

Although not all mutagens are carcinogenic nor vice versa, the relationship between these two activities is nevertheless so close that mutagenesis tests are performed frequently as a rapid screening of chemicals for their potential carcinogenicity. To improve the reliability of the results, a battery of these tests is usually conducted (e.g., U.S. ISGC, 1986). Weisburger and Williams (1981) recommended the following short-term in vitro tests: (1) bacterial mutagenesis, (2) mammalian mutagenesis, (3) mammalian cell DNA repair, (4) chromosome integrity, and (5) cell transformation. The results of these tests are also useful in defining the mechanism of action.

Tests for Promoters and Cocarcinogens

Mouse skin has long been used as a model for testing promoters, as discussed in an earlier section. More recently, tests for promoters in other organs, such as colon, mammary gland, liver, pancreas, and urinary bladder, have been developed (Pereira, 1983). A cocarcinogen would increase the tumor incidence induced by a genotoxic carcinogen whether it is administered before, during, or after the genotoxic carcinogen.

Limited Carcinogenicity Tests

Limited carcinogenicity tests have been recommended by Williams and Weisburger (1993), because of certain advantages. These tests are superior to the mutagenesis tests in that the end point is tumor formation. Furthermore, the duration of these tests is much shorter than that of the long-term carcinogenicity studies.

Skin Tumors in Mice   Mouse skin responds to topical application of chemicals, such as polycyclic aromatic hydrocarbons, and crude products, such as tars from coal and petroleum, by the formation of papillomas and carcinomas. This procedure, introduced by Berenblum and Shubik (1947), has been widely used. Mouse skin responds positively apparently because it has the enzymes that convert the substances into active metabolites.

Some chemicals act as initiator and as promoter; they may therefore be referred to as complete carcinogens. Others act mainly or exclusively as initiators. Their carcinogenicity is revealed only after the application of a promoter. Results obtained in the mouse skin test reported in the literature on the effects of chemicals as initiators and as promoters have been compiled by Pereira (1982).

Pulmonary Tumors in Mice   Strain A mice spontaneously have an essentially 100% lung tumor incidence by 24 mo of age. Positive results from carcinogens can be obtained in about 24 wk when few controls have tumors. With some chemicals, the test can be completed in 12 wk (Shimkin and Stoner, 1975).

Altered Foci in Rodent Liver   It has been demonstrated that distinct liver foci appear before the development of hepatocarcinoma. These foci are resistant to iron accumulation, a phenomenon that can be identified histochemically. There are also abnormalities in certain enzymes, which can be demonstrated histochemically. The latter alteration occurs in rats but not in mice. These foci can be detected within 3 wk of exposure and occur in large numbers in 12–16 wk (Goldfarb and Pugh, 1982).

Breast Cancer in Female Rats   Polycyclic hydrocarbons can induce breast cancers in young female Sprague-Dawley and Wister rats. The tumors can develop in less than 6 mo (Huggins et al., 1959).

BIOMARKERS

Carcinogenesis, as noted earlier, involves three major steps: initiation, promotion, and conversion and progression. Identification of biomarkers for these steps is in various stages of development. The interest in these markers stems from their potential usefulness in exploring the mode of action of carcinogens, in determining exposure to carcinogens, and in early diagnosis of cancer.

Biomarkers of Exposure and Initiation

Initiation is associated with covalent binding of electrophilic carcinogens or their reactive metabolites to DNA. The carcinogen–DNA adduct can be demonstrated and quantified to indicate exposure and effect of the carcinogen. This procedure has been applied to situations wherein human exposure to a particular carcinogen is suspected, for example, in the determination of exposure to aflatoxin B_1 and its relationship to hepatocellular carcinoma (Qian et al., 1994).

Biomarkers of Promotion

Promotion has been most extensively studied in skin carcinogenesis. A variety of biochemical changes have been noted in initiated as well as normal cells on treatment with promoters, the most active of which is TPA (12-*O*-tetradecanoyl phorbol 13-acetate). Other examples are Mirex and benzoyl peroxide. The changes include accumulation of plasminogen activator and increased prostaglandin synthesis. A liver tumor initiated by acetylaminofluorene (AAF) has been shown to be promotable by phenobarbital, DDT, polychlorinated biphenyls (PCB), and TCDD. Growth factors, protein kinase C, TPA- and dioxin-responsive elements in genes, and interaction of promoters with oncogenes and/or suppressor genes are being studied to determine their role as markers of preneoplasia in the liver.

Tumor Markers

α-Fetoprotein (AFP) is a product of fetal liver and hepatocarcinoma. AFP had therefore been used to screen large populations for hepatocellular carcinomas, allowing early detection and treatment. However, it has been shown to be nonspecific. Human chorionic gonadotropin (HCG) is a sensitive marker and can be used to detect cancer at a subclinical phase. Mammary carcinomas are often associated with abnormal levels of biochemical parameters such as carcinoembryonic antigen, ferritin, and C-reactive protein. Unfortunately, these changes generally appear only when the tumor has become metastatic, hence too late to be of value in the early diagnosis of cancer. Nevertheless, these are useful in evaluating the effect of clinical treatment and in following remissions and relapses. PSA (prostate-specific antigen) has recently been shown to be a useful biomarker of prostate cancer.

Biomarkers of Susceptibility

Individuals with certain genetic disposition may be more susceptible to carcinogenesis. For example, those with xeroderma pigmentosa are prone to skin cancer, and cigarette smoke is more likely to induce lung cancer in individuals of the debriquine hydroxylation or the α-1-antitrypsin phenotype.

EVALUATION

Preliminary Assessment

Chemical Structure   A number of chemicals are known to be carcinogenic. A list of known and suspected human carcinogens is presented in Appendix 7-1. In addition, a large number of chemicals have been shown to be carcinogenic in animals (see Genotoxic Carcinogens). While chemicals that have structures similar to any of these or other carcinogens/ mutagens are not necessarily carcinogens, they should be assigned high priority in carcinogenicity testing programs. In fact, certain chemical structures have been shown to be correlated with carcinogenicity (e.g., Ashby and Tennant, 1988).

Mutagenicity   Mutagenic agents produce heritable genetic changes essentially through their effects on DNA. The mutagenicity tests also provide information on the mode of action as well as on the question as to whether metabolic activation is required for the mutagenicity. While positive results from these tests do not constitute positive evidence that the chemical is carcinogenic, they do indicate that extensive testing is required. Furthermore, the mutagenesis data are useful in the risk assessment of the chemical in question. On the other hand, negative results do not establish the safety of the chemical.

Limited Carcinogenicity Tests   The end point in these tests is tumor formation. Therefore, certain chemicals, such as cocarcinogens that yield negative results in mutagenesis tests, may be positive in these tests. Positive results from more than one of these limited carcinogenicity tests may be considered unequivocal qualitative evidence of carcinogenicity.

Definitive Assessment

Data from well-designed and properly executed long-term carcinogenicity studies generally provide a sound basis for assessment of the carcinogenic potential.

General Considerations   Results from these studies are generally more reliable than those from the rapid screening tests. However, the conclusiveness of the results depends on a number of factors. For example, too few animals surviving until tumor development may preclude statistical analysis of the data. This event may occur as a result of insufficient animals placed in each dosage group and/or excessive mortality resulting from improper husbandry or from competing toxicity of the chemical given at inordinately high dose levels.

The thoroughness of the postmortem examination also plays an important role. This applies to the gross as well as the microscopic examinations. Tumors in tissues and organs may be overlooked if they are subjected only to a curscry inspection. Special techniques may be required for proper examination of certain organs, such as the urinary bladder. Concomitant events such as stones and parasites in the bladder must be looked for and their presence or absence recorded.

Tumor Incidence As noted at the beginning of the chapter, carcinogenesis may manifest in one of the four forms or any combination thereof. An appreciable increase in the tumor-bearing animals is the most common form. The occurrence of unusual tumors is an important phenomenon if there are a significant number of them; when one or only a few of them are detected, further critical examination is required. Shortening of the latency period is readily noted with dermal and subcutaneous tumors. The latency of visceral tumor is, in practice, equivalent to the survival of the tumor-bearing animals because the tumor development is, in general, positively diagnosed only at autopsy. An increase in the number of tumors per animal without a concomitant increase in the number of tumor-bearing animals usually indicates cocarcinogenicity only.

The tumors in the experimental animals may not be at the same stage of development. The stages may include, for example, atypical hyperplasia, benign tumors, carcinomas in situ, invasion of adjacent tissues, and metastasis to other parts of the body. Although tumors of the same type but at different stages should be separately tabulated, they should be combined for statistical analysis.

Dose-Response Relationship As a rule, a positive dose-response relationship is apparent. However, there may be a lower tumor incidence in the high-dose group. This phenomenon usually results from poor survival among these animals, which succumb to competing toxic effects of the chemical.

Reproducibility of the Results The confidence in a carcinogenicity study is enhanced if the results are produced in another strain of animals. Reproducibility in another species is even more significant. However, if negative results are obtained in another species, this fact may not nullify the positive findings but does justify further investigation. For example, there may be differences in their biotransformation of the chemical or variations in the precise composition of the product used. On the other hand, the positive findings in one experiment may well be considered spurious when several other identical experiments all yielded negative results.

Evaluation of Safety / Risk

The various approaches used in the evaluation of the safety/risk of carcinogens are discussed in chap. 22. The following points, however, are worthy of emphasizing.

First, while the tests just enumerated are a valuable basis for risk/safety assessment, other data relating to the mechanism of action and influences of modifying factors are also essential (U.S. ISGC, 1986). The significant differences between genotoxic and epigenetic carcinogens are also considered valid reasons for assessing their risks differently: It is generally assumed that genotoxic carcinogens exhibit no threshold, whereas nongenotoxic carcinogens induce cancer secondary to other biological effects, which are likely to show no-effect dose levels. However, a chemical, such as chloroform, may act as an epigenetic as well as a genotoxic carcinogen.

Furthermore, there are chemicals with carcinogenicity secondary to noncarcinogenic biologic or physical effects that are elicited only at dose levels that could never be approached in realistic human exposure situations. There has been general consensus that there are threshold doses for such secondary carcinogens (Lu, 1976; Munro, 1988). The U.S. ISGC (1986) also cautions that extremely high doses of a toxicant may exhibit qualitatively different distribution, detoxication, and elimination of the toxicant. The response at such doses therefore may not be applicable to more realistic exposure conditions. Furthermore, evidence of extensive tissue damage, disruption of hormonal function, formation of urinary stones, and saturation of DNA repair function should be carefully reviewed (U.S. ISGC, 1986).

Carcinogens also differ in the potency and latent periods. Some carcinogens are active in a particular species, whereas others affect several species and strains of animals. All these factors must be taken into account in evaluating the safety/risk of carcinogens.

Finally, it is important to bear in mind that chemicals differ tremendously in their value to humans. For example, the use of a food color can often be suspended on the basis of suggestive carcinogenicity data. On the other hand, life-saving drugs, even when there is evidence of their carcinogenicity in humans, may still be used clinically. There are also environmental carcinogens, including those in food, that cannot be eliminated with present technology (see also Ames, 1989).

REFERENCES

Ames, B. N. 1989. What are the major carcinogens in the etiology of human cancer? Environmental pollution, natural carcinogens, and the causes of human cancer: Six errors. In

Important advances in oncology, 1989, eds. V. T. Da Vita, Jr., et al. Philadelphia: J. P. Lippincott.

Anderson, R. I., Bishop, W. E., and Campbell, R. L. 1985. A review of the environmental mammalian toxicology of nitrilotriacetic acid. *CRC Crit. Rev. Toxicol.* 15:1–102.

Ashby, J., and Tennant, R. W. 1988. Chemical structure, *Salmonella* mutagenicity and extent of carcinogenicity among 222 chemicals tested in rodents by the U.S. NCI/NTP. *Mutat. Res.* 204:17–115.

Berenblum, I., and Shubik, P. 1947. A new quantitative approach to the study of the stages of chemical carcinogenesis in the mouse's skin. *Br. J. Cancer* 1:383–391.

Berenblum, I., and Shubik, P. 1949. An experimental study of the initiating stage of carcinogenesis, and a re-examination of the somatic cell mutation theory of cancer. *Br. J. Cancer* 3:109–118.

Bishop, J. M. 1987. The molecular genetics of cancer. *Science* 235:305–311.

Butterworth, B. E., and Goldworthy, T. L. 1991. The role of cell proliferation in multistage carcinogenesis. *Proc. Soc. Exp. Biol. Med.* 198:683–687.

Chou, I.-N. 1989. Distinct cytoskeletal injuries induced by As, Cd, Co, Cr, and Ni compounds. *Biomed. Environ. Sci.* 2:358–365.

Goldfarb, S., and Pugh, M. B. 1982. The origin and significance of hyperplastic hepatocellular islands and nodules in hepatic carcinogenesis. *J. Am. Coll. Toxicol.* 1:119–144.

Greenblatt, M.S., Bennett, N.P., Hollstein, M., and Harris, C. C. 1994. Mutations in the p53 tumor suppressor gene: Clues to cancer etiology and molecular pathogenesis. *Cancer Res.* 55: 4855–5878.

Huggins, C., Briziarelli, G., and Sutton, H., Jr. 1959. Rapid induction of mammary carcinoma in the rat and the influence of hormones on the tumors. *J. Exp. Med.* 109:25–41.

International Agency for Research on Cancer. 1987. *Monographs for carcinogenic chemicals: Overall evaluation of carcinogenicity: An updating of IARC monographs*, vols. 1–42. Suppl. 7. Lyon, France: IARC.

Klaunig, J. E. 1991. Alterations in intercellular communication during the stage of promotion. *Proc. Soc. Exp. Biol. Med.* 198:688–692.

Lake, B. G. 1995. Mechanisms of hepatocarcinogenicity of peroxisome-proliferating drugs and chemicals. *Annu. Rev. Pharmacol. Toxicol.* 35:483–507.

Lu, F. C. 1976. Threshold doses in chemical carcinogenesis: Introductory remarks. *Oncology* 33:50.

McClain, R. M. 1989. The significance of hepatic microsomal enzyme induction and altered thyroid function in rats: Implications for thyroid gland neoplasia. *Toxicol. Pathol.* 17: 294–306.

Mermelstein, R., Marrow, P. E., and Christian, M. S. 1994. Organ or system overload and its regulatory implications. *J. Am. Col. Toxicol.* 13:143–147.

Munro, I. C. 1988. Risk assessment of carcinogens: Present status and future directions. *Biomed. Environ. Sci.* 1:51–58.

Neumann, H. G. 1983. The dose-response of DNA interactions of aminostilbene derivatives and other chemical carcinogens. In *Developments in science and practice of toxicology*, eds. A. W. Hayes and T. S. Miya, pp. 135–144. New York: Elsevier Science.

Organization for Economic Cooperation and Development. 1981. OECD Guidelines for Testing of Chemicals. Paris: OECD.

Pereira, M. A. 1982. Mouse skin bioassay for chemical carcinogens. *J. Am. Coll. Toxicol.* 1: 47–82.

Pereira, M. A., ed. 1983. International Symposium on Tumor Promotion. *Environ. Health Perspect.* 50:3–330.

Pitot, H. C., Beer, D., and Hendrich, S. 1988. Multistage carcinogenesis: The phenomenon underlying the theories. In *Theories of carcinogenesis,* ed. O. H. Iversen, pp. 159–177. Washington, DC: Hemisphere.

Qian, G.-S., Ross, R. K., Yu, M. C., Yuan, J.-M., Gao, Y.-T., Henderson, B. E., Wogan, G. N., and Groopman, J. D. 1994. A follow-up study of urinary markers of aflatoxin ex-

posure and liver cancer risk in Shanghai, China. *Cancer Epidemiol. Biomarkers Prevent.*
3:3–10.
Rashko, D., and Brand, G. 1983. Chromosomal aberrations in foreign body tumorigenesis of
mice. *Proc. Soc. Exp. Biol. Med.* 172:382–388.
Reddy, J. K., and Lalwani, N. D. 1983. Carcinogenesis by hepatic peroxisome proliferators:
Evaluation of the risk of hyperlipidemic drugs and industrial plasticizers to humans. *CRC
Crit. Rev. Toxicol.* 12:1–58.
Ryffel, B. 1992. The carcinogenicity of cyclosporin. *Toxicology* 73: 1–22.
Shimkin, M. B., and Stoner, G. D. 1975. Lung tumors in mice: Application to carcinogenesis
bioassay. *Adv. Cancer Res.* 21:2–58.
Sunderman, F. W., Jr. 1984. Recent advances in metal carcinogenesis. *Ann. Clin. Lab. Sci.* 14:
93–122.
Swenberg, J. A., Short, B., Borghoff, S., Strasser, J., and Charbonneau, M. 1989. The com-
parative pathobiology of $\alpha_{2\mu}$-globulin nephropathy. *Toxicol. Appl. Pharmacol.* 97: 35–46.
Trosko, J. E., and Chang, C. C. 1988. Chemical and oncogene modulation of gap junctional
intercellular communication. In *Tumor promoters: Biological approaches for mechanistic
studies and assay systems*, eds. R. Langenbach et al., pp. 97–111. New York: Raven
Press.
U.S. Environmental Protection Agency. 1986. Guidelines for carcinogen risk assessment. *Fed.
Reg.* 51:33,992, Sept. 24.
U.S. Interagency Staff on Carcinogens. 1986. Chemical carcinogens: A review of the science
and its associated principles. U.S. Interagency Staff on Carcinogens. *Environ. Health
Perspect.* 67:201–282.
van Duuren, B. L. 1982. Cocarcinogens and tumor promoters and their environmental impor-
tance. *J. Am. Coll. Toxicol.* 1:17–27.
Weinberg, R. A. 1989. Oncogenes, antioncogenes, and the molecular bases of multistep car-
cinogenesis. *Cancer Res.* 49:3713–3721.
Weisburger, J. H., and Williams, G. M. 1981. Basic requirements of health risk analysis: The
decision point approach for systematic carcinogen testing. *Proc. Third Life Sciences
Symp. Health Risk Analysis*, pp. 401–407. Philadelphia: Franklin Press.
Williams, G. M., and Weisburger, J. H. 1993. Chemical carcinogenesis. In *Casarett and Doull's
toxicology*, eds., M. O. Amdur, J. Doull, and C. D. Klaassen, pp. 127–200. New York:
McGraw-Hill.
World Health Organization. 1969. Principles for the Testing and Evaluation of Drugs for
Carcinogenicity. WHO Tech. Rep. Ser. 426.

ADDITIONAL READING

World Health Organization. 1993. Biomarkers and Risk Assessment: Concepts and Principles.
Environ. Health Criteria 155. Geneva: WHO.

APPENDIX 7-1   CARCINOGENIC CHEMICALS

An IARC Working Group (IARC, 1987) concluded that the following
agents are carcinogenic to humans:

Aflatoxins
Aluminum production
4-Aminobiphenyl
Analgesic mixtures containing phenacetin
Arsenic and arsenic compounds*
Asbestos
Auramine, manufacture of
Azathioprine
Benzene
Benzidine
Betel quid with tobacco
N,N-Bis(2-chloroethyl)-2-naphthylamine (Chlornaphazine)
Bis(chloromethyl)ether and chloromethyl methyl ether (technical grade)
Boot and shoe manufacture and repair
1,4-Butanediol dimethanesulfonate (Myleran)
Chlorambucil
1-(2-Chloroethyl)-3-(4-methylcyclohexyl)-1-nitrosourea (Methyl-CCNU)
Chromium compounds, hexavalent*
Coal gasification
Coal-tar pitches
Coal tars
Coke production
Cyclophosphamide
Diethylstilbestrol
Erionite
Estrogen replacement therapy
Estrogens, nonsteroidal*
Estrogens, steroidal*
Furniture and cabinet making
Hematite mining, underground, with exposure to radon
Iron and steel founding
Isopropyl alcohol manufacture, strong-acid process
Magenta, manufacture of
Melphalan
8-Methoxypsoralen (Methoxsalen) plus ultraviolet radiation
Mineral oils, untreated and mildly treated
MOPP (combined therapy with nitrogen mustard, vincristine, procarbazine, and prednisone) and other combined chemotherapy including alkylating agents
Mustard gas (sulfur mustard)
2-Naphthylamine
Nickel and nickel compounds*

* This evaluation applies to the group of chemicals as a whole and not necessarily to all individual chemicals within the group.

† There is also conclusive evidence that these agents have a protective effect against cancers of the ovary and endometrium.

Oral contraceptives, combined†
Oral contraceptives, sequential
The rubber industry
Shale oils
Soots
Talc containing asbestiform fibers
Tobacco products, smokeless
Tobacco smoke
Treosulphan
Vinyl chloride

APPENDIX 7-2 PROBABLE CARCINOGENIC CHEMICALS

An IARC Working Group (IARC, 1987) concluded that the following are probably carcinogenic to humans:

Acrylonitrile
Adriamycin
Androgenic (anabolic) steroids
Benz[a]anthracene
Benzidine-based dyes
Benzo[a]pyrene
Beryllium and beryllium compounds
Bischloroethyl nitrosourea (BCNU)
Cadmium and cadmium compounds
1-(2-Chloroethyl)-3-cyclohexyl-1-nitrosourea (CCNU)
Cisplatin
Creosotes
Dibenz[a,h]anthracene
Diethyl sulfate
Dimethylcarbamoyl chloride
Dimethyl sulfate
Epichlorohydrin
Ethylene dibromide
Ethylene oxide
N-Ethyl-N-nitrosourea
Formaldehyde
5-Methoxypsoralen
4,4′-Methylene bis(2-chloroaniline) (MOCA)
N-Methyl-N'-nitro-N-nitrosoguanidine (MNNG)
N-Methyl-N-nitrosourea
Nitrogen mustard
N-Nitrosodiethylamine
Nitrosodimethylamine
Phenacetin

Polychlorinated biphenyls
Procarbazine hydrochloride
Propylene oxide
Silica, crystalline
Styrene oxide
Tris(1-aziridinyl)phosphine sulfide (Thiotepa)
Tris(2,3-dibromopropyl) phosphate
Vinyl bromide
Some 200 other chemicals have been recognized by IARC as possible human carcinogens.

Mutagenesis

CHAPTER 8 CONTENTS

INTRODUCTION

Mutagenesis can occur as a result of interaction between mutagenic agents and the genetic materials of organisms. While spontaneous mutation and natural selection are the major means of evolution, a number of toxicants, in recent decades, have been found to be mutagenic to a variety of organisms.

Health Hazards

The eventual effects of human exposure to these mutagenic substances cannot be predicted at present. However, some of the spontaneous abortions, stillbirths, and heritable diseases have been shown to be related to changes in DNA molecules and to chromosomal aberrations. There are approximately one thousand dominant gene mutations responsible for various illnesses, including the hereditary neoplasms such as bilateral retinoblastoma, and about the same number of recessive gene disorders such as sickle-cell anemia, cystic fibrosis, and Tay–Sachs disease. In addition, abnormal chromosomal numbers are associated with such diseases as Down's syndrome, Klinefelter's syndrome, and Edward's syndrome. These have been estimated to occur with an incidence of 0.5% among the live births in the United States. The true effects of any additional mutagen in the environment can only manifest after a lapse of several generations. The seriousness of this matter therefore warrants the extensive investigations in the various fields of mutagenesis.

A number of human diseases are the result of defects of the DNA repair systems. For example, patients with xeroderma pigmentosa are deficient in excision repair in the skin; they are susceptible to ultraviolet light and many chemical carcinogens and thus are prone to developing skin tumors. Those with ataxia telangiectasia have such deficiencies in the lymphoid system and are known to be susceptible to x-rays and the carcinogen methyl nitronitrosoguanidine. Fanconi's anemia is associated with defective DNA repair in the blood and skeleton. The afflicted persons are susceptible to mitomycin C and psoralens.

In addition, tests for mutagenicity in recent years have become more widely used because of their value as a rapid screening for carcinogenicity (see chap. 7). This development stems mainly from the fact that most mutagens have been found to be carcinogens. Furthermore, these tests, with a variety of end points, are useful in the elaboration of the mode of action of carcinogens. It is also worth noting that various chromosomal abnormalities have been detected in human tumors. The following are some examples:

Neoplasm	Abnormality of chromosome
Chronic myelogenous leukemia	Translocation of chromosomes 9 and 12
Acute monocytic leukemia	Loss of long arm of chromosome 11
Small-cell lung cancer	Loss of small arm of chromosome 6
Acute lymphoblastic leukemia	Extra chromosome 6
Retinoblastoma	Deletion of chromosome 13

Categories of Mutagenesis and Their Tests

It is well known that DNA, consisting of nucleotide bases, plays a key role in genetics. First, it transmits the genetic information from one generation of cells to the next through self-replication. This is done by the separation of the double strands of the DNA molecule and the synthesis of new daughter strands. Second, the genetic information coded in the DNA molecule is expressed through the transcription of a complementary RNA strand from one strand of DNA, which serves as a template, and the subsequent translation of the information from the RNA to the amino acids in proteins. Every set of three nucleotide bases, a codon, specifies an amino acid. Derangement of the bases therefore alters the amino acid content of the protein synthesized.

In earlier studies, mutagenic activity was demonstrated mainly in fruit flies and onion root tips because of the simpler techniques involved. More recently, many new test systems have been developed. They range in complexity from microorganisms to intact mammals. The use of such widely different organisms is based on the fact that all double-stranded DNA shares the same biochemical characteristics, which are listed in Table 8-1.

At present, there are more than a hundred test systems. A number of exemplary tests are outlined in this chapter under four major categories, namely, gene mutation, chromosomal effects, DNA repair and recombination, and others, which are designed to confirm carcinogenicity. Because of the brevity of their description, at least one reference is cited for each test. Additional references and more details are given elsewhere on these and other tests (U.S. EPA, 1994; OECD, 1987).

It is worth noting that gene mutation may be detected in all organisms including bacteria. On the other hand, effects related to chromosomes (aberration, aneuploidy, and DNA repair) can only be detected in higher organisms, that is, those with chromosomes.

GENE MUTATION

Gene mutations involve additions or deletions of base pairs or substitution of a wrong base pair in the DNA molecules.

Table 8-1 Basic Biochemical Characteristics of All Double-Stranded DNA

1 DNA consists of two different purines (guanine, adenine) and two different pyrimidines (thymine and cytosine).

2 A nucleotide pair consists of one purine and one pyrimidine [adenine/thymine (A-T) or guanine/cytosine (G-C)].

3 Nucleotide pairs are connected into a double-helix molecule by sugar-phosphate backbone linkages and hydrogen bonding.

4 The A-T base pair is held by two hydrogen bonds, while the G-C is held by three.

5 The distance from each base pair to the next in a molecule is 3.4 Å, producing 10 nucleotide pairs per turn of the DNA helix.

6 The number of adenine molecules must equal the number of thymine molecules in a DNA molecule. The same relationship exists for guanine and cytosine molecules. However, the ratio of A-T to G-C base pairs may vary in DNA from species to species.

7 The two strands of the double helix are complementary and antiparallel with respect to the polarity of the two sugar-phosphate backbones, one strand being 3'-5' and the other being 5'-3' with respect to the terminal OH group on the ribose sugar.

8 DNA replicates by a semiconservative method in which the two strands separate and each is used as a template for the synthesis of a new complementary strand.

9 The rate of DNA nucleotide polymerization during replication is approximately 600 nucleotides per second. The helix must unwind to form templates at a rate of 3600 rpm to accommodate this replication rate.

10 The DNA content of cells is variable (1.8×10^9 Da for *Escherichia coli* to 1.9×10^{11} Da for human cells).

Source: Brusick (1987, p. 15).

Substitutions consist of transitions and transversions. The former involve the replacement of a purine (adenine, guanine) by another or a pyrimidine (cytosine, thymine) by another. With transversion, a purine is replaced by a pyrimidine, or vice versa.

When the number of base pairs added or deleted is not a multiple of three, the amino acid sequence of the protein coded distal to the addition or deletion will be altered. This phenomenon is called frame-shift mutation and is likely to affect the biologic property of the protein. Figure 8-1 clearly illustrates the effects of a deletion and an addition of a nucleotide base.

In addition, a mutagenic chemical, or a part of it, may be incorporated into the DNA molecule. For example, a number of electrophilic compounds react with DNA forming covalent addition products, known as "DNA adducts." Thus, acetylaminofluorene (AAF) binds specifically to the carbon at the 8-position of guanine. For a partial list of such chemicals, see the discussion of procarcinogens in Categories of Carcinogens, chap. 7. Alkylating agents such as ethylnitrourea and diethyl sulfate, donate an alkyl group to DNA.

These various changes in the DNA molecule may cause the substitution of a new amino acid in the subsequently coded protein molecule or result in a different sequence of amino acids in the protein synthesized. Furthermore, a protein synthesis termination codon may be formed, giving rise to a shortened protein. While the first type of effect may or may not result

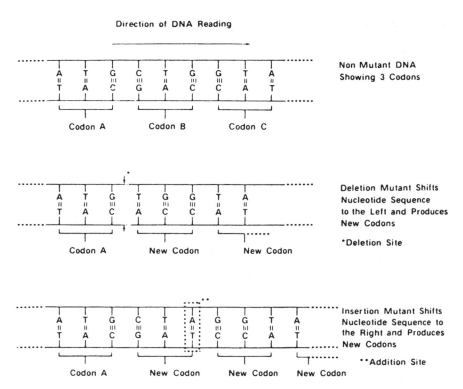

Figure 8-1 Frame-shift mutation resulting from deletion or insertion of a nucleotide base. A series of new codons is formed distal to the deletion or insertion, and hence new amino acids in the protein are synthesized (from Brusick, 1987).

in a modification of the biologic property of the protein molecule, the latter two types almost invariably do.

Microbial Tests In Vitro

These involve prokaryotic and eukaryotic microorganisms.

Prokaryotic Microorganisms Such microorganisms consist of various strains of bacteria. For the detection of point mutations the commonly used bacteria are *Salmonella typhimurium* and *Escherichia coli*. Most bacterial systems are intended to detect reverse mutation. For example, the Ames test (Ames, 1971) measures the reversion of histidine-dependent mutants of *S. typhimurium* to the histidine-independent wild type. The mutants are incubated in a medium that contains insufficient histidine to permit visible growth. If the toxicant added to the culture medium is capable of inducing reverse mutation, then the bacteria can become histidine-independent and grow appreciably in the histidine-deficient medium. It is customary to use several strains because of their specificity. Their mutation to histidine independency results from either frame-shift or base-pair substitution; different mutagens may affect one strain but not the other.

A number of strains of *S. typhimurium* have been rendered more sensitive to the effects of mutagens through alterations in the permeability of their cell walls (deficient in lipopolysaccharide) and in their DNA excision repair capabilities (through a specific deletion in the DNA molecule) and through the bearing of an ampicillin resistance factor (Ames et al., 1975; McCann et al., 1975). These various strains (e.g., TA 98, 100, 1537) may be susceptible to different mutagens.

Since many mutagens are inactive before bioactivation, the test can be carried out with a bioactivating system included in the in vitro procedure. The bioactivating system usually consists of the microsomal fraction (containing the mixed-function oxidase system) of the liver of the rat or other animals, although the human liver is also used for special purposes. The activity of the microsomal enzyme is usually enhanced by pretreating the animal with an inducing agent, such as 3-methylcholanthrene, phenobarbital, or polychlorinated biphenyls (PCB). Appropriate cofactors are also added to the mixture prior to incubation.

Strains of *E. coli* that are tryptophan-dependent are also used to detect reverse mutation. Mutagenic changes will result in a tryptophan-independent strain (Ames et al., 1975).

Eukaryotic Microorganisms Certain strains of *Saccharomyces, Schizosaccharomyces, Neurospora,* and *Aspergillus* have been developed to detect mainly reverse mutations and, to a limited extent, forward mutations. Like the bacterial systems, these systems in general also include bioactivating enzymes and cofactors. For example, a type of mutant of *Saccharomyces cerevisiae* requires adenine and produces red-pigmented colonies, whereas the wild type microorganisms are adenine-independent and produce white colonies. Thus the reverse mutation can be determined by the prevalence of white colonies (Brusick and Mayer, 1973).

Microbial Tests In Vivo (Host-Mediated Assay)

In this type of test, the microorganisms are injected into the peritoneal cavity of the host mammal (usually the mouse). They can also be injected into the circulatory system or the testes. The toxicant is injected into the host, usually prior to the introduction of the microorganisms. After a few hours elapse, the host is sacrificed. The microorganisms are then collected and examined for manifestations of mutation. These assays have the advantage of incorporating the biotransformation of the toxicant in the host mammal but have the drawback that the microorganisms can only be kept in the host for a relatively short time. Apart from microorganisms, cells from multicellular animals can also be used in the host-mediated assay (Gabridge and Legator, 1969). Despite its theoretical advantage, the procedure has been found to be insensitive to certain types of carcinogens and hence is unsuitable as a routine screening procedure (Simmons et al., 1979).

A modified procedure involves pretreatment of the host with a toxicant, collecting the urine from the host, and injecting the urine, which may contain a high concentration of the metabolite(s) of the toxicant, back into the host. This modified procedure demonstrates positive mutagenicity with 2-acetylaminofluorene, which yields negative results with the regular host-mediated assay (Durston and Ames, 1974).

Insects

The fruit fly *Drosophila melanogaster* is the most commonly used insect. It is well characterized genetically. It has an advantage over microorganisms in that it metabolizes toxicants in a manner that is similar to mammals. Furthermore, it is superior to mammals in two respects, namely, its generation time is only 12–14 d, and it can be tested in sufficient numbers at much lower cost.

The sex-linked recessive lethal test measures the lethal effect on the F_2 males after exposing the males of the parental generation. It is the preferred procedure because the X chromosome represents about 20% of the total genome, and it is capable of screening for point mutation and short deletions at about 800 loci on the X chromosome (Lee et al., 1983).

Mammalian Cells in Culture

The commonly used systems include cells from mouse lymphoma, human lymphoblasts, and cells from the lung, ovary, and other tissues of Chinese hamsters. These cells usually maintain a near-diploid chromosome number, grow actively, and have high cloning efficiency. Both forward and reverse mutations can occur, and the mutants respond selectively to nutritional, biochemical, serologic, and drug-resistant growth manipulations.

For example, cells from mouse lymphoma, which are heterozygous at the thymidine kinase locus ($TK+/-$), may undergo forward mutation via the action of a mutagen and become $TK-/-$. Both genotypes $TK+/-$ and $TK-/-$ can grow in a normal medium, but $TK-/-$ can also grow in a medium containing 5-bromo-2'-deoxyuridine (BrdU). The mutagenicity of a toxicant can thus be determined by comparing the growth of the lymphoma cells in the presence and absence of the toxicant both in a medium containing BrdU and in a normal medium (DeMarini et al., 1989).

In Chinese hamsters, as in humans, the use of preformed hypoxanthine and guanine is controlled by an X-linked gene. Mutant cells at these loci are deficient in the enzyme hypoxanthine-guanine phosphoribosyl transferase and can be identified by their resistance to toxic purine analogs, such as 8-azaguanine or 6-thioguanine, that kill the cells that utilize these analogs (DeMarini et al., 1989).

These cell lines are generally deficient in metabolizing enzymes. Therefore, such enzyme systems are often added (*microsome-mediated*). Alternatively, these cells can be cocultivated with other cells that possess greater ability to biotransform toxicants. Such a *cell-mediated* system involves the use of freshly isolated hepatocytes as a feeder system (Williams, 1979). It offers an additional advantage of having capabilities to conjugate as well as to degrade toxicants.

Gene Mutation Tests in Mice

Mouse Spot Test   This test is designed to detect gene mutation in somatic cells. Basically it involves treating pregnant mice whose embryos are heterozygous at specific coat color loci and examining the newborn for any mosaic patches in the fur. Such patches indicate the formation of clones of mutant cells that are responsible for the color of the fur. This test is relatively inexpensive and takes only a few weeks to complete. Although it may yield false-positive results, it has not yet yielded false-negative results. The spot test is therefore a useful prescreen for heritable germinal mutations in mammals (Russell, 1978).

Specific Locus Test   The specific locus test was developed by Russell (1951) for determining the mutagenicity of ionizing radiation in the germ cells. This procedure was later adapted to assess the mutagenicity of chemicals (Searle, 1975). It has the advantage of directly detecting in intact mammals the mutagenic effects of toxicants in the germ cells, but it usually requires a very large number of animals.

It involves exposing nonmutant mice to the chemical and subsequently mating them to a multiple-recessive stock. Mutant offspring have altered phenotypes expressed in hair color, hair structure, eye color, ear length, and other traits. Some mutants are mosaic rather than whole animal. Mutation can also be detected by the rejection or acceptance of skin grafts made between first-generation offspring. It can be further characterized immunogenetically (Russell and Shelby, 1985).

CHROMOSOMAL EFFECTS

The effect of a toxicant on chromosomes may be large enough to be visible microscopically, and manifest as structural aberrations or as changes in their number. The former, *aberrations*, include deletions, duplications, and translocations. The latter, *aneuploidy*, involve a decrease or increase in the number of the chromosomes. Some of the effects are heritable.

The mode of action underlying these effects may involve molecular cross-linkage, which may cause an arrest of the synthesis of DNA, thereby leaving a gap in the chromosome. An unsuccessful repair of the DNA damage may also be responsible. Nondisjunction (failure of a pair of chromosomes to separate during mitotic division) can lead to mosaicism. A nondisjunction during gametogenesis (meiotic nondisjunction) gives rise to daughter cells that contain either one extra chromosome or one less than normal. The former is known as *trisomy* and the latter *monosomy*.

A number of test systems have been developed to determine the chromosomal effects. The following are the major systems.

Insects

Drosophila melanogaster has an advantage in that the chromosomes of some of its cells are superior in size and morphology. In addition, the chromosomal effects can be readily confirmed genetically, such as the sex-linked recessive lethalility. The chromosomal effects include loss of X and Y chromosomes, and translocations of fragments between second and third chromosomes.

Effects on the sex chromosome can also be detected by phenotypic changes, such as body color and color and shape of the eye (National Research Council, 1983).

Cytogenetic Studies with Mammalian Cells

In Vitro Tests For cytogenetic tests, the commonly used cells are derived from Chinese hamster ovaries and human lymphocytes. These cells are cultured in suitable media. They are then exposed to different concentrations of the test chemical in the presence or absence of a bioactivator system (usually the microsomal fraction of the rat liver homogenate). The test generally includes two positive control mutagens, namely, ethylmethane sulfonate, which is direct-acting, and dimethylnitrosamine, which requires bioactivation. After an appropriate incubation period, the cell division is arrested by the addition of colchicine. The cells are then mounted, stained, and scored (Preston et al., 1981).

An example of scoring of aberrations is shown: chromatid gap, chromatid break, chromosome gap, chromatid deletion, fragment, acentric fragment, translocation, triradial, quadriradial, pulverized chromosome, pulverized chromosomes, pulverized cells, ring chromosome, dicentric chromosome, minute chromosome, greater than 10 aberrations, polyploid, and hyperploid (Brusick, 1987).

In Vivo Tests Mammalian cells used in the in vivo study of chromosomal effects include germ cells and somatic tissues. The chemical to be tested is administered to intact animals, such as rodents and humans. The somatic tissues commonly used are bone marrow and peripheral lymphocytes. A classic protocol using bone marrow from mice, rats, or hamsters has been provided by the Ad Hoc Committee of the Environmental Mutagen Society and the Institute for Medical Research (1972). The scoring is the same as in the in vitro test.

The *micronucleus* test is a somewhat simpler in vivo procedure. It involves the use of polychromatic erythrocyte stem cells of CD-1 mice. Six hours after two treatments with the test chemical, given 24 h apart, the animals are killed and the bone marrow is collected from both femurs. An increase in micronucleated cells over the controls (about 0.5%) is considered positive (Schmid, 1976). Many other types of cells may also be used. These micronuclei represent fragments of chromosome and chromatid resulting from spindle/centromere dysfunction.

For tests on *germ cells*, the male animal is usually used. In order to allow cells of different stages of spermatogenesis to be exposed, the chemical is given daily for 5 d and the animals sacrificed 1, 3, and 5 wk following the last dose. The sperm are collected surgically from the caudae epididymides. After mounting and staining, the incidence of abnormal spermheads is determined, and it is compared with the negative and positive controls (Wyrobek and Bruce, 1975).

Sister Chromatid Exchange (SCE)

This test measures a reciprocal exchange of DNA between two sister chromatids of a duplicating chromosome. The exchange takes place because of a breakage and reunion of DNA during its replication. The test can be done with mouse lymphoma cells, Chinese hamster ovary cells, and human lymphocytes. It may also be done in vivo, by collecting cells from treated animals. The procedure involves labeling of cells with 5-BrdU (5-bromodeoxyuridine), and after two cycles of replication, the cells are stained with a fluorescent-plus-Giemsa technique. The frequency of sister chromatid exchanges per cell and per chromosome is scored and compared. The exchange is visible because in one chromatid the semiconservative replication of DNA results in a substitution of BrdU in one polynucleotide strand, and in the other chromatid the BrdU is substituted in both polynucleotide strands (Wolff, 1977).

While the mechanism underlying SCE is not fully understood, it shows that a chemical has attacked the chromosomes or impaired their replication. The test has the advantage of being simple to perform. Furthermore, its end point is often observed at concentrations much lower than those required with other tests (NRC, 1983).

Dominant Lethal Test in Rodents

This test is designed to demonstrate toxic effects on germ cells in the intact male animal, usually the mouse or rat. The effects can manifest in the mated females as dead implantations and/or preimplantation losses (the difference between the number of corpora lutea and the number of implantations). These effects are generally due to chromosomal damages, which lead to developmental errors that are fatal to the zygote. However, other cytotoxic effects can also cause early fetal death (see also chap. 17).

Heritable Translocation Test in Mice

This test is intended to detect the heritability of chromosomal damages. The damages, consisting of reciprocal translocation in the germ line cells of the treated male mice, are transmitted to the offspring. By mating the male F1 progeny with untreated female mice, the chromosomal effects are revealed by a reduction of viable fetuses. The presence of these reciprocal translocations can be verified by the presence of translocation figures among the double tetrads at meiosis (Adler, 1980).

DNA REPAIR AND RECOMBINATION

These biologic processes are not mutations per se, but they occur after DNA damage. These phenomena therefore indicate the existence of DNA damages, which are caused essentially by mutagens. There are three main types of DNA damages that can be repaired: missing, incorrect, or altered bases; interstrand cross-links; and strand breaks.

Bacteria

Among *E. coli* there are those with normal DNA polymerase I enzyme, which is capable of repairing DNA damage, and those deficient in this enzyme. Mutagens induce DNA damage and thereby impair the growth of the *E. coli* that is deficient in the repair enzyme, whereas the growth of those with this enzyme is not affected. The DNA repair-efficient strain is included to rule out the effect of cytotoxicity (Rosenkranz et al., 1976).

Similarly, there are also recombination efficient and deficient strains of *Bacillus subtilis*. Damage to DNA is repaired in the former strain through recombination but not in the latter. Mutagens will thus inhibit the growth of the latter but not the former.

Yeasts

Various eukaryotic microorganisms, such as *Saccharomyces cerevisiae*, have been used to test the mutagenicity of chemicals by the induced mitotic crossing-over and mitotic gene conversion. These effects on DNA results in the growth of colonies with different colors (Zimmermann et al., 1984).

Mammalian Cells

Unscheduled DNA synthesis (UDS) is an indication of DNA repair. It can be detected in human cells in culture. The synthesis is determined by the amount of radioactive thymidine incorporated per unit weight of DNA over the control value. This is done both in the presence and absence of an added activator system (Stich and Laishes, 1973). Such synthesis can also be determined in primary rat liver cells. The extent of DNA synthesis is determined using an autoradiographic method. Since these cells have sufficient metabolic activity, there is no need to add an activator system (Mitchell et al., 1983).

Because of their greater relevance to genetic risk, germ cells have also been used in UDS tests: Male mice are treated with a suspected mutagen, and [^{3}H]thymidine ([^{3}H]-dT) is injected intratesticularly. Any incorporation of [^{3}H]-dT into the DNA of meiotic and postmeiotic germ cells (see chap. 17, Introduction) indicates the production of repairable damage to the DNA (Russell and Shelby, 1985).

OTHER TESTS

As noted in chap. 7, a number of related tests are used to determine carcinogenicity.

In Vitro Transformation of Mammalian Cells

Cells from the BALB/3T3 mouse are commonly used in this test. Others include Syrian hamster embryo cells, mouse 10T1/2 cells, and human cells. Normally these cells will grow in the culture medium to form a monolayer. Those treated with a carcinogen, however, will reproduce without being attached to a solid surface and grow over the monolayer. The appearance of such multilayered colonies indicates malignant transformation. This end point can be confirmed by injecting these cells into syngeneic animals. In general, malignant tumors will develop if the cells have undergone transformation (Kakunaga, 1973). Therefore, in general, positive results from this test are especially significant.

Nuclear Enlargement Test

HeLa cells are grown in culture medium and treated with different concentrations of the chemical on test. After an appropriate duration, the cells are harvested and counted. They are then stripped of their cytoplasmic material and the size of the nucleus is determined with a particle counter. An increase in the nuclear size indicates carcinogenicity of the chemical (Finch et al., 1980).

EVALUATION

Need for Mutagenesis Studies

There is little doubt about the seriousness of mutagenesis. As stated earlier, many hereditary diseases are apparently associated with chromosomal aberrations, and dominant and recessive gene mutations. In addition, mutagenesis may contribute to the etiology of such common diseases as diabetes mellitus, epilepsy, schizophrenia, essential hypertension, cataracts, aging, heart disease, and certain cancers. Finally, the close relationship between mutagens and carcinogens must be borne in mind.

Thus, there is an enormous challenge to the toxicologist in identifying the mutagens to which humans are exposed and in defining their risks. So far, achievement in this area has been limited. New test systems are still being developed, and the validity and limitations of the existing tests are still being studied. Nevertheless, the current knowledge in this field does provide a basis for a rational approach to the screening of toxicants for their mutagenic/carcinogenic potential.

Selection of Test Systems

Since mutagens affect the genetic material in different ways, they may yield negative results in one test although positive in others. To rule out false-negatives (and false-positives), it is advisable to conduct several tests, preferably of different categories. The Organization for Economic Cooperation and Development (OECD, 1987) recommended a series of tests for screening, confirmation, and risk assessment (Table 8-2).

The Committee on Chemical Environmental Mutagens of the National Research Council recommended a mutagen assessment program (National Research Council, 1983). It suggests that the mutagenesis tests be placed in three tiers. Tier I consists of (1) the *Salmonella*/microsome gene-mutation test, (2) a mammalian cell gene-mutation test, and (3) a mammalian cell chromsomal breakage test. If all tests are negative, the chemical is considered a presumed mammalian nonmutagen. If two of these tests are positive, it is classified as a presumed mammalian mutagen. If only one is positive, then the Tier II test (*Drosophila* sex-linked lethal mutation) is conducted. For further screening of the most crucial chemicals, supplemental tests are done. A specific-locus test is recommended for chemicals

Table 8-2 Utility and Application of Assays

A. Assays that may be used for mutagen and carcinogen screening
    Salmonella typhimurium reverse mutation assay
    Escherichia coli reverse mutation assay
    Gene mutation in mammalian cells in culture
    Gene mutation in *Saccharomyces cerevisiae*
    In vitro cytogenetics assay
    Unscheduled DNA synthesis in vitro
    In vitro sister chromatid exchange assay
    Mitotic recombination in *Saccharomyces cerevisiae*
    In vivo cytogenetics assay
    Micronucleus test
    Drosophila sex-linked recessive lethal test
B. Assays that confirm in vitro activity
    In vivo cytogenetics assay
    Micronucleus test
    Mouse spot test
    Drosophila sex-linked recessive lethal test
C. Assays that assess effects on germ cells and that are applicable for estimating ge-
    netic risk
    Dominant lethal assay
    Heritable translocation assay
    Mammalian germ cell cytogenetic assay

Source: OECD (1987).

with a potential mutagenicity in mammalian germ cells, and a dominant lethal test should be done for those having chromosomal effects (see also WHO, 1990).

Many chemicals have been tested for genotoxicity (mutagenicity, carcinogenicity, and reproductive toxicity) using a multiplicity of tests. To facilitate the task of a "weight-of-evidence" analysis of the genotoxicity of the chemicals and an analysis of the merit of the tests used in generating the data, a method has been proposed by the International Commission for Protection Against Environmental Mutagens and Carcinogens (1992). The method begins with the classification and coding of the tests. An abbreviated version of the classification is shown in Appendix 8-1.

Significance of Results

Relation Between Mutagenicity and Carcinogenicity   A number of investigators have shown the relation between carcinogens and mutagens. For example, McCann et al. (1975) reported on their study of 300 substances for mutagenicity in the *Salmonella*/microsome test. The results were compared with the reported carcinogenicity or noncarcinogenicity of these substances. The authors demonstrated a high correlation between these toxic effects: 90% (156/175) of carcinogens are mutagenic in the test. Few noncarcinogens showed any degree of mutagenicity.

Of the 18 carcinogens that yielded false-negative results, some have been shown to require other metabolic activation (e.g., cycasin and 1,2-dimethylhydrazine are not carcinogenic in germ-free animals, indicating the need for activation by intestinal flora). Others such as aminotriazole, thioacetamide, and thiourea are goitrogenic and cause thyroid tumors via a nonmutagenic mechanism (see also chap. 7). Still others, such as auramine, are carcinogenic only because of their impurities. The mutagenicity of diethylstilbestrol could not be properly tested in this system because of its toxicity to the bacteria.

More recently, Mason et al. (1990) compiled information on the correlation between carcinogenicity in rodents and mutagenicity as determined by *S. typhimurium*. The correlations varied between 55 and 93%.

Heritable Effects At present there is no direct correlation between laboratory tests for heritable mutations and human experience. Nevertheless, if a substance has been shown to be mutagenic in a variety of test systems including heritable mutations in intact mammals, it must be considered as a mutagen in humans unless there is convincing evidence to the contrary. Furthermore, for many chemicals, such as food additives, pesticides, cosmetics, and most drugs, where human exposure can be avoided, much less information will be sufficient to warrant suspension of their use (see Flamm, 1977). At present no reliable method is available for estimating risks associated with mutagens by their strength (National Research Council, 1983).

As mentioned earlier, the study of mutagenesis is a new discipline. The rapidly accumulating knowledge in this field will, in all probability, affect the interpretation of the significance of the mutagenicity testing results as well as the selection of the test systems for screening toxicants.

REFERENCES

Ad Hoc Committee of the Environmental Mutagen Society and the Institute of Medical Research. 1972. Chromosome methodologies in mutagen testing. *Toxicol. Appl. Pharmacol.* 22:269–275.

Adler, I. D. 1980. New approaches to mutagenicity studies in animals for carcinogenic and mutagenic agents. I. Modification of heritable translocation test. *Teratogen. Carcinogen. Mutagen.* 1:75–86.

Ames, B. N. 1971. The detection of chemical mutagens with enteric bacteria. In *Chemical mutagens: Principles and methods for their detection*, ed. A. Hollander, vol. 1, pp. 267–282. New York: Plenum Press.

Ames, B. N., McCann, J., and Yamasaki, E. 1975. Methods for detecting carcinogens and mutagens with the *Salmonella*/mammalian-microsome mutagenicity test. *Mutat. Res.* 31: 347–364.

Brusick, D. J. 1987. *Principles of genetic toxicology*, 2nd ed. New York: Plenum Press.

Brusick, D. J., and Mayer, V. W. 1973. New developments in mutagenicity screening techniques with yeast. *Environ. Health Perspect.* 6:83–96.

DeMarini, D. M., Brockman, H. E., deSerres, F. J., et al. 1989. Specific-locus induced in eukaryotes (especially mammalian cells) by radiation and chemicals: A perspective. *Mutat. Res.* 220:11–29.

Durston, W. E., and Ames, B. N. 1974. Simple method for the detection of mutagens in urine: Studies with the carcinogen 2-acetylaminofluorene. *Proc. Natl. Acad. Sci. USA* 71: 737–741.

Finch, R. A., Evans, I. M., and Bosmann, H. B. 1980. Chemical carcinogen in vitro testing: A method for sizing cell nuclei in the nuclear enlargement assay. *Toxicology* 15:145–154.

Flamm, W. G. (Chairman, DHEW Working Group on Mutagenicity Testing). 1977. Approaches to determining the mutagenic properties of chemicals: Risk to future generations. *J. Environ. Pathol. Toxicol.* 1:301–352.

Gabridge, M. G., and Legator, M. S. 1969. A host-mediated microbial assay for the detection of mutagenic compounds. *Proc. Soc. Exp. Biol. Med.* 130:831–834.

International Commission for Protection Against Environmental Mutagens and Carcinogens. 1992. A method for combining and comparing short-term genotoxicity test data. The basic system. *Mutat. Res.* 266:7–25.

Kakunaga, T. 1973. A quantitative system for assay of malignant transformation by chemical carcinogens using a clone derived from BALB/3T3. *Int. J. Cancer* 12:463–473.

Lee, W. R., Abrahamson, S., Valencia, R., et al. 1983. The sex-linked recessive lethal test for mutagenesis in *Drosophila melanogaster*: A report of the U.S. EPA Gene-Tox Program. *Mutat. Res.* 123:183–279.

Mason, J. M., Langenbach, R., Sheldby, M. D., Zeigler, E., and Tennant, R. W. 1990. Ability of short term tests to predict carcinogenesis in rodents. *Annu. Rev. Pharmacol. Toxicol.*, 30:149–268.

McCann, J., Choi, E., Yamasaki, E., and Ames, B. N. 1975. Detection of carcinogens as mutagens in the *Salmonella*/microsome tests assay of 300 chemicals. *Proc. Natl. Acad. Sci. USA* 72:5135–5139.

Mitchell, A. D., Casciano, D. A., Meltz, M. L., Robinson, D. E., San, R. H. C., Williams, G. M., and von Halle, E. S. 1983. Unscheduled DNA synthesis tests: A report of the U.S. Environmental Protection Agency Gene-Tox Program. *Mutat. Res.* 123:363–410.

National Research Council. 1983. *Identifying and estimating the genetic impact of chemical mutagens.* A report of the Committee on Chemical Environmental Mutagens, National Research Council. Washington, DC: National Academy Press.

Organization for Economic Cooperation and Development. 1987. OECD Guidelines for Testing Chemicals. Washington, DC: OECD Publications and Information Center.

Preston, R. J., Au, W., Bender, M. A., et al. 1981. Mammalian in vivo and in vitro cytogenetic assays: A report of the U.S. EPA Gene-Tox Program. *Mutat. Res.* 87:143-188.

Rosenkranz, H. S., Gutter, G., and Spek, W. J. 1976. Mutagenicity and DNA-modifying activity: A comparison of two microbial assays. *Mutat. Res.* 41:61–70.

Russell, L. B. 1978. Somatic cells as indictors of germinal mutations in the mouse. *Environ. Health Perspect.* 24:113–116.

Russell, L. B., and Shelby, M. D. 1985. Tests for heritable genetic damage and for evidence of gonadal exposure in mammals. *Mutat. Res.* 154:69–84.

Russell, W. L. 1951. X-ray-induced mutations in mice. *Cold Spring Harbor Symp. Quant. Biol.* 16:327–336.

Schmid, W. 1976. The micronucleus test. *Mutat. Res.* 31:9–15.

Searle, A. G. 1975. The specific locus test in the mouse. *Mutat. Res.* 31:277–290.

Simmons, V. F., Rozenkranz, H. S., Zeiger, E., and Poirier, L. A. 1979. Mutagenic activity of chemical carcinogens and related compounds in the intraperitoneal host-mediated assay. *J. Natl. Cancer Inst.* 62:911–918.

Stich, H. F., and Laishes, B. A. 1973. DNA repair and chemical carcinogens. *Pathobiol. Annu.* 3:341–376.

U.S. Environmental Protection Agency. 1994. Health Effects Test Guidelines, Title 40, Part 798. Washington, DC: U.S. EPA.

Williams, G. M. 1979. The status of in vitro test systems utilizing DNA damage and repair for the screening of chemical carcinogens. *J. Assoc. Off. Anal. Chem.* 63:857–863.

Wolff, S. 1977. Sister chromatid exchange. *Annu. Rev. Genet.* 11:183–201.

World Health Organization. 1990. *Summary Report on the Evaluation of Short-Term Tests for Carcinogenesis.* Environmental Health Criteria 109. Geneva: WHO.

Wyrobek, A. J., and Bruce, W. R. 1975. Chemical induction of sperm abnormalities in mice. *Proc. Natl. Acad. Sci. USA* 72:4425–4429.

Zimmermann, F. K., von Borstel, R. C., von Halle, E. S., et al. 1984. Testing of chemicals for genetic activity with *Saccharomyces cerevisiae*: A report of the U.S. EPA Gene-Tox Program. *Mutat. Res.* 133:199–244.

ADDITIONAL READING

Kilby, B. J., Legator, M., Nichols, W., and Ramel, C. 1984. *Handbook of mutagenicity test procedures.* Amsterdam: Elsevier.

Appendix 8-1 Mutagenesis Tests Proposed by International Commission for Protection Against Environmental Mutagens and Carcinogens (1992)

A. In vitro family

A1	Primary DNA damage—prokaryotes (*B. subtilis, E. coli,* other DNA repair-deficient bacteria)
A2	Primary DNA damage—lower eukaryotes (*Saccharomyces cerevisiae*: gene conversion, homozygosity by recombination or gene conversion)
A3	Primary DNA damage—mammalian cells (unscheduled DNA synthesis: human fibroblasts, lymphocytes, transformed cells, other cells; rat hepatocytes; other animal cells)
A4	Gene mutation—prokaryotes [*S. typhimurium,* strains 1535, 1537, 1538, 98, 100; *E. coli* WP2 reverse mutation, *E. coli* K12 forward or reverse mutation, *E. coli* (excluding K12) forward mutation, *B. subtilis* multigene test]
A5	Gene mutation—lower eukaryotes (*Saccharomyces cerevisiae* forward, reverse mutation; *Schizosaccharomyces pombe,* forward mutation; *Neurospora crassa,* forward–reverse mutation)
A6	Gene mutation—mammalian cells (Chinese hamster ovary cells; lung V-79 cells: ouabain, HPRT; mouse L5178Y cells, TK locus, all other loci; other animal cells)
A7	Aneuploidy—lower eukaryotes (*Saccharomyces cerevisiae*)

Appendix 8-1 (Continued)

A8	Sister-chromatid exchange—mammalian cells (human fibroblasts, lymphocytes, other cells; Chinese hamster cells, Syrian hamster cells, mouse cells, rat cells, transformed cells, other cells)
A9	Chromosome aberration—mammalian cells (human fibroblasts, lymphocytes, other cells; Chinese hamster cells, Syrian hamster cells, rat cells, transformed cells, other animal cells)
A10	Transformation—mammalian cells. (Syrian hamster embryo cells, mouse cells, Fischer rat embryo cells, other established cell lines)

B. In vivo family: Somatic cells

B1	DNA repair, somatic—mammalian (unscheduled DNA synthesis, mouse cells, rat cells, rat hepatocytes, other animal cells)
B2	Gene mutation, somatic—insect (*Drosophila melanogaster*)
B3	Spot test, somatic—mammal (mouse spot test)
B4	Sister chromatid exchange, somatic—mammal (human lymphocytes, other cells, animal cells)
B5	Micronuclei, somatic—mammal (hamster, mouse, rat)
B6	Chromosome aberration, somatic—mammal (human bone marrow cells, lymphocytes; animal bone marrow cells, leukocytes; other animal cells)

B. In vivo family: Germ cells

B7	Heritable damage—insect (*Drosphila melanogaster* heritable translocation, dominant lethal, sex-linked recessive lethal)
B8	Heritable specific-locus test—mammal (mouse specific-locus test)
B9	Dominant lethal—mammal (mouse, rat)
B10	Heritable translocation—mammal (mouse)
B11	Chromosomal aberrations, germ cells—mammal (oocytes or embryos, spermatogonia, spermatocytes)
B12	Sperm morphology—mammal (mouse, rat)

Note: Each test is assigned a code. For example, A2 *S. cerevisiae* gene conversion is assigned SCG, and homozygocity, SCH.

Teratogenesis

CHAPTER 9 CONTENTS

INTRODUCTION

Historical Background

Teratogenesis is the formation of congenital defects. This type of illness has been known for decades and is an important cause of morbidity and mortality among newborns. For example, Murphy (1928) reviewed 320 human pregnancies and found 14 cases of children with small head circumference and mental retardation. Their mothers had been exposed to therapeutic radiation early in the pregnancy. Hale (1933) reported anophthalmia in the offspring of a sow deprived of vitamin A before pregnancy and during the first month of gestation. Warkany and Schraffenberger (1944) reported malformations resulting from nutritional deficiencies. Gregg (1941) suggested a relationship between the exposure of pregnant women to German measles and the blindness, deafness, and death among their offspring.

A connection was not suspected to exist between congenital malformation and chemicals because there was a tendency among toxicologists to assume that the natural protective mechanisms, such as detoxication, elimination, and placental barrier, were sufficient to shield the embryo from maternal exposure to chemicals. On the other hand, it was not unexpected that the natural protective mechanisms were ineffective against ionizing radiation, viruses, and nutritional deficiencies.

A new era in teratology was initiated as a result of the clinical use of thalidomide, a sedative-hypnotic. This drug, first introduced in the late 1950s in Germany, was found to be relatively nontoxic in experimental animals and in humans. Thus, while the therapeutic dose was 100 mg, ingestion of 14,000 mg by a person with suicidal intent did not result in death. It was used, among other indications, for the relief of morning sickness. In 1960, a few cases of phocomelia were reported. In the following year, there were many more cases. Phocomelia is a very rare type of congenital malformation, with shortening or absence of limbs. The causative agent in these cases was soon traced to the ingestion of thalidomide by the mothers, mainly between the third and eighth week of pregnancy. The use of the drug was promptly prohibited. In spite of that action, about 10,000 such malformed babies were born in a number of countries (Lenz and Knapp, 1962; Lenz, 1964). Because of the severity of the defects, elaborate prostheses were designed and utilized and special rehabilitation programs were instituted. Nevertheless, the profound, tragic effect on the malformed individuals and the traumatic impact on the families and society were so great that all feasible steps were instituted in an attempt to prevent another occurrence of such a man-made teratogenesis. One of these steps was to subject numerous drugs, food additives, pesticides, environmental contaminants, and other chemicals to various types of testing to determine their potential teratogenicity.

Some toxic effects on the fetus are not observable at birth. They may manifest as *delayed developmental toxicity.*

Embryology

After fertilization, the ovum undergoes a precise sequence of cell proliferation, differentiation, migration, and organogenesis. The embryo then passes through a set of metamorphoses and a period of fetal development before birth.

Predifferentiation Stage   During this stage the embryo is not susceptible to teratogenic agents. These agents either cause death of the embryo by killing all or most of the cells, or have no apparent effect on the embryo. Even when some mildly harmful effects have been produced, the surviving cells can compensate and form a normal embryo. This resistant stage varies from 5 to 9 d depending on the species.

Embryonic Stage   This is the period when the cells undergo intensive differentiation, mobilization, and organization. It is during this period that most of the organogenesis takes place. As a result, the embryo is most susceptible to the effects of teratogens. This period generally ends some time from the 10th to the 14th day in rodents and in the 14th week of the gestation period in humans. Furthermore, not all organs are susceptible at the same time of the pregnancy. Figure 9-1 shows that the rat embryo is

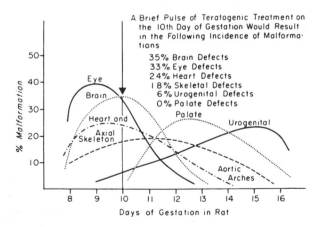

Figure 9-1 Expected incidences of malformation of different organs and systems the susceptibilities of which vary according to the days of gestation. A brief exposure to a teratogen on the 10th day of gestation is expected to induce a variety of malformations, with their incidences shown here. (Reprinted from Wilson, 1965, by permission of the University of Chicago Press.)

most susceptible between days 8 and 12 for most organs, but the palate and urogenital organs are more susceptible at a later stage.

Fetal Stage This stage is characterized by growth and functional maturation. Teratogens are thus unlikely to cause morphologic defects during this stage, but they may induce functional abnormalities. Although morphologic defects are in general readily detected at birth or shortly thereafter, functional abnormalities, such as central nervous system (CNS) deficiencies, may not be diagnosed for some time after birth.

TERATOGENS AND THEIR EFFECTS

Many chemical and physical agents may affect the conceptus. The effect may result in one or more of the following manifestations: death, malformations, growth retardation, and functional disorder.

Death may be detected by the difference between the number of corpora lutea and the number of implantations, or the number of resorptions and/or the number of dead fetuses.

Malformations may involve external and/or internal structures. Minor abnormalities, or deviations, generally do not affect the survival of the fetus. Examples are supernumary ribs and decreased or abnormal sternal ossification.

Major malformations, such as spina bifida or hydrocephalus, are incompatible with survival, growth and fertility.

Minor anomalies are of doubtful significance. Examples are curly tail, straight legs, malrotated limbs and paws, wristdrop, protruding tongue, enlarged atria and/or ventricles, abnormal pelvic development, and translucent skin.

Growth retardation and *functional disorders* are observed shortly or much later after birth. They are generally referred to as developmental effects.

Various agents are known to be teratogenic in humans. These include radiation, certain infections, nutritional imbalance, and certain drugs and chemicals. Table 9-1 lists many such agents and is adapted from Shepard (1986) with additional information from Cordier et al. (1992) and Sylvester et al. (1994). This list is not exhaustive because of the difficulties involved in confirming the teratogenicity of an agent in humans. Furthermore, the teratogenic effect of an agent may not be observed if the conceptus is miscarried. These difficulties can be minimized in animal experimentation. The teratogens that are confirmed in animals are listed in Appendix 9-1, adapted from Shepard (1986).

MODE OF ACTION OF TERATOGENS

Various chemicals have been shown to be teratogenic in humans and/or animals. In view of the great diversity of the properties of these agents, it

Table 9-1   Known Human Teratogens

Ionizing radiation	Drugs and chemicals
Therapeutic	Thalidomide
Radioiodine	Abamectin
Atomic weapon	Alcohol
	Aminopterin
Infections	Androgenic hormone
Rubella	Anesthetics
Cytomegalovirus infection	Antithyroid drugs
Herpes simplex	Busulfan
Syphilis	Caffeine
Toxoplasmosis	Chlorobiphenyls
	Coumarin anticoagulants
Metabolic imbalances'	Cyclophosphamide
Cretinism	Diethylstilbestrol
Diabetes	Dinocap
Phenylketonuria	Halothane
Virilizing tumors	Isotretinoin
Hyperthermia	Lithium
	Methimazole
	Organic mercury compounds
	Organic solvents
	Phenytoin
	Procymidone
	Tetracyclines
	Trimethadione
	Valproic acid

is not surprising that many different mechanisms are involved in their teratogenic effects.

Interference with Nucleic Acids

Many agents interfere with nucleic acid replication, transcription, or RNA translation. Their effects may result in cell death or somatic mutation in the embryo. Structural or functional defects may occur where enough cells are so affected. Ionizing radiation and genotoxic carcinogens are likely to act through this mechanism. Although some chemicals, such as carbon tetrachloride and nitrosamines, also yield metabolites that react with nucleic acids, their reactive metabolites are too unstable to reach the embryo. Therefore, these toxicants are carcinogenic but not potent teratogens.

Deficiency of Energy Supply and Osmolarity

Certain teratogens can affect the energy supply for the metabolism of the organism by restricting the availability of substrates either directly (e.g., dietary deficiencies) or through the presence of analogs or antagonists of vitamins, essential amino acids, and others such as 6-aminonicotinamide, which also interfere with glycolysis. In addition, hypoxia and agents inducing hypoxia (CO, CO2) can be teratogenic by depriving the metabolic process of the required oxygen and probably also by the production of osmolar imbalances. These can induce edema and hematomas, which in turn can cause mechanical distortion and tissue ischemia.

Inhibition of Enzymes

Inhibitors of enzymes, such as 5-fluorouracil, can induce malformation through interference with differentiation or growth, by inhibiting thymidylate synthetase. 6-Aminonicotinamide, which inhibits glucose-6-phosphate dehydrogenase, is also a potent teratogen.

Oxidative Stress

Teratogens such as phenytoin undergo bioactivation and induce lipid peroxidation, protein oxidation, and protein degradation in both maternal and embryonic tissues. These biochemical changes may be responsible for the teratogenesis (Liu and Wells, 1995).

Others

Hypervitaminosis A may be associated with ultrastructural damage to cellular membranes in rodent embryos, a mechanism that may explain the teratogenicity of vitamin A. Physical agents that can cause malformations include radiation, hypothermia and hyperthermia, and mechanical trauma.

It should be noted that the mode of action of many teratogens is as yet uncertain. Furthermore, a potential teratogen may or may not exert teratogenic effects, depending on such factors as bioactivating mechanism, stability of the reactive metabolites, ability to cross the placental barrier, and detoxifying capability of the embryonic tissues. Appropriate experimental testing for the teratogenicity of toxicants is therefore essential.

TERATOGENS OF SPECIAL INTEREST

Thalidomide, as noted earlier, is otherwise a relatively safe drug but induced an episode of unprecedented tragic congenital malformation. This episode broadened the scope of teratology. Unfortunately, after some 25 years of intensive study, the mechanism underlying its teratogenicity remains to be confirmed. The proposed mechanisms include interference with folic acid or glutamic acid metabolism, depurination of DNA, and acylation of polyamines. In addition to these biochemical investigations, a number of target tissues have been studied without definitive answer. These are limb mesenchyme tissue, mesonephric-limb tissue, and the developing neural crest tissue (Manson and Wise, 1993). A detailed account of the 24 different approaches that have been explored is provided by Stephens (1988).

Diethylstilbestrol (DES) was used in the 1940s to 1970s to prevent threatened abortion. Unfortunately, a few of the young adult female offspring (usually at age 19–22 yr) of these mothers developed adenocarcinoma of the vagina and cervix; more of them developed other disorders of the vagina and cervix (Poskanzer and Herbst, 1977). In addition, abnormal structural and functional disorders of the genital organs were observed in some male offspring (Bibbo et al., 1977).

TESTING PROCEDURES

Animals

Rats, rabbits, mice, and hamsters are the commonly used animals, because of their ready availability, easy handling, larger litter size, and short gestational period. The use of nonhuman primates has also been suggested because of their phylogenetic proximity to humans. There are advantages and disadvantages of various species of animals for use in teratology. On balance, it would appear that rabbits and nonhuman primates offer more advantages (Schardein et al., 1985).

The animals should be young, mature, and healthy. Prima gravida females are preferred. With rats, at least 20 females are placed in each dose group; with rabbits, 12 females are used per dose (U.S. EPA, 1994). Smaller numbers of large animals such as dogs and nonhuman primates are used.

Because of the simplicity of the technique, the developing chick embryo had been widely used in the 1960s. However, it is now generally accepted that this model yields too many false-positives associated with its lack of a placenta and its susceptibility to such nonspecific factors as pH, specific gravity, and osmotic pressure.

Administration of the Chemical

Dosage   At least three dosage levels are used. The higher dosage should include some maternal (and/or fetal) toxicity, such as reduction in body weight. The lowest dosage should induce no observable ill effect. One or more doses should be appropriately interspersed between the two extremes.

In addition, two control groups are included. One of these is given the vehicle or physiologic saline, and the other receives a substance of known teratogenic activity. These groups will provide information on the incidence of spontaneous malformations and the sensitivity of the specific lot of animals under the existing experimental conditions. In addition to these contemporary controls, data from historical controls are also useful.

Route and Timing   The test substances should be administered by the route that simulates the human exposure situations. For food additives and contaminants, the chemical is preferably incorporated in the animal feeds. Oral drugs are generally administered by gastric gavage.

The timing of administering the chemical is important, as illustrated by the experiment of Tuchmann-Duplessis (1965) with 6-mercaptopurine, which produced either nervous and ocular defects or skeletal anomalies, depending on the timing (Fig. 9-1). However, for routine teratologic studies, it is customary to administer the chemical during the entire period of organogenesis when the embryo is most susceptible. This period varies from one species to another. Such periods for some species of animals and related information are included in Table 9-2.

Observations

Pregnant Animals   The animals should be examined daily for gross signs of toxicity, and any female that shows signs of impending abortion or premature delivery (e.g., vaginal bleeding) should be sacrificed and examined.

Fetuses   Fetuses are usually surgically removed from the mother about 1 d prior to the expected delivery. This procedure is intended to avoid cannibalism and to permit counting of resorption sites and dead fetuses.

The following observations are to be made and recorded:

Number of corpora lutea
Number of implantations
Number of resorptions
Number of dead fetuses
Number of live fetuses
Sex of each live fetus
Weight of each live fetus

Table 9-2   Teratogenesis Studies on Various Animals

	Rat	Mouse	Hamster	Rabbit
Age of dam at start	100–120 d	60–90 d	60–90 d	Adult virgin
Period of dosing[a]	d 6–15	d 6–15	d 5–12	d 6–18
Cesarean section[a]	d 20	d 17	d 14	d 29
Positive control	ASA,[b] 250 mg/kg	ASA, 150 mg/kg	ASA, 250 mg/kg	6-aminonicotinamide, 2.5 mg/kg

[a]Day 0 is when sperm is found in the vagina or, in the rabbit, the day of copulation or artificial insemination.

[b]ASA, acetylsalicylic acid, is a potent teratogen in certain laboratory animals, although only capable of inducing bleeding in human fetuses and only after large doses.

Length (crownrump) of each live fetus
Abnormalities of each fetus

Detailed Examinations These are performed to determine the different types of abnormalities. Each fetus is examined for external defects. In addition, about two-thirds of randomly sampled fetuses are examined for skeletal abnormalities after staining with alizarin red (Dawson, 1926). The remaining one-third of the fetuses are examined for visceral defects after fixation in Bouin's fluid and sectioned with a razor blade (Wilson, 1965). With larger animals, such as dogs, pigs, and nonhuman primates, the skeletal structure is generally examined with x-rays instead of staining.

Delayed Effects With toxicants that are suspected of having effects on the fetal central nervous system or genitourinary system, a sufficient number of pregnant females are allowed to deliver their pups. These pups are nursed either by their biologic mothers, thus possibly being exposed to the toxicants via the milk, or by foster mothers. In the latter case, the potential effects of postnatal exposure are eliminated.

Neuromotor and behavioral tests may be used to detect CNS effects. In evaluating two known teratogens, Goldey et al. (1994) measured motor activity, acoustic startle, T-maze delayed alternation, and total and regional brain weight, as well as glial fibrillary acidic protein. Male rats exposed to TCDD in utero and lactationally may exhibit altered androgenic status, including reduced sperm count and testosterone levels (Mably et al., 1992).

EVALUATION OF TERATOGENIC EFFECTS

Categories and Relative Significance

Resorption is a manifestation of death of the conceptus. If there is an appreciable increase in the number of resorptions in the treated group, it may be necessary to alter the testing procedure to differentiate embryotoxicity from teratogenicity, for example, by lowering the dose used to reduce the toxicity or shorten the exposure period of the dams.

Fetal toxicity may manifest as reduced body weight on the nonviable fetus. This type of data is often useful as corroborating evidence in assessing the teratogenicity of the toxicant in question. With rabbits, the viability of the fetus, if in question, may be determined by incubating it for 24 h. With rodents, it may be advisable to repeat the test but allow the dams to deliver the pups.

Aberrations may be incompatible with survival. These are known as major *malformations*. Examples are hydrocephalus and spina bifida. Minor *anomalies*, for example, curly tail, wristdrop, and protruding tongue, are generally not life-threatening.

Sources of Error

1   The animals used may exhibit an excessive number of spontaneous malformations or may be resistant to teratogenic effects. These errors can usually be assessed by the response of the animals to the negative and positive control agents.

2   Poor animal husbandry and mishandling of the animals may also result in an increased incidence of malformations.

3   The food consumption of the dams can be affected by the toxicant. This fact may then alter the body weight of the mothers and indirectly affect the fetuses.

4   Excessively large doses can result in many resorptions but few or no malformations. On the other hand, if the doses are too small, there may not be any evidence of teratogenicity.

5   Some teratogenic effects may be overlooked if only a cursory examination is carried out.

Analysis of the Results

In comparing the treated and control groups, the proper experimental unit is the litter rather than the individual fetuses, since each dam is an experimental unit (Weil, 1970). In other words, the numbers of litters with malformed fetuses, resorptions, or dead fetuses are the parameters to be used in statistical analysis. However, an increase in the average number of fetuses with defects per litter may provide corroborative evidence of teratogenicity.

If the results indicate a relationship between the doses and the response (incidence of malformation), it is generally justifiable to conclude that the agent is teratogenic under the specific experimental conditions.

Extrapolation to Humans

The results obtained in teratogenesis studies in animals cannot be readily extrapolated to humans. The lack of a suitable animal model is evidenced by the fact that the most potent human teratogen, thalidomide, which is effective at a dose of 0.5–1.0 mg/kg, has no teratogenic effects in rats and mice at 4000 mg/kg. Only moderate embryopathy is noted in rabbits. On the other hand, acetylsalicylic acid has a long history of safe use in human pregnancy but is a potent teratogen in rats, mice, and hamsters.

On the other hand, the fact that many chemicals have been shown to be teratogenic in animal models but not in humans may be due partly to lower human susceptibility and lower levels of human exposure, but it may also be due to inadequate epidemiological studies. Furthermore, it is to be noted that the teratogenic effects of a chemical may manifest as low pregnancy rate, stillbirths, or poor viability of the neonates.

The value of animal teratogenicity studies to the assessment of human health hazards was shown by Frankos (1985). Analyzing the Food and Drug Administration (FDA) data, he noted that 37 of the 38 known human teratogens were positive in at least one laboratory animal test species, and that 130 of the 165 chemicals showing no teratologic findings were negative in at least one laboratory animal test species.

In view of the foregoing, it is prudent to carry out appropriate animal tests on all chemicals to which women of childbearing age may be exposed. If positive results are obtained with a substance, especially when this is so in more than one species of animal, exposure of women of childbearing age to this substance should be avoided, if possible. In assessing the teratogenic effects of a chemical, not only the incidence but also the severity of the aberrations should be taken into account (Khera, 1981).

IN VITRO TESTS

While these tests are not in routine use as yet, they show promise either as screening procedures, in pinpointing target organs, or in elaborating the mode of action of teratogens. Some of these tests are briefly described next; some details and references are provided by Saxén (1981) and the In Vitro Teratology Task Force (1987). The latter critically reviewed the literature on in vitro teratological research using (1) mammalian whole embryo, (2) rodent limb bud culture system, (3) embryonic organs in culture, (4) cells in culture, and (5) nonmammalian model systems. The nonmammalian systems that have been used include hydra, planarians, crickets, fish, amphibians, and *Drosophila*. A few of these are outlined in the following sections.

Cell Culture

Cell cultures may be grown in suspension, as a monolayer, or in various supporting materials. Teratogenic effects can be determined by a variety of end points.

One type of end point involves analysis of the protein synthesized by the cultured cells, such as those from chick embryo. To ensure that the influences of bioactivation and placental barrier are taken into account, the cell culture is exposed to the chemical and its metabolites extracted from the amniotic fluid of pregnant mice that had been given the chemical.

Certain tumor cells in culture attach rapidly to a specially coated surface. It was found that chemicals shown to be teratogenic in animals generally inhibit the attachment of these cells. Another end point is alteration of cell differentiation by teratogenic chemicals. The alteration may be determined biochemically and morphologically.

Organ Culture

Metanephric kidney, developing tooth, and a number of other organs have been used for this purpose. The metanephric model is derived from 11-d mouse embryo metanephric mesenchyme and grown on a porous filter. An embryonic spinal cord is fixed on the opposite side of the filter as the inductor. It is removed after 24 h, when the induction has taken place. The tissue then differentiates into glomeruli, proximal tubules, and distal tubules. A number of chemicals have been shown to reduce the number of tubules developed.

Unlike cell culture, organ cultures are too complex for use as a prescreen but appear useful for the study of the mode of action and target site of suspect chemicals.

Hydra Culture

Johnson and Gabel (1982) described a procedure using cultures of *Hydra attenuata* raised in laboratory conditions. Exposure of the adult hydra and artificial embryos (composed of randomly reaggregated cells of dissociated hydra) to chemicals causes various morphologic changes and death. The ratio of the lethal concentration in the embryo to that in the adult has been determined for several chemicals. These ratios show a good correlation with the ratios of the teratologic doses and the toxic doses in adult rodents. The procedure, therefore, also appears promising as a prescreen.

A much more extensive discussion of tests involving cultures of specific organs, tissues, whole embryos, and a variety of invertebrates is provided by the World Health Organization (1984).

REFERENCES

Bibbo, M., Gill, W., Azizi, F., Blough, R., Fnag, V., Rosenfield, R., Schumacher, G., Sleeper, K., Sonek, M., and Wild, G. 1977. Follow-up study of male and female offspring of DES-exposed mothers. *Obstet. Gynaecol.* 49:1–8.

Cordier, S., Ha, M.-C., Ayme, S., and Goujard, J. 1992. Maternal occupational exposure and congenital malformations. *Scand. J. Work Environ. Health* 18:11–17.

Dawson, A. B. 1926. A note on the staining of the skeleton of cleared specimens with Alizarin Red S. *Stain Technol.* 1:123–124.

Frankos, V. H. 1985. FDA perspectives on the use of teratology data for human risk assessment. *Fundam. Appl. Toxicol.* 5:615–625.

Goldey, E. S., O'Callaghan, J. P., Stanton, M. E., Barone, S., Jr., and Crofton, K. M. 1994. Developmental neurotoxicity: Evaluation of testing procedures with methylagomethanol and methylmercury. *Fundam. Appl. Toxicol.* 23:447–464.

Gregg, N. M. 1941. Congenital cataract following German measles in the mother. *Trans. Ophthalmol. Soc. Aust.* 3:35–46.

Hale, F. 1933. Pigs born without eyeballs. *J. Hered.* 24:105–106.

In Vitro Teratology Task Force. 1987. Report of the Task Force, organized by Center for Food Safety and Applied Nutrition, FDA. *Environ. Health Perspect.* 72:201–249.

Johnson, E. M., and Gabel, B. E. G. 1982. Application of the hydra assay for rapid detection of developmental hazards. *J. Am. Coll. Toxicol.* 1(3):57–71.

Khera, K. S. 1981. Common fetal aberrations and their teratologic significance: A review. *Fundam. Appl. Toxicol.* 1:13–18.

Lenz, W. 1964. Chemicals and malformation in man, and congenital malformations. Papers and discussions presented at the Second International Medical Conference, New York.

Lenz, W., and Knapp, K. 1962. Thalidomide embryopathy. *Arch. Environ. Health* 5:100–105.

Liu, L., and Wells, P. G. 1995. Potential molecular targets mediating chemical teratogenesis: In vitro peroxidase-catalyzed phenytoin metabolism and oxidative damage to proteins and lipids in marine maternal hepatic microsomes and embryonic 9000 g supernatant. *Toxicol. Appl. Pharmacol.* 34:71–80.

Mably, T. A., Moore, R. W., and Peterson, R. E. 1992. In utero and lactational exposure of male rats to 2,3,7,8-tetrachlorodibenzo-*p*-dioxin: 1. Effects on androgenic status. *Toxicol. Appl. Pharmacol.* 114:97–107.

Manson, J. M., and Wise, L. D. 1993. Teratogens. In *Casarett and Doull's toxicology*, eds. M. O. Amdur, J. Doull, and C. D. Klaassen, pp. 226–254. New York: McGraw-Hill.

Murphy, D. P. 1928. Ovarian irradiation: Its effect on the health of subsequent children: Review of the literature, experimental and clinical, with a report of 320 human pregnancies. *Surg. Gynecol. Obstet.* 47:201–215.

Poskanzer, D., and Herbst, A. 1977. Epidemiology of vaginal adenosis and adenocarcinoma associated with exposure to stilbestrol in utero. *Cancer* 39:1892–1895.

Saxén, L. 1981. Tests in vitro for teratogenicity. In *Tests for toxicity*, ed. J. W. Gorrod, pp. 185–196. London: Taylor & Francis.

Schardein, J. L., Schwartz, B. B., and Kenel, M. F. 1985. Species sensitivities and prediction of teratogenic potential. *Environ. Health Perspect.* 61:55–62.

Shepard, T. H. 1986. *Catalog of teratogenic agents*, 5th ed. Baltimore: Johns Hopkins University Press.

Stephens, T. D. 1988. Proposed mechanisms of action in thalidomide embryopathy. *Teratology* 38:229–239.

Sylvester, G. C., Khoury, M. J., Lu, X.-P., and Erickson, J. D. 1994. First-trimester anesthesia exposure and the risk of central nervous system defects: A population based case-control study. *Am. J. Public Health* 84:1757–1760.

Tuchmann-Duplessis, H. 1965. Design and interpretation of teratogenic tests. In *Embryopathic activity of drugs*, eds. J. M. Robson, F. M. Sullivan, and R. L. Smith. Boston: Little, Brown.

U.S. Environmental Protection Agency. 1994. Health Effects Test Guidelines/Code of Federal Regulations, Title 40, Part 789. Washington, DC: U.S. EPA.

Warkany, J., and Schraffenberger, E. 1944. Congenital malformations induced in rats by maternal nutritional deficiency. VI. Preventive factor. *J. Nutr.* 27:477–484.

Weil, C. 1970. Selection of the valid number of sampling units and a consideration of their combination in toxicological studies involving reproduction, teratogenesis or carcinogenesis. *Food Cosmet. Toxicol.* 8:177–182.

Wilson, J. G. 1965. Methods for administering agents and detecting malformations in experimental animal. In: *Teratology: Principles and techniques*, eds. J. G. Wilson and J. Warkany, pp. 251–277. Chicago: University of Chicago Press.

World Health Organization. 1984. Principles for Evaluating Health Risks to Progeny Associated with Exposure to Chemicals During Pregnancy. Environmental Health Criteria 30. Geneva: WHO.

Appendix 9-1   Teratogens in Animal Models

1 Physical agents: hypothermia and hyperthermia, hypoxia, radiation
2 Agents producing hypoxia: carbon monoxide, carbon dioxide
3 Infections: rubella viruses, syphilis
4 Dietary deficiency or excess: vitamins A, D, and E, ascorbic acid, nicotinamide, trace metals (Zn, Mn, Mg, Co)
5 Vitamin antagonists: antifolic drugs, 6-aminonicotinamide
6 Hormone deficiency or excess: cortisone, hydrocortisone, thyroxine, vasopressin, insulin, androgens, estrogens
7 Natural toxins: aflatoxin B_1, ochratoxin A, ergotamine, nicotine
8 Heavy metals: methylmercury, phenylmercuric acetate, lead, thallium, strontium, selenium
9 Solvents: benzene, carbon tetrachloride, 1,1-dichloroethane, dimethyl sulfoxide, propylene glycol, xylene
10 Insecticides, herbicides, fungicides
11 Azo dyes: trypan blue, Evans blue, Niagara blue
12 Antibiotics: dactinomycin, penicillin, streptomycin, tetracyclines
13 Sulfonamides: sulfanilamide, hypoglycemic sulfonamides
14 Drugs and chemicals: caffeine, carbutamide, chlorcyclizine, chlorpromazine and derivatives, diphenylhydantoin, hydroxyurea, imipramine, meclizine, nitrosamines, pilocarpine, quinine, rauwolfia, thalidomide, triparanol, veratrum alkaloids, vinca alkaloids

Part Three

Target Organs and Systems

Toxicology of the Immune System

CHAPTER 10 CONTENTS

GENERAL CONSIDERATIONS

The function of the immune system is to protect the host against foreign organisms (virus, bacteria, fungus), "foreign cells" (neoplasm), and other foreign substances. Its importance is evidenced by the seriousness of immunodeficiency: Patients with this disorder are prone to be affected by infection and tumors. Immunodeficiency can be congenital or acquired; the latter is also known as AIDS (acquired immunodeficiency syndrome).

The immune system is composed of several types of organs, cells, and noncellular components. The functions of the individual components are in general interrelated. Thus, upon encountering a foreign substance, a cascade of reactions usually appears between different types of cellular and humoral components. These reactions involve the recognition, memory, and response to the foreign substance, and are designed for its elimination or control.

Various toxicants are known to suppress immune function. This effect will lead to lowered host resistance to bacterial and viral infections, and to parasitic infestation, as well as lowered control of neoplasm. In addition, certain toxicants may provoke exaggerated immune reactions leading to local or systemic reactions. Furthermore, it may even result in "autoimmune reactions."

This chapter briefly describes the components of the immune system and their functions, major immunotoxicants, and appropriate testing procedures.

COMPONENTS OF THE SYSTEM

The immune system consists of a network of organs including the bone marrow, thymus, spleen, and lymph nodes. From these organs, various lymphocytes and other cells with different immune functions are derived.

Some of the components are involved in specific immune responses, and others in nonspecific responses. Both types of cells are derived from the pluripotent cells in the bone marrow (Fig. 10-1). From these cells are generated the lymphoid stem cells. Some of these cells are processed through the thymus and become T cells (T lymphocytes); others go through

Figure 10-1 Cells involved in specific and nonspecific defense mechanisms and their precursors.

the "bursal equivalent" tissues (including bone marrow, lymph nodes, lymphoid tissues in the gut such as appendix, cecum, and Peyer's patches) to become B cells (B lymphocytes). Still others are released from the bone marrow without further processing. These are known as natural killer (NK) cells. Unlike the T cells and B cells, NK cells are involved in nonspecific defense against neoplasms and certain other foreign substances.

Other pluripotent stem cells give rise to myeloid stem cells, from which are derived monocytes, mast cells, and polymorphonuclear (PMN) cells. Monocytes then become macrophages, which are involved in specific and nonspecific immune reactions. In addition, there are three types of PMN cells, namely, neutrophils, eosinophils, and basophils. These cells are involved in nonspecific defense mechanisms.

T Cells

As noted already, the T cells, after passing through the thymus, enter the blood and constitute 70% of the circulating lymphocytes. Some settle in thymus-dependent areas of the spleen and lymph nodes. These small and medium-sized lymphocytes have a life span of up to 5 yr.

On contact with macrophage-processed antigen, the T cells undergo proliferation and differentiation. Some of these cells become "activated" and responsible for mediating cellular immunity. Others become T memory cells, which can be activated by combining with antigens, or become *helper* or *suppressor* cells. Once activated, helper T cells will proliferate and secrete lymphokines. The lymphokines will cause the B cells to become plasma cells. Suppressor T cells suppress both the formation of antibodies by B cells and the ability of T cells to mount cellular immune responses.

The activated T cells react either directly with cell-membrane-associated antigens or by releasing various soluble factors known as lymphokines. There are a large number of lymphokines (see next section).

B Cells

Other stem cells undergo changes in certain tissues as already noted to become B cells (B lymphocytes). They enter the blood to constitute 30% of the lymphocytes. Some of them have a life span of 15 d, and others months to years.

The primary immune response is initiated by the contact of antigen with B cells, which then differentiate and proliferate. Some of these become *memory* cells, which retain the surface immunoglobulin receptors, whereas others become *plasma* cells. The cells are mature and capable of synthesizing small amounts of immunoglobulin M (IgM). Exposure of the memory cells to the same antigen at a later time results in the secondary immune response. This response differs from the primary type in that not only do all the processes proceed much more rapidly but the immunoglobulins are of the IgG class and in greater quantities.

Other Types of Cells

Other lymphocytes lack the characteristic surface markers of the T cells and the B cells, but they participate in the nonspecific immune system functions. These are the null cells. Some of these, the *natural killer* (NK) cells, have spontaneous (without prior sensitization) cytolytic activity against other cells, especially leukemia and carcinoma cells. On the other hand, *killer cells* (KC), a subpopulation of T cells, can mediate antibody-dependent cellular cytotoxicity in the presence of antibodies.

Macrophages are also derived from the stem-cell pool in the bone marrow. After their release, they appear in the bloodstream as monocytes and in the tissues as histiocytes. On contact with a foreign body, they engulf the foreign body and become activated macrophages. These cells are rich in cytoplasmic hydrolytic enzymes. Most bacterial cells are readily digested by these enzymes. Macrophages can also be activated, as noted earlier, by certain lymphokines produced by T cells.

Macrophages also participate in the T-cell- and B-cell-mediated specific immune reactions by the following mechanism: Much of the antigen is engulfed by macrophages and processed by these cells. A portion of the antigen is not engulfed by macrophages, but attached to their surface. The nearby T cell will then produce cellular immunity or enhance the T-dependent B cells to produce antibody.

Langerhans cells are also derived from bone marrow and are located in the skin. They serve to process dermal antigens and initiate contact allergy and rejection of skin graft.

Among the *polymorphonuclear cells*, neutrophil PMNs have phagocytic activity. The eosinophils possess cytotoxic function, and basophils (which become mast cells in tissues) release histamine and other substances, thereby initiating local reactions to a foreign substance inducing immediate hypersensitivity.

Humoral Components

Immunoglobins are proteins produced by plasma cells (derived from B cells). They have specific antibody activities. Their specificity is determined by the amino acid sequence and the tertiary surface configuration. There are five major types of immunoglobins. Their characteristics and functions are outlined in Table 10-1.

Interleukins (cytokines) are proteins produced by activated T cells (lymphokines) or monocytes/macrophages (monokines) in response to an-

Table 10-1   Characteristics of Immunoglobulins

Class	Molecular weight	Mean survival $T_{1/2}$ (d)	Mean serum concentration (mg/dl)	Major function
IgG	150,000	23	720–1500	Most prevalent; major antibody for toxins, viruses, and bacteria
IgA	170,000	6	90–325	In secretions from mucosa; for early antibacterial and antiviral defense
IgM	900,000	5	45–150	Major antibody after exposure to most antigens
IgD	180,000	3	3	Present on B-cell surface, functions as an antigen receptor
IgE	200,000	2	0.03	Fixed on mast cells, responsible for immediate-type hypersensitivity

tigenic or mitogenic stimulation. They promote the proliferation of T cells, B cells, and hematopoietic stem cells. A notable one, interleukin-2 (IL-2), may promote the growth of antigen-activated T cells from immune donors in long-term T-cell culture. IL-2 has therefore been investigated for possible use in the management of cancer and AIDS. A list of interleukin functions has been compiled by Sharma and Reddy (1987).

The complement system consists of 20 soluble plasma and body fluid proteins. These proteins complement a variety of immune functions, such as adherence of antibody-coated bacteria to macrophages, modulation of immune response, and lysis of cells. Immunotoxicants can activate or inhibit the complements. Macrophages are capable of synthesizing certain important cytokines, such as tumor necrosis factor and growth factors; the latter play a central role in the fibrotic lung lesions in humans exposed to asbestos and silica (see chap. 11).

IMMUNOTOXICANTS

Major Immunotoxicants

A variety of substances have been found to affect the immune system. They may be placed in five categories as follows:

   1 Antineoplastic drugs: cyclophosphamide, nitrogen mustards, 6-mercaptopurine, azathioprine, methotrexate, 5-fluorouracil, actinomycin, doxorubicin.

2   Heavy metals, organometals, etc.: beryllium, nickel, chromium, gold, methylmercury, platinum, organic tin compounds, sodium arsenite and arsenate, and arsenic trioxide.

3   Pesticides: pyrethroids, chlordane, DDT, dieldrin, methylparathion, carbofuran, maneb, hexachlorobenzene (HCB), carbaryl, 2, 4-D, paraquat, diquat.

4   Halogenated hydrocarbons: 2,3,7,8-tetrachlorodibenzo-*p*-dioxin (TCDD), polychlorinated biphenyls (PCB), polybrominated biphenyls (PBB), trichloroethylene, chloroform, pentachlorophenol.

5   Miscellaneous compounds: benzo[a]pyrene, methylcholanthrene, diethylstilbestrol, benzene, corticosteroids, TPA, penicillin, sulfites, subtilisin formaldehyde, toluene diisocyanates.

The effects of toxicants on the immune system are complex; some suppress the cell-mediated immunity, others the humoral immunity, and still others may even stimulate certain immune functions (Table 10-2).

Effects on Immune Functions

Immunosuppression   Most of the immunotoxicants suppress immune functions. An extensively studied immunotoxicant is TCDD. Its effect on the immune function is one of the most sensitive targets for toxicity. It suppresses all the specific immune functions tested, while sparing the

Table 10-2   Effects of In Vivo Exposure to Chemicals on Immune Function and Host Resistance

Parameters	DES	BaP	TPA
Resistance to *Listeria* challenge	D	NE	I
Resistance to tumor challenge	D	NE	D
Trichinella expulsion	D	D	NE
Thymus weight	D	NE	D
Delayed hypersensitivity	D	NE	NE
Lymphocyte responses[a]	D	D[b]	D
T-cell quantification	D	—	D
Spontaneous lymphocyte cytotoxicity	NE	NE	D
Antibody plaque response	D	D	D
Immunoglobulins M, G, and A levels	NE	NE	D
Macrophage phagocytosis	I	NE	I
Macrophage cytostasis	I	NE	I
RES clearance time	I	NE	I
Bone marrow cellularity[c]	D	D	NE

Source: Data from Dean et al. (1982), copyright 1982, American Society for Pharmacology and Experimental Therapeutics.

Note: DES, diethylstilbestrol; BaP, benzo[a]pyrene; TPA, 12-*O*-tetradecanoylphorbol 13-*o*-acetate; D, decreased; I, increased; NE, no effect; —, not tested.

[a]Lymphocyte responses to phytohemagglutinin, concanavalin A, lipopolysaccharide, and mixed lymphocyte culture.
[b]Decreased, except the response to mixed lymphocyte culture.
[c]Colony-forming units, multipotent cells, and granulocyte/macrophage progenitors.

nonspecific functions, such as the NK cell activity and macrophage functions. Its immunotoxicity is apparently mediated through binding to the Ah receptors on lymphoid cells (Luster et al., 1989).

Other immunosuppressants have more restricted activities. For example, antineoplastic drugs such as cyclosporin adversely affect B cells; T cells that have undergone antigenic differentiation may also be affected. Metals such as lead and mercury impair both humoral and cell-mediated host resistance. In addition, gold may also induce glomerular nephritis through an autoimmune mechanism resulting in deposits in the glomeruli. Nickel may suppress immune functions through a variety of mechanisms, with its major clinical effect being hypersensitivity. Organochlorine pesticides impair immune functions mainly in neonatal animals. Carbaryl depresses antibody response and phagocytosis by granulocytes. Corticoids depress immune functions as well as inflammatory responses.

Immunodysfunction Certain agents cause hypersensitivity reactions or allergies. There are four types of such reactions. With the first type, the reactions are immediate (usually within 15 min), resulting from a second or subsequent exposure to an antigen. The first exposure to that antigen induces the production of IgE antibodies. Subsequent exposure to the same antigen triggers the release of existing histamine, heparin, serotonin, etc., and the release of newly formed SRS-A (slow-reacting substances of anaphylaxis), prostaglandins, etc. These substances induce a variety of clinical manifestation, such as asthma, rhinitis, urticaria, and anaphylaxis. Allergenic agents are diverse in nature: Notable examples are metals (nickel, beryllium, platinum compounds), therapeutic agents (penicillin), food additives [sulfites, monosodium glutamate (MSG), tartrazine, benzoates], pesticides (pyrethrum), and industrial chemicals such as toluene diisocyanate (TDI).

Type IV is a delayed hypersensitivity reaction. The latent period is usually between 12 and 48 h. The reaction is mediated by T cells (rather than antibodies) and characterized by perivascular infiltration of monocytes, lymphocytes, and lymphoblasts (resulting from local transformation of lymphocytes). Clinically, this is seen with contact dermatitis and granulomatous reactions. A commonly encountered hypersensitivity inducer is nickel, which also induces immediate immune reaction. Others include beryllium, chromium, formaldehyde, thimerosol (a mercurial compound widely used as an antimicrobial agent), and TDI.

Type II and type III hypersensitivity reactions are less common. Type II is characterized by cytolysis through IgG and/or IgM. The targets are usually erythrocytes, leukocytes, platelets, and their progenitors. The result of the cytolysis is hemolytic anemia, leukopenia, or thrombocytopenia. The offending agents include gold salts, chlorpromazine, phenytoin, sulfonamides, and TDI. Type III, also known as Arthus reactions, are mediated mainly by IgG. The antigen–antibody complexes, after combining with complement, are deposited in the vascular endothelium. Depending on the site, the damaged blood vessels may cause lupus erythematosus (e.g., procainamide) and glomerular nephritis (e.g., gold) (Dean and Murray, 1993).

Autoimmunity With autoimmune diseases, the immune system produces autoantibodies to endogenous antigens, thus damaging normal tissues. Hemolytic anemia is an example of such disorders with phagocytosis of antibody-sensitized erythrocytes leading to hemolysis and anemia. Certain chemicals and metals have been reported to induce such diseases. For example, the pesticide dieldrin has been shown to cause hemolytic anemia. Exposure to gold and mercury has been associated with a type of glomerular nephritis that is considered an autoimmune disease (Dean et al., 1982).

In addition, a number of drugs are known to be toxic through their effects on the cellular or humoral immunity, inducing either *hypersensitivity reactions* or *autoimmune diseases.* Clinically these conditions manifest as anaphylaxis, asthma, dermatitis, urticaria, hepatitis, nephritis, hemolytic anemia, neutropenia, thrombocytopenia, etc. (see also chaps. 11–14). A compilation of such drugs (Pohl et al., 1988) is reproduced as Appendix 10-1.

The mode of action of these drugs appears to be mediated through covalent binding of the drug or its metabolite to tissue macromolecules. The target specificity may be related to differences in tissue distribution of the conjugates. In general, the incidence of these side effects is low. The low incidence might be due to complex genetic makeup, which determines the levels of activating and detoxicating enzymes (Pohl et al., 1988; Park and Kiteringham, 1990).

TESTING PROCEDURES

As noted earlier, the immune system is composed of a variety of cellular and humoral components and has numerous activities. An immunotoxicant can affect any one or more of these components and activities. It is therefore necessary to have an array of tests for use. As a result, many tests have been developed. While more investigation is required to define the optimum conditions and procedures and to compare their relative significance in terms of human health, the following tests appear to be in common use.

Immunocompetence Tests in Intact Animals

These tests are designed to study the effects of chemicals on host resistance/susceptibility to bacterial, viral, and parasitic diseases as well as to bacterial endotoxins and tumor cells. In general, mice are used because of the large number of animals required.

The test chemical is given to the animals by an appropriate route, preferably mimicking the human exposure. Usually three dose groups plus a control group are included in the test. The duration of the dosing is generally 14 or 90 d. After this pretreatment, the animals are given a suitable quantity of the challenging agent. The quantity of the agent is selected on the basis that 10–20% of the mortality or morbidity is induced in the control animals. Increased mortality or morbidity indicates decreased host resistance. A list of various infectious agents has been compiled by Bradley and Morahan (1982).

Cell-Mediated Immunity

This can be studied in intact animals or with cells in vitro. In the intact animals, usually mice, the commonly used procedure is to determine the *delayed hypersensitivity* response to a specific antigen. The antigen, such as sheep erythrocytes or keyhole limpet hemocyanin, is injected into a footpad or an ear of the animal. Four days later, a challenging dose of the antigen is given at the sensitized site. The extent of the swelling or the amount of localized radioactivity from a radiolabeled substance, such as ^{125}I-labeled human serum albumin or tritiated thymidine, is measured (Luster et al., 1982; Munson et al., 1982; Sanders et al., 1982).

In vitro tests are conducted on cells collected from animals pretreated with the test chemical. Such tests include lymphocyte proliferation and lymphocyte subpopulation. The *lymphocyte proliferation* assay is done by culturing, in the presence of mitogens, lymphocytes collected from the spleen of pretreated animals. Mitogens such as phytohemagglutinin and concanavalin A are capable of inducing proliferation of normal T lymphocytes, whereas lipopolysaccharides, such as the cell membrane of gram-negative bacteria, affect B lymphocytes. Immunosuppressive agents inhibit lymphocyte proliferation. The extent of proliferation can be determined by the incorporation of tritiated thymidine into DNA (Luster et al., 1982).

Lymphocytes, as noted earlier, consist of T cells, B cells, and null cells, and the T-cell population is composed of T-memory, T-helper, T-suppressor, and T-killer cells. Techniques for their enumeration include the use of immunofluorescence, rosette formation, histochemistry, cell electrophoresis, cytolysis, and fluorescence-activated cell sorting (Norbury, 1982).

Humoral Immunity

A commonly used procedure, the plaque assay, involves quantitative determination of plaque-forming cells (PFC) of the IgM class: Four days after the mouse has been sensitized to an antigen (e.g., sheep erythrocytes), the spleen is removed and a cell suspension is made. A quantity of the antigen, along with a suitable complement, is added to the suspension. The mixture is then spread on a slide and the number of plaques is counted. This represents the primary humoral immune response. To determine the secondary immune response, the mouse is given on d 10 a second dose of the antigen. On d 15 the spleen is removed and the procedure is repeated with an additional step of incubation with rabbit anti-mouse IgG to develop the IgG-producing plaques. Reduced plaques indicate immunosuppression (Spyker-Cranmer et al., 1982). Instead of sheep erythrocytes, which are T-dependent antigens, lipopolysaccharides, which are T-independent antigens, may be used.

The levels of various immunoglobulins (IgG, IgM, IgA) in the serum may be directly measured. The techniques for their measurement have been reviewed by Davis and Ho (1976). The number of B cells in the spleen also provides information on the status of humoral immunity (Dean et al., 1982). The procedures and advantages of the enzyme-linked immunosorbent assay (ELISA) in testing chemicals for immunotoxicity have been elaborated by Vos et al. (1982).

Macrophage and Bone Marrow

The functions of macrophages can be tested in a number of ways: (1) the number of resident peritoneal cells, (2) phagocytosis, (3) lysosomal enzymes, (4) cytostasis of tumor target cells, and (5) reticuloendothelial system uptake of ^{132}I-triolein. Parameters of bone marrow activity include (1) cellularity, (2) colony-forming units of pluripotent cells, (3) colony-forming units of granulocyte/macrophage progenitors, and (4) iron incorporation in the bone marrow and spleen (Dean et al., 1982).

Others

A variety of pathotoxicologic data are also useful indicators of immune function: (1) hematology profile—erythrocyte count, leukocyte count, differential cell count; (2) serum proteins—albumin, globulin, albumin/globulin ratio; (3) weights—body, spleen, thymus, and adrenals; and (4) histology—thymus, adrenal, lung, kidney, heart, spleen, and cellularity of spleen and bone marrow. For example, thymic atrophy appears to be a very sensitive indicator of immunotoxicity. A paucity of lymphoid follicles and germinal centers in the spleen is indicative of B-cell deficiency, whereas T-cell deficiency is characterized by lymphoid hypoplasia in the paracortical areas (Dean et al., 1982).

Because of the multiplicity of the tests, "tier approaches" have been proposed. The National Toxicology Program's tier testing is summarized

Table 10-3   NTP Tier Testing for Chemical-Induced Immunotoxicity in Mice

Parameter	Testing
	Tier 1
Hematology	White blood cell count and differential count
Weights	Body, spleen, thymus, kidney, liver
Histology	Spleen, thymus, lymph node cellurity
Humoral immunity	PFC to T-cell-dependent and -independent antigens
Cell-mediated immunity	Lymphocyte transformation with concanavalin A
Nonspecific immunity	Natural killer cell function
	Tier 2
T and B cells	Enumeration of these cells in spleen
Humoral immunity	Quantitation of IgG response to sheep red blood cells (RBCs)
Cellular immunity	T-cell cytolysis of tumors
Nonspecific immunity	Macrophage function
Host resistance	Syngeneic tumors: PYB6 sarcoma, B16 F10 melanoma
	Bacterial models: *Listeria*, streptococci
	Virus: influenza
	Parasite: *Plasmodium yoelii*

Source: Adapted from Luster et al. (1988).

in Table 10-3. Toxicants testing positive in Tier 1 tests can be further evaluated with tests selected from Tier 2.

EVALUATION

A number of immunotoxicants have been investigated with the tests listed in Table 10-3. Analysis of the results demonstrated the following: (1) No single test per se was adequate in predicting impaired host resistance. (2) On the other hand, whenever the host resistance was impaired, one or more immune function tests were affected. (3) Most immune tests yielded useful results; total white blood cell count and PFC response to lipopolysaccharide, however, were relatively poor indicators of host resistance. (4) Host resistance depended not only on the extent of immunosuppression but also on the quantity of infectious agents administered (Luster et al., 1993).

REFERENCES

Bradley, S. G., and Morahan, P. S. 1982. Approaches to assessing host resistance. *Environ. Health Perspect.* 43:65–71.

Davis, N. C., and Ho, M. 1976. Quantitation of immunoglobulins. In *Manual of clinical immunology*, eds. N. R. Rose and H. Friedman. Washington, DC: American Society of Microbiology.

Dean, J. H., and Murray, M. J. 1993. Toxic responses of the immune system. In *Casarett and Doull's toxicology*, eds. M. O. Amdur, J. Doull, and C. D. Klaassen, pp. 282–333. New York: Macmillan.

Dean, J. H., Luster, M. I., Boorman, G. A., and Lauer, L. D. 1982. Procedure available to examine the immunotoxicity of chemicals and drugs. *Pharmacol. Rev.* 34:137–148.

Luster, M. I., Dean, J. H., and Boorman, G. A. 1982. Cell-mediated immunity and its application in toxicology. *Environ. Health Perspect.* 43:31–36.

Luster, M. I., Munson, A. E., Thomas, P. T., Hosapple, M. P., Fenters, J. D., et al. 1988. Development of a Testing Battery to Assess Chemical-Induced Immunotoxicity: National Toxicology Program's Guidelines for Immunotoxicity Evaluation in Mice. *Fundam. Appl. Toxicol.* 10:2–19.

Luster, M. I., Ackermann, M. F., Germolec, D. R., and Rosenthal, G. J. 1989. Perturbations of the immune system by xenobiotics. *Environ. Health Perspect.* 81:157–162.

Luster, M. I., Portier, C., Pait, D. G., Rosenthal, G. J., et al. 1993. Risk assessment in immunotoxicology. II. Relationship between immune and host resistance tests. *Fundam. Appl. Toxicol.* 21:71–82.

Munson, A. E., Sanders, V. M., Douglas, K. A., Sain, L. E., Kauffmann, B. M., and White K. L. 1982. In vivo assessment of immunotoxicity. *Environ. Health Perspect.* 43:41–52.

Norbury, K. C. 1982. Immunotoxicology in the pharmaceutical industry. *Environ. Health Perspect.* 43:53–59.

Park, B. K., and Kiteringham, N. 1990. Drug-protein conjugation and its immunological consequences. *Drug Metab. Rev.* 22:87–144.

Pohl, L. R., Satoh, H., Christ, D. D., and Kenna, J. G. 1988. The immunologic and metabolic basis of drug hypersensitivities. *Annu. Rev. Pharmacol.* 28:367–387.

Sanders, V. M., et al. 1982. Humoral and cell-mediated immune status in mice exposed to trichloroethylene in the drinking water. *Toxicol. Appl. Pharmacol.* 62:358–368.

Sharma, R. P., and Reddy, R. V. 1987. Toxic effects of chemicals on the immune system. In *Handbook of toxicology*, eds. T. J. Haley and W. O. Berndt, pp. 555–591. Washington, DC: Hemisphere.

Spyker-Cranmer, J. M., Barnett, J. B., Avery, D. L., and Cranmer, M. F. 1982. Immunoteratology of chlordane: Cell-mediated and humoral immune responses in adult mice exposed in utero. *Toxicol. Appl. Pharmacol.* 62:402–408.

Vos, J. G., Krajnac, E. I., and Beekhof, P. 1982. Use of the enzyme-linked immunosorbent assay (ELISA) in immunotoxicity testing. *Environ. Health Perspect.* 43:115–121.

ADDITIONAL READING

Barrell, R., Flaherty, D. K, and Sauers, L. J. 1992. *Toxicology of the immune system.* New York: Van Nostrand Reinhold.

Vanderlaan, M., Stanker, L. H., Watkins, B. D., and Roberts, D. W. 1991. *Immunoassays for trace chemical analysis.* Washington, DC: American Chemical Society.

Appendix 10-1   Drug Toxicities in Which Specific Humoral and Cellular Immunity Have Been Implicated

		Immunity	
Drug	Toxicity[a]	Humoral	Cellular
Acetaminophen	T	+	
Salicylates	A, As, U	+	
Muscle relaxants: alcuronium, gallamine, decamethonium, succinylcholine, tubocurarine	A	+	
Thiopentone	A	+	
Floxacillin	H		+
Erythromycin	H		+
Diphenylhydantoin	H, SS	+	
Chlorpropamide	HA	+	
Allopurinol	D, U		+
Practolol	O	+	
Amoxicillin	HA	+	
Penicillins	As, SS, D, U, A	+	+
Ethinylestradiol	Th	+	
Alprenolol	D		+
Mianserin	T, N	+	
Cyclophosphamide	A, U	+	
Cloxacillin	H	+	
Tolbutamide	HA	+	
Captopril	U, D, Ne	+	+
Cephamandole	T	+	
Quinine, quinidine	T	+	
Nomifensine	HA	+	
Methyldopa	HA, N, H	+	
Cianidanol	HA	+	
Amodiaquin	N	+	
Probenecid	HA	+	
Penicillamine	N	+	
Chlorhexidine	A	+	
Tienilic acid	H	+	
Procainamide	DLE	+	
Hydralazine	DLE	+	
Halothane	H	+	+

Source: Pohl et al. (1988). Reproduced with permission from the *Annual Review of Pharmacology and Toxicology*, vol. 28, copyright 1988 by Annual Reviews, Inc.

[a]A, anaphylaxis; As, asthma; D, dermatitis; H, hepatitis; HA, hemolytic anemia; Ne, nephritis; N, neutropenia; O, oculomucocutaneous syndrome; SS, serum sickness; T, thrombocytopenia; Th, thrombosis; U, urticaria; DLE, drug-induced lupus erythematosus.

Respiratory System: Inhalation Toxicology

CHAPTER 11 CONTENTS

INTRODUCTION

With industrialization, the respiratory system of humans is increasingly exposed to airborne toxicants. Their health effects and a number of testing procedures are briefly described in this chapter.

Structure

The respiratory tract is a complex system, both in structure and in function. It consists of the nasopharynx, the tracheal and bronchial tract, and the pulmonary acini, which are composed of respiratory bronchioles, alveolar ducts, and alveoli. The nasopharynx serves to remove large particles from the inhaled air, add moisture, and moderate the temperature. The tracheal and bronchial tract serves as the conducting airway to the alveoli.

Functions

The pulmonary acini are the sites where oxygen and carbon dioxide are exchanged between the blood and the air and are the main sites of absorption of toxicants that exist in the form of gases and vapors. The alveoli are lined with epithelial cells, especially those of type I. These cells have a very thin cytoplasm (0.1–0.2 m), but each covers a relatively large surface (2290 μm^2). The cuboidal (63 μm^2) type II cells can undergo mitosis and, in time, mature to type I cells. In addition, there are endothelial cells, macrophages, and fibroblasts.

Apart from its vital function in the exchange of oxygen and carbon dioxide, the respiratory system also regulates the blood concentrations of angiotensin, biogenic amines, and prostaglandins. Furthermore, it can excrete toxicants that have been absorbed from the lungs or via other routes.

Defense Mechanisms

The trachea and bronchi are lined with ciliated epithelium and covered with a thin layer of mucus secreted by certain cells in the epithelial lining. This lining, with the cilia and mucus, can move particles deposited on the surface up to the mouth. The particle-containing mucus can then be eliminated from the respiratory tract by spitting or swallowing.

The respiratory tract has various cytochrome P-450 enzyme systems, which may detoxify certain toxicants. However, many toxicants may be activated by these enzyme systems. They are concentrated in the Clara cells and, to a lesser extent, in the type II cells (Dormons and Van Bree,

1995). The Clara cells are located at the boundary where alveolar ducts branch from bronchioles.

Apart from clearance and detoxication, the respiratory tract also possesses mechanisms to phagocytize and contain toxicants, notably solid particles. The main effector is the macrophage. Similar to the enzyme systems, the macrophage may also aggravate the toxic effects (Brain, 1992).

TOXICANTS AND THEIR EFFECTS

Many toxicants are known to adversely affect the respiratory system in humans and animals. Those that pose serious occupational hazards are listed in Appendix 11-1.

Inhalable toxicants exist in the form of gases, vapors, liquid droplets, and solid particulate matters. Gases and vapors are readily absorbed. The droplets and particulate matters may also be absorbed. However, they vary in size, and their sizes have marked effect on the extent of absorption. In general, large particles (10 μm) do not enter the respiratory tract. Very small particles (0.01 μm) are likely to be exhaled. The optimal size of particle for retention is between 1 and 3 μm; see also chap. 2.

A toxicant may exert systemic effects after its absorption from the respiratory tract and distribution to other tissues, or it may induce local effects on the respiratory tract, or both. A toxicant may also affect the respiratory tract after exposure from other routes.

Systemic Effects

Many chemicals can be absorbed from the inspired air. After absorption, they are carried by the circulating blood to various parts of the body and exert their effects, such as general anesthesia.

Toxic gases can be absorbed from various parts of the respiratory tract including the nasopharynx. The main site of absorption, however, is the alveoli, and the principal mechanism of absorption is simple diffusion. In addition, liquid aerosols and solid particulate matter can also be absorbed via different mechanisms. Further details regarding the uptake of toxicants are given in chap. 2.

Effects on Lungs

Various pulmonary effects have been observed. These are briefly described under five categories. Additional details and references have been provided by Gordon and Amdur (1993).

Local Irritation Ammonia and chlorine are classic examples of irritant gases. They cause bronchial constriction and edema, which result in dyspnea, but chronic effects are rare. Arsenicals induce irritation on acute exposure; after prolonged exposure they can cause formation of lung cancer.

Cellular Damage and Edema   Toxic gases, such as ozone and oxides of nitrogen, can cause cellular damage, perhaps through peroxidation of cellular membranes. Edema ensues as a result of the increased permeability through the damaged membrane. The edematous fluid, however, accumulates in the airway instead of in the interstitial space, as is the case with other tissues. Such effects are also observed after inhalation of toxicants that exist in small particles, such as nickel carbonyl and certain beryllium and boron compounds.

Cellular damage usually affects type I cells in the alveoli. Death of these cells leads to proliferation of type II cells, which then flatten and become type I cells. However, more extensive damage will result in the exudation of fibrin-rich protein, neutrophils, and debris into the alveoli. These eventually become fibrous tissue.

Certain organic solvents, such as perchloroethylene and xylene, are rapidly absorbed after inhalation and distributed to various parts of the body including the liver, which is the major site of biotransformation. Part of the solvent reenters the lung through circulation and may form reactive metabolites, leading to covalent binding with macromolecules there. This process in turn produces cellular damage and edema.

Ipomeanol is a toxin produced by the mold *Fusarium solani*, grown on sweet potatoes. This toxin is interesting in that it causes necrosis of one type of cell only, namely, the Clara cells. These cells bioactivate the toxin to a reactive metabolite that binds to the macromolecules and causes cellular necrosis. This is followed by edema, congestion, and hemorrhage in the lungs. Death may ensue (Timbrell, 1991).

Fibrosis (Pneumoconiosis)   Pulmonary fibrosis is a serious, debilitating disease. *Silicosis*, with a history that goes back for thousands of years, is caused by crystalline forms of silica (silicon dioxide). Of the crystalline forms, quartz is the most stable. On heating, such as in volcanic eruption and mining, quartz may become tridymite or cristobalite. Both of these forms are more fibrogenic than quartz. The toxic effect stems from the rupture of the lysosomal membrane in a macrophage. The released lysosomal enzymes digest the macrophage, and this process, in turn, releases the silica from the lysed macrophage. Thus the process is repeated. It has been suggested that the damaged macrophage releases factors that stimulate the fibroblasts and the formation of collagen (Brain, 1980). Other cells, such as fibroblasts and epithelial cells, in response to macrophage inflammatory proteins, may also play a role in the fibrotic changes (Driscoll et al., 1993). Kuhn et al. (1995) suggest that cytokine is involved in the fibrosis and its increase precedes deterioration of pulmonary function, and hence may serve as a biomarker for initiating intervention in exposed workers.

Another major cause of pulmonary fibrosis is *asbestos*. Asbestos refers to a large number of fibrous hydrated silicates of magnesium, calcium, and others. In addition, some of these mineral fibers, such as the blue asbestos (crocidolites), can cause bronchogenic carcinoma and mesothelioma. The white variety (chrysotile) appears to have no effect on the incidence of mesothelioma. The potency of asbestos seems related to the chemical and physical properties. Fibers of 5 μm in length and 0.3 μm in diameter appear to be most potent. Various types of man-made refractory ceramic fibers have been used in place of asbestos. In the rat, they also induce fibrosis and carcinoma, but appear to be less carcinogenic than asbestos (Mast et al., 1995).

Other fibrogenic substances include coal dust, kaolin, talc, aluminum, beryllium, and carbides of tungsten, titanium, and tantalum (see Appendix 11-1).

Emphysema is also a debilitating disease. It may be induced by cigarette smoking or exposure to aluminum, cadmium oxide, or oxides of nitrogen, ozone, and others. It has been suggested that the elastic fibers surrounding and supporting the alveoli and bronchi may be damaged by the elastase released from polymorphonuclear granulocytes under certain conditions (Spitznagel et al., 1980).

Allergic Response   This type of response is usually induced by pollens, spores of molds, bacterial contaminants, cotton dust, and so forth. Detergents containing enzymes derived from *Bacillus subtilis* have been reported to cause asthma among workers. A common chemical used in plastic industry, toluene diisocyanate (TDI), as other isocyanates, also produces hypersensitivity reaction. It is probable that this reactive chemical binds with proteins in the blood or lungs to form antigen, which stimulates antibody formation. The major response is bronchoconstriction triggered by the reaction between the antigens and circulating or fixed antibodies (Karol and Jin, 1991). Long-term exposure may result in other pulmonary effects such as chronic bronchitis and fibrosis.

Lung Cancer   Cigarette smoke contains a number of carcinogens, cocarcinogens, and irritants. These substances initiate and promote carcinogenesis. Furthermore, many other substances may induce *oxidative stress,* and thereby adversely affect health (Appendix 11-2). Some details of this topic have been outlined by Halliwell and Cross (1994). It is well established that cigarette smoking is the leading cause of lung cancer in many countries and that it greatly increases the incidence of lung cancers among asbestos workers (chap. 5). Other causes of lung cancer include arsenic, chromates, nickel, uranium, and coke oven emissions.

Asbestos has been well known for its carcinogenicity in the respiratory tract in humans and animals. Man-made refractory ceramic fibers appear to be carcinogenic also, but only at maximum tolerated doses. Much investigation is in progress to determine their health hazards, if any, in humans. One important approach is to assess their persistence, which is a determinant of their toxicity (Bignon et al., 1994).

Effects on Upper Respiratory Tract

Large airborne particles in the inhaled air are mainly deposited in the nasal passages. They may cause hyperemia, squamous- or transitional-cell metaplasia, hyperplasia, ulceration, and, in certain cases, carcinoma. For example, nickel subsulfide, nickel oxide, and nickel usually exist in large particles during their production and mining; therefore, their effects are mainly on the nasal passage (NAS, 1975). The larynx is also a site of chemical carcinogenesis, for example, with asbestos and chromium. Inhalation of gases and vapors such as sulfur dioxide and toluene may cause irritation of trachea and bronchi. Other toxic effects include deciliation, goblet-cell hyperplasia, and squamous metaplasia.

Effects After Other Routes of Exposure

Paraquat, a herbicide, causes lung damages not only after exposure by inhalation but also after ingestion (Clark et al., 1966). Its storage in the lungs and its inherent toxicity are apparently the reasons for its pulmonary effects after noninhalation routes. In contrast, a closely related herbicide, diquat, although also toxic to cultured lung cells, is not toxic to the lungs either after inhalation or after ingestion. It is interesting that diquat is not retained by the lungs (see also chap. 19).

A number of drugs are known to induce pulmonary fibrosis in humans. These include bleomycin, busulfan, cyclophosphamide, gold salts, melphalan, methotrexate, and mitomycin. In these cases, there is an increase in interstitial collagen and in the number of type II cells. Methotrexate and streptomycin have been reported to cause pulmonary eosinophilia. Phenylbutazone and oxyphenylbutazone may cause pulmonary edema.

In addition, a number of amphiphilic drugs, such as chloroquine and triparanol, are known to interact with the phospholipids in certain cells to form myeloid bodies and pulmonary foam cells in humans and animals. These bodies and cells lead to alteration of cell activities and later to impairment of respiratory functions (Hruban, 1984).

TESTING PROCEDURES

The local and systemic effects of toxicants resulting from exposure via the respiratory tract are usually studied by mixing or suspending the toxicants in the air to be inhaled by the test subject. In exceptional cases the material on test is deposited, in liquid or solid form, in the respiratory tract.

Exposure Facilities

The systemic and local effects of toxicants administered to animals through the respiratory tract generally require elaborate facilities. The test animal may be placed in whole-body exposure chambers or exposed through the head or the nose only. Other systems have been designed to study the effects of toxicants through lung-only or partial lung exposure. The advantages and disadvantages of these approaches have been discussed by Phalen (1976).

Whole-Body System   Such a system typically consists of a chamber wherein the test animal is kept. The chamber is equipped with windows for observation of the test animal, and is connected to an air inlet and an air outlet. The toxicant, in the form of vapor or aerosol, is mixed with clean air and introduced into the chamber through the inlet. The outlet is usually connected to a filtering system to remove the toxicant from the exhaust before being released to the atmosphere. Typical systems have been described by Drew and Laskin (1973) and Phalen (1976). More recently, the design, operation, and characterization of a large, chronic inhalation exposure facility, with four 12.6-m^3 exposure chambers, have been described (Schreck et al., 1981). Equipment for generating and controlling atmospheres in inhalation chambers has been described and compared by Rampy (1981) and Davies et al. (1987).

Head- and Nose-Exposure Systems   These systems have the advantages of (1) avoiding absorption of the toxicant deposited on the fur, either directly through the skin or indirectly through the gastrointestinal tract when the animal grooms itself and (2) requiring a more limited quantity of the test material. However, the animals must be restrained. Moreover, fitting the head or nostrils of the animals to the apparatus requires some skill and time. A number of such systems have been developed and the references to their descriptions are also given in a World Health Organization (WHO) document (1978). Many of these systems have been used to study the effects of cigarette smoke in various species of animals, including donkeys. A more recent article describes a method for chronic nose-only exposure of laboratory animals to inhaled aerosols of man-made fibers (Smith et al., 1981).

Choice of Animals

The commonly used experimental animals are rats, dogs, and monkeys. Others include mice, hamsters, guinea pigs, rabbits, miniature pigs, and donkeys. The choice should be based on a number of criteria. It may be noted that monkeys are distinctly different from humans in terms of respiratory tract, in spite of their phylogenetic proximity. Horses, and presumably donkeys also, are very similar to humans in this respect. Other factors, which may be more important, are the similarity of their biochemical and physiologic responses to those of humans and an abundance of experimental results, which permits comparison between the toxicities of various chemicals.

It has been well documented in epidemiologic studies that people with preexisting cardiopulmonary diseases are at special risk during air pollution episodes (see chap. 21). To simulate this condition, papain-induced emphysematous animals have been used (Gross et al., 1965).

Doses

Definition of Dose   In general, the dose is the amount of a substance that is administered to an organism. The amount is readily ascertained when the substance is given by a route such as oral, subcutaneous, intravenous, or intraperitoneal. This definition is not applicable to exposure by inhalation, because the amount that is retained in the animal depends on the concentration of the toxicant in the inhaled air as well as the duration of the exposure. In other words, the dose might be expressed as the product of the concentration (C) and the time (t). It has been recognized that for a fixed $C \times t$ product the response will be the same. However, this rule is not valid when either C or t is an extreme value. For example, if C is too small, generally no response will be elicited no matter how long the animal is exposed to it.

In most inhalation studies the retained doses are not estimated. Instead, the duration of exposure is kept constant, but the test animals are exposed to different concentrations of a toxicant. For example, in acute median lethality studies, the animals are exposed, as a rule, for 4 h. In longer term studies either a *continuous* (23 h/d) or an *intermittent* (8 h/d, 5 d/wk) exposure scheme is adopted, with the former being designed to simulate the exposure to environmental pollutants and the latter, industrial situations.

Selection of Doses In acute lethality studies, one concentration should be aimed at causing the death of about 50% of the animals. At least two other concentrations are selected, one killing more than 50% but less than 90%, and the other killing 10–50% of the animals.

In longer term studies, at least three concentrations should be selected. The highest concentration is intended to cause some toxic effects but no deaths, and the lowest concentrations should have no observable effects.

Maintenance of Preselected Concentrations The nominal concentration is determined by dividing the amount of the agent used in the system that generates the airborne toxicant by the air flow through the exposure chamber. The actual concentration, which is often not the same as the nominal concentration, is determined by actual analysis of samples of the chamber air taken near the breathing zone of the animals. Since the actual concentrations usually vary through an exposure period, it is necessary to analyze a number of samples taken at appropriate time intervals. The exposure facility should be so designed as to minimize the range of variations. A number of references on exposure systems, generating systems, and sampling methods are provided by WHO (1978).

Duration of Exposure

For acute LC_{50} determinations (LC_{50} is the concentration that will cause the death of 50% of the animals at a specified duration of exposure), the duration of exposure is usually between 1 and 4 h. In short-term studies the duration is usually 30 or 90 d, and in long-term studies it is 1 yr or more. The repeated exposures are either on a continuous or intermittent basis, as discussed earlier.

Observations and Examinations

General These include body weight and food consumption, general observations, laboratory tests, and postmortem examinations. Some details on these are given in chap. 6.

Respiratory Functions Tests on these functions are often carried out because of their greater sensitivity than morphologic changes and because of their ability to detect reversible effects. As a result, these tests are often used in studies in humans. Similar tests in animals would therefore allow a more valid comparison between humans and the experimental animals with respect to their relative susceptibility to the toxic effects of the substance being tested.

Respiratory frequency is a sensitive indicator of local irritation and is often concentration related. Certain gases, such as ozone and nitrogen dioxide, increase the frequency, whereas others, such as sulfur dioxide and formaldehyde, decrease it.

Mechanics of respiration can be measured in terms of pulmonary flow resistance and pulmonary compliance. An increase in pulmonary flow resistance can result from bronchoconstriction, swelling of the respiratory mucosa, or an increase in mucous secretion. Pulmonary compliance is decreased by fibrosis, and it is increased in emphysema because of loss of supportive connective tissue. References to their measurements are given in a WHO document (1978).

Respiratory efficiency can be estimated by measuring oxygen and carbon dioxide in the blood or by measuring the rate at which inhaled carbon monoxide is taken into the blood (O'Neil and Raub, 1984).

Morphologic and Biochemical Changes   As described earlier, various morphologic changes can result from inhalation exposure to toxicants. These include local irritation, cellular damage, edema, fibrosis, and neoplasms. In addition, toxicants can cause a number of other types of morphologic changes such as inflammation, hyperplasia, and emphysema, as shown in Appendix 11-1.

Some examinations are especially useful. For example, lung-weight increases are indicators of vascular congestion, edema, or increase in connective tissue. Bronchoalveolar lavage (BAL) can provide information on the cell number, type, and morphology as well as on noncellular components, especially the enzyme content. Furthermore, the collagen content can be estimated by determining hydroxyproline or prolylhydroxylase in lung tissues (see Tyler et al., 1985). See also the U.S. Environmental Protection Agency guide on inhalation toxicity (1994).

EVALUATION

Analyses of the data relating to the effects and the dose are essentially the same as those following other routes of administration, with the exception that the dose is generally handled differently.

As noted earlier, while the retained dose after exposure by inhalation can be estimated, the common practice is to use the concentration instead. Thus, the results of acute medial lethality studies are expressed as LC_{50}. The LC_{50} values of various compounds can be compared, provided the same duration of exposure was used in the inhalation studies.

The determination of the dose-effect and the dose-response relationships can also be done in the conventional manner, using concentrations instead of doses. The procedure employed in the estimation of the no-observed-adverse-effect level, as described in chap. 6, can also be adopted in inhalation studies.

Although the concentration can be readily expressed with gases and vapors, the *effective* concentration of aerosols is influenced by the particle size, which can greatly influence the deposition, penetration, and absorption of the material. Thus, when reporting inhalation studies, it is necessary to provide information on the median particle size and their geometric standard deviations (chap. 2).

IN VITRO TESTS

In order to conduct more definitive studies on the effects of toxicants on the respiratory system, various in vitro systems have been developed.

Isolated Perfused Lung

Lungs isolated from rabbits or rats are perfused with heparinized blood at a constant pressure and ventilated with positive pressure through the trachea or negative pressure from outside of the lung. A constant blood flow can be maintained over a period of several hours. The system is especially useful in determining nonrespiratory functions of the lung. For example, the levels of the endogenous hormones and vasoactive amines can be readily determined in the exudate. Furthermore, the pulmonary metabolism of a toxicant can be ascertained by adding it to the perfusate and analyzing the exudate for the toxicant and its metabolite. Some details and references are provided by Anderson and Eling (1976) and Roth (1980).

Tracheal Explants and Lung Organ Culture

The effects of toxic gases and vapors can be assessed on the trachea removed from animals, such as rats, that have been exposed to toxicants. When incubated in a tissue culture medium the trachea will continue to secrete mucous glycoproteins. The rate of secretion can be affected by exposure to toxicants. For example, tracheal explants taken from rats exposed to ozone at 0.8 ppm showed an increased rate of secretion, but those from rats exposed to 0.5 ppm ozone or 1.1 mg/m^3 sulfuric acid did not. Exposure to the combination, however, induced significantly greater rates of secretion (Last and Kaizer, 1980).

Isolated Cells

Various types of cells from the respiratory system have been isolated and cultured. These include the epithelial cells of the trachea and the lung tissue as well as the endothelial cells. Isolated cultured cells show promise of becoming useful tools in toxicology of the respiratory system. Reiser and Last (1979), for example, pointed out the importance of pulmonary alveolar macrophages and fibroblasts in the development of fibrosis in chronic silicosis. They also noted the likelihood of involvement of other cell types, the precise role of which awaits further studies with isolated cells.

REFERENCES

Anderson, M. W., and Eling, T. E. 1976. Studies on the uptake, metabolism, and release of endogenous and exogenous chemicals by the use of the isolated perfused lung. *Environ. Health Perspect.* 16:77–81.

Bignon, J., Saracci, R., and Touray, J. C. 1994. Biopersistence of respirable synthetic fibers and minerals. *Environ. Health Perspect.* 102(suppl. 5).

Brain, J. D. 1980. Macrophage damage in relation to the pathogenesis of lung diseases. *Environ. Health Perspect.* 35:21–28.

Brain, J. D. 1992. Mechanisms, measurement and significance of lung macrophage function. *Environ. Health Perspect.* 97:5–10.

Clark, D. G., McElligott, T. F., and Hurst, E. W. 1966. The toxicity of paraquat. *Br. J. Ind. Med.* 23:126–132.

Davies, D. W., Walsh, L. C. III, Hiteshaw, M. E., Mnache, M. G., Miller, F. J., and Grose, E. C. 1987. Evaluating the toxicity of urban pattern of oxidant gases. I. An automated chronic gaseous animal inhalation exposure facility. *J. Toxicol. Environ. Health* 21:89–97.

Dormans, J. A. M. A., and Van Bree, L. 1995. Function and response of type II cells to inhaled toxicants. *Inhal. Toxicol.* 7:319–342.

Drew, R. T., and Lasken, S. 1973. Environmental inhalation chambers. In *Methods of animal experimentation*, ed. W. I. Gray, pp. 1–42. New York: Academic Press.

Driscoll, K. E., Hassenbein, D. G., Carter, J., et al. 1993. Macrophage inflammatory proteins 1 and 2: Expression by rat alveolar macrophages, fibroblasts, and epithelial cells and in rat lung after minimal dust exposure. *Am. J. Respir. Cell Mol. Biol.* 8:311–318.

Gordon, T., and Amdur, M. O. 1993. Responses of the respiratory system to toxic agents. In *Casarett and Doull's toxicology: The basic science of poisons*, 4th ed., eds. M. O. Amdur, J. Doull, and C. D. Klaassen, pp. 383–406. New York: McGraw-Hill.

Gross, P., Pfitzer, E. A., Tolker, E., Babyak, M. A., and Kaschak, M. 1965. Experimental emphysema: Its production with papain in normal and silicotic rats. *Arch. Environ. Health* 11:50–58.

Halliwell, B., and Cross, C. E. 1994. Oxygen-derived species: Their relation to human disease and environmental stress. *Environ. Health Perspect.* 102(suppl. 10):5–12.

Hruban, Z. 1984. Pulmonary and generalized lysosomal storage induced by amphiphilic drugs. *Environ. Health Perspect.* 55:53–76.

Karol, M. H., and Jin, R. 1991. Mechanism of immunotoxicity to isocyanates. *Chem. Res. Toxicol.* 4:503–509.

Kuhn, D. C., Stauffer, J. L., Gaydos, L. J., and Demers, L. M. 1995. Inflammatory and fibrotic mediator release by alveoli macrophages from coal miners. *J. Toxicol. Environ. Health* 45:9–21.

Last, J. A., and Kaizer, T. 1980. Mucus glycoprotein secretion by tracheal explants: Effect of pollutants. *Environ. Health Perspect.* 35:131–137.

Mast, R. W., McConnell, E. E., Anderson, R., et al. 1995. Studies on the chronic toxicity (inhalation) of four types of refractory ceramic fiber in male Fischer 344 rats. *Inhal. Toxicol.* 7:425–467.

Menzel, D. B., and Amdur, M. O. 1986. Toxic responses of the respiratory system. In *Casarett and Doull's toxicology: The basic science of poisons*, 3rd ed., eds. C. D. Klaassen, M. O. Amdur, and J. Doull. New York: Macmillan.

National Academy of Sciences. 1975. *Nickel*. Washington, DC: NAS.

O'Neil, J. J., and Raub, J. A. 1984. Pulmonary function testing in small laboratory animals. *Environ. Health Perspect.* 56:11–22.

Phalen, R. F. 1976. Inhalation exposure of animals. *Environ. Health Perspect.* 16:17–24.

Rampy, L. W. 1981. Generating and controlling atmospheres in inhalation chambers. In *Scientific considerations in monitoring and evaluating toxicological research*, ed. E. J. Gralla, pp. 57–69. Washington, DC: Hemisphere.

Reiser, K. M., and Last, J. A. 1979. Silicosis and fibrogenesis: Fact and artifact. *Toxicology* 13:51–72.

Roth, J. A. 1980. Use of perfused lung in biochemical toxicology. *Rev. Biochem. Toxicol.* 1: 287–309.

Schreck, R. M., Chan, T. L., and Soderholm, S. C. 1981. Design operation and characterization of large volume exposure chambers. In *Proceedings of the Inhalation Toxicology and Technology Symposium*, ed. B. K. J. Leong, pp. 29–52. Ann Arbor, MI: Ann Arbor Science.

Smith, D. M., Ortiz, L. W., Anchuleta, R. F., Spalding, J. F., Tillery, M. I., Ettinger, H. J., and Thomas, R. G. 1981. A method for chronic nose-exposures of laboratory animals to inhaled fibrous aerosols. In *Proceedings of Inhalation Toxicology and Technology Symposium*, ed. B. K. J. Leong, pp. 89–105. Ann Arbor, MI: Ann Arbor Science.

Spitznagel, J. K., Moderzakowski, M. C., Pryzwansky, K. B., and MacRae, E. K. 1980. Neutral proteases of human polymorphonuclear granulocytes: Putative mediators of pulmonary damage. *Environ. Health Perspect.* 35:29–38.

Timbrell, J. A. 1991. *Principles of biochemical toxicology*. London: Taylor & Francis.

Tyler, W. S., Dungworth, D. L., Plopper, C. G., Hyde, D. M., and Tyler, N. K. 1985. Structural evaluation of the respiratory system. *Fundam. Appl. Toxicol.* 5:405–422.

U.S. Environmental Protection Agency. 1994. Health Effect Testing Guidelines. Code of Federal Regulations Title 40, Part 798.

World Health Organization. 1978. Inhalation exposure. In *Principles and methods for evaluating the toxicity of chemicals. Part I.* Environmental Health Criteria 6. Geneva: WHO.

ADDITIONAL READING

Kennedy, G. L., Jr., and Valentine, R. 1994. Inhalation toxicology. In *Principles and methods of toxicology*, ed. A. W. Hayes, pp. 805–838. New York: Raven Press.

McClellan, R. O., and Henderson, R. F. 1995. *Concepts in inhalation toxicology*. Washington, DC: Taylor & Francis.

Appendix 11-1 Site of Action and Pulmonary Disease Produced by Selected Occupationally Inhaled Toxicants

Toxicant	Common name of disease	Acute effect	Chronic effect
Aluminum dust	Aluminosis	Cough, shortness of breath	Interstitial fibrosis
Aluminum abrasives	Shaver's disease, corundum smelter's lung, bauxite lung	Alveolar edema	Fibrotic thickening of alveolar walls, interstitial fibrosis and emphysema
Ammonia		Immediate upper and lower respiratory tract irritation, edema	Chronic bronchitis
Arsenic		Bronchitis	Lung cancer, bronchitis, laryngitis
Asbestos	Asbestosis		Pulmonary fibrosis, pleural calcification, lung cancer, pleural mesothelioma
Beryllium	Berylliosis	Severe pulmonary edema, pneumonia	Pulmonary fibrosis, progressive dyspnea, interstitial granulomatosis, cor pulmonale
Cadmium oxide		Cough, pneumonia	Emphysema, cor pulmonale
Carbides of tungsten, titanium, tantalum	Hard metal disease	Hyperplasia and metaplasia of bronchial epithelium	Fibrosis, peribronchial and perivascular fibrosis
Chlorine		Cough, hemoptysis, dyspnea, tracheobronchitis, bronchopneumonia	
Chromium (VI)		Nasal irritation, bronchitis	Lung tumors and cancers
Coal dust	Pneumoconiosis		Pulmonary fibrosis
Coke oven emissions			Tracheobronchial cancers
Cotton dust	Byssinosis	Tightness in chest, wheezing, dyspnea	Reduced pulmonary function, chronic bronchitis
Hydrogen fluoride		Respiratory irritation, hemorrhagic pulmonary edema	
Iron oxides	Siderotic lung disease:	Cough	
	Silver finisher's lung		Subpleural and perivascular aggregations of macrophages
	Hematite miner's lung		Diffuse fibrosis-like pneumoconiosis
	Arc welder's lung		Bronchitis
Isocyanates		Cough, dyspnea	Asthma, reduced pulmonary function

Appendix 11-1 (Continued)

Toxicant	Common name of disease	Acute effect	Chronic effect
Kaolin	Kaolinosis		Pulmonary fibrosis
Nickel		Pulmonary edema, delayed by 2 days (NiCO)	Squamous-cell carcinoma of nasal cavity and lung
Oxides of nitrogen		Pulmonary congestion and edema	Emphysema
Ozone		Pulmonary edema	Emphysema
Phosgene		Edema	Bronchitis
Perchloroethylene		Pulmonary edema	
Silica	Silicosis, pneumoconiosis		Pulmonary fibrosis
Sulfur dioxide		Bronchoconstriction, cough, tightness in chest	
Talc	Talcosis		Pulmonary fibrosis
Tin	Stanosis		Widespread mottling of x-ray without clinical signs
Vanadium		Upper airway irritation and mucus production	Chronic bronchitis

Source: Adapted from Menzel and Amdur (1986).

Appendix 11-2   Mechanisms Underlying the Oxidative Stress Induced by Cigarette Smoke

1 Smoke contains many free radicals, especially peroxyl radicals, that might attack biological molecules and deplete antioxidants, such as vitamin C and α-tocopherol.

2 Smoke contains oxides of nitrogen, including the unpleasant nitrogen dioxide (NO_2^-).

3 The tar phase of smoke contains hydroquinones. These are lipid-soluble and can redox-cycle to form O_2^- and H_2O_2. They can enter cells and may even reach the nucleus to cause oxidative DNA damage. Some hydroquinones may release iron from the iron-storage protein ferritin in lung cells and respiratory tract lining fluids.

4 Smoking may irritate lung macrophages, activating them to make O_2^-.[a]

5 Smokers' lungs contain more neutrophils than the lungs of nonsmokers, and smoke might activate these cells to make O_2^-.[a]

6 Smokers often eat poorly and drink more alcohol than nonsmokers and have a low intake of nutrient antioxidants.

Source: Halliwell and Cross (1994).
[a]The effects of cigarette smoke on phagocytes are dose related. Low levels may stimulate them, but high levels may poison them and so depress their activity.

Toxicology of the Liver

CHAPTER 12 CONTENTS

GENERAL CONSIDERATIONS

The liver is the largest and metabolically the most complex organ in the body. It is involved in the metabolism of nutrients as well as most drugs and toxicants. The latter type of substances can usually be detoxified, but some of them can be bioactivated and become more toxic.

Hepatocytes (hepatic parenchymal cells) comprise the bulk of the organ. They are responsible for the liver's central role in metabolism. These cells lie between the blood-filled sinusoids and the biliary passages. Kupffer cells line the hepatic sinusoids and constitute an important part of the reticuloendothelial system of the body. The blood is supplied through the portal vein and hepatic artery, and it is drained through the central veins and then the hepatic vein into the vena cava. The biliary passages begin as tiny bile canaliculi formed by adjacent parenchymal cells. The canaliculi coalesce into ductules, interlobular bile ducts, and larger hepatic ducts. The main hepatic duct joins the cystic duct from the gallbladder to form the common bile duct, which drains into the duodenum (Fig. 12-1).

The toxicology of liver is complicated by the variety of liver injuries and by the different mechanisms through which the injuries are induced. The types of injury, the underlying mechanisms, and the morphologic and biochemical changes are described and discussed.

The liver is often the target organ for a number of reasons. Most toxicants enter the body via the gastrointestinal tract, and after absorption they are carried by the hepatic portal vein to the liver. The liver has a high concentration of binding sites. It also has a high concentration of xenobiotic-metabolizing enzymes (mainly cytochrome P-450), which render most toxicants less toxic and more water soluble, and thus more readily excretable. But in some cases the toxicants are activated to be capable of inducing lesions (see also chap. 3). The fact that hepatic lesions are often centrilobular has been attributed to the higher concentration of cytochrome P-450 there. In addition, the relatively lower concentration of glutathione there, compared to that in other parts of the liver, may also play a role (Smith et al., 1979).

TYPES OF LIVER INJURY

Toxicants can induce a variety of toxic effects on different organelles in the cells in liver (as shown in Table 12-1), exhibiting different types of liver injury as described next.

These liver injuries are mediated through a number of biochemical reactions, such as lipid peroxidation, covalent binding, inhibition of protein synthesis, disturbance of biliary production and/or flow, immunologic reaction, and perturbation of calcium homeostasis.

Fatty Liver (Steatosis)

A fatty liver is one that contains more than 5% lipid by weight. The presence of an excess stainable fat in such liver is demonstrable histochemically. The lesion can be acute, such as that induced by ethionine, phosphorus, or tetracycline. Ethanol and methotrexate can cause either acute or chronic lesions. Some toxicants, such as tetracycline, produce many small fat droplets in a cell, whereas others, such as ethanol, induce large fat droplets, which displace the nucleus.

Although lipid accumulation in the liver is the common end point of these toxicants, the underlying mechanisms are varied. One of the mech-

Central Vein
Parenchymal Cell
Kupffer Cell
Sinusoid

Bile Canaliculus

Hepatic Artery
Portal Vein
Bile Ductule

Figure 12-1 Schematic structure of the liver indicating the relation between parenchymal cells and vascular and ductal systems (from Klaassen and Watkins, 1984).

anisms is an increased synthesis of triglyceride and the other lipid moieties. However, the most common mechanism is impairment of the release of hepatic triglyceride to the plasma. Since hepatic triglyceride is secreted only when it is combined with lipoprotein [forming *very low density lipoprotein* (VLDL)], accumulation of hepatic lipid can occur as a result of a number of mechanisms: (1) inhibition of the synthesis of the protein moiety of lipoprotein, (2) depressed conjugation of triglyceride with lipo-

Table 12-1 Effects of Toxicants on Subcellular Organelles in Liver Cells

Organelle	Effect	Examples of toxicants
Plasma membrane	Enzyme leakage	Acetaminophen, carbon tetrachloride, phalloidin
Nucleus	Neoplasia	Aflatoxin, beryllium, cycasin, dimethylnitrosamine, tannic acid
Mitochondria	Swelling	Carbon tetrachloride, cycasin, dimethylnitrosamine, ethanol, phosphorus
Lysosomes	Accumulation	Beryllium, carbon tetrachloride, ethionine, phosphorus
Peroxisomes	Proliferation	Clofibrate, trichlorethylene, high-fat diet
Endoplasmic reticulum	Degranulation; proliferation	Carbon tetrachloride, dimethyl- nitrosamine, ethionine, phosphorus
Cytoskeleton	Derangement	Cytochalasin B, phalloidin
Bile canaliculi	Dilatation	Lithocholate, taurocholate

Source: Adapted from de la Iglesia et al. (1982), Stott (1988), and Plaa (1993).

proteins, and (3) loss of potassium from hepatocytes, resulting in an interference of transfer of the VLDL across the cell membrane (Plaa, 1993).

Liver Necrosis

Liver necrosis involves the death of hepatocytes. The necrosis can be focal (central, mid-zonal, peripheral) or massive. It is usually an acute injury. A number of chemicals have been demonstrated or reported to cause liver necrosis. It is a serious toxic manifestation but is not necessarily critical because of the remarkable regenerating capacity of the liver.

Cell death occurs along with rupture of the plasma membrane. No ultrastructural changes of the membrane per se have been detected prior to its rupture. There are, however, a number of changes that precede the cell death. Early morphologic changes include cytoplasmic edema, dilatation of endoplasmic reticulum, and disaggregation of polysomes. There is an accumulation of triglycerides as fat droplets in the cells. Late changes are progressive swelling of mitochondria with cristae disruption, cytoplasmic swelling, dissolution of organelles and nucleus, and rupture of plasma membrane (see Bridges et al., 1983).

The biochemical changes are complex, and various hepatotoxicants apparently act through different mechanisms. One of them appears to be inhibition of protein synthesis. Among other hepatotoxicants, ethionine and carbon tetrachloride (CCl_4) have been shown to exhibit this effect. However, CCl_4 acts primarily through its reactive metabolite, the trichloromethyl radical $^{\cdot}CCl_3$ (Recknagel and Glende, 1973), which covalently binds with proteins and unsaturated lipids and induces lipid peroxidation. Subcellular membranes are rich in such lipids and are therefore susceptible (see Table 12-1). The chemical alterations in the plasma membrane may be the cause of its rupture.

Recknagel et al. (1982), however, suggested that microsomal lipid peroxidation might lead to a depression of microsomal Ca^{2+} pump resulting in an early disturbance of liver cell Ca^{2+} homeostasis, which might then induce cell death. In addition, Shah et al. (1979) suggested that the toxicity of CCl_4 might be mediated through another metabolite, namely, phosgene.

A number of chemically related compounds, such as chloroform, tetrachloroethane, and carbon tetrabromide, as well as phosphorus, appear to act in similar ways. Acetaminophen also induces liver necrosis but apparently not through lipid peroxidation (Kamiyama et al., 1993). At low doses, its reactive metabolite conjugates with sulfate and glutathione. With increasing doses the level of glutathione reduces, and the covalent binding of the chemical to the proteins rises, as dramatically shown in Fig. 3-2. Bromobenzene is also bioactivated in the liver. Its 3,4-epoxide covalently binds to proteins and lipids and causes necrosis (see also chap. 3). Other examples include isoniazid and iproniazid, both of which undergo bioactivation and form metabolites that bind with macromolecules and cause necrosis (Mitchell et al., 1976).

Disturbance of Ca^{2+} homeostatis may also play an important role through an activation of molecular oxygen resulting in an oxidative stress as discussed in chap. 4 (Thomas and Reed, 1989). The important role of oxidative stress is also discussed in chap. 11.

The main biochemical changes include loss of regulation of cellular Ca^{2+} and depletion of glutathione. However, there is a complex process involving mitochondrial damage, lysosomal enzyme leakage, inhibition of protein synthesis, binding to macromolecules, and oxidative stress (Kulkarni and Byczkowski, 1994).

Cholestasis

This type of liver damage, usually acute, is less common than fatty liver and necrosis, and it is more difficult to induce in animals with the possible exception of the steroids. The cholestatic agents appear to act through several mechanisms. For example, ANIT (α-naphthylisocyanate) can induce cholestasis, hyperbilirubinemia, and inhibition of microsomal mixed-function oxygenases. Reduction of biliary excretory activity of the canalicular membrane appears to be the predominant mechanism for the cholestasis. Furthermore, ANIT seems to alter ductular cell permeability. More recently, it has been shown that platelets seem to contribute to ANIT-induced liver injury (Bailie et al., 1994).

A number of anabolic and contraceptive steroids as well as taurocholate, chlorpromazine, and erythromycin lactobionate have been found to cause cholestasis and hyperbilirubinemia associated with canalicular bile plugs. Ethinyl estradiol and chlorpromazine seem to impair the permeability of the biliary tract, thus reducing bile salt-independent bile flow (Plaa and Priestly, 1976; Plaa, 1993).

Cirrhosis

Cirrhosis is characterized by the presence of septae of collagen distributed throughout most of the liver. Separated by these fibrous sheaths, clusters of hepatocytes appears as nodules.

The pathogenesis is not fully understood, but in a majority of cases, cirrhosis seems to originate from single-cell necrosis associated with a deficiency in the repair mechanism. This condition then leads to fibroblastic activity and scar formation. Inadequate blood flow in the liver may be a contributing factor.

Several chemical carcinogens and long-term administration of CCl_4 can induce cirrhosis in animals. The most important cause of human cirrhosis is chronic ingestion of alcoholic beverages. The mechanism is not fully understood, but ethanol may damage mitochondria and increase local production of reactive oxygen species. These may lead to steatosis, necrosis, and cirrhosis. This pathologic condition can be induced in animals only with ethanol in combination with diets deficient in choline, proteins, methionine, vitamin B12, and folic acid. Since this type of nutritional deficiency is common in alcoholism, Hartroft (1975) suggested the nutritional deficiency as the primary cause. Lieber and DiCarli (1976) were able to induce cirrhosis in baboons with ethanol alone and claimed, therefore, that alcohol has direct hepatotoxicity.

Viral-Like Hepatitis

A clinical syndrome indistinguishable from viral hepatitis has been known to be associated with various drugs. In general, they have the following characteristics (Plaa, 1993): (1) Such liver injuries are not demonstrable in animals. (2) The effects in humans do not seem to be related to the dose. (3) The latent period varies greatly. (4) The toxicity is manifest in only a few susceptible individuals. (5) The histologic picture is more variable. (6) The patients usually show other signs of hypersensitivity and sometimes respond to a challenge dose. (7) Fever, rash, and eosinophilia are present in many cases.

The clinical picture may vary from patient to patient. For example, among those with halothane-induced hepatotoxicity, 50% of the patients had signs of typical immunologic reaction: fever, eosinophilia, and prior exposure to this anesthetic. Others did not exhibit these signs and the livers of fatal cases showed lesions similar to those induced by CCl_4 (Lewis and Zimmerman, 1989).

Halothane may induce a mild hepatotoxicity that is reproducible in animals. In addition, it may act through an immune-mediated mechanism to produce the viral-like liver toxicity, which is more severe and delayed in onset (Hubbard et al., 1988).

Carcinogenesis

Hepatocellular carcinoma and cholangiocarcinoma are the most common types of primary malignant neoplasms of the liver. Others include angiosarcoma, glandular carcinoma, trabecular carcinoma, and undifferentiated liver cell carcinoma. The significance of adenoma, focal basophilic hyperplasia, and hyperplastic nodule is as yet uncertain, whereas bile duct hyperplasia is likely to be a physiologic response to toxic exposure (Newberne, 1982).

As discussed in chap. 7, a large number of toxicants are known to induce liver cancers in animals. However, the carcinogenicity of these chemicals in humans with respect to liver has not been well established

(Wogan, 1976). On the other hand, the role of vinyl chloride in causing angiosarcoma in humans is beyond doubt.

HEPATOTOXICANTS

Some of the liver injuries described earlier, namely, steatosis, necrosis, cirrhosis, and neoplasia, have a number of common features. (1) These injuries are relatively easily produced in experimental animals. (2) Many toxicants can induce several types of such injuries. For example, steatosis, necrosis, and cirrhosis can result from exposure to CCl_4 (and related chemicals such as chloroform), aflatoxins, and phosphorus. Aflatoxins and dioxins can induce necrosis, cirrhosis, and neoplasm. Steatosis and cirrhosis are seen after exposure to ethanol, and bromobenzene is known to induce necrosis and cirrhosis.

Cholestasis is induced mainly by certain bile salts, α-naphthylisocyanate, certain anabolic and contraceptive steroids, manganese, and a number of drugs. Some of these drugs and other substances are also known to induce viral-like hepatitis. For example, p-aminosalicylic acid, chlorpromazine, erythromycin, and phenytoin (diphenylhydantoin) appear to produce viral-like hepatitis through a type of hypersensitivity reaction. On the other hand, iproniazid, isoniazid, and hydrazine derivatives induce this effect perhaps through a metabolic abnormality.

Examples of the various types of hepatotoxicants are listed in Appendix 12-1.

TESTING PROCEDURES

Animals

The animals most commonly used are rats and mice. This is because of their ready availability, small size, low cost, ease in handling, and the relative abundance of toxicologic data. Furthermore, determinations of toxicities on the liver are often a part of short-term and long-term studies, which are usually carried out in rats and mice. Sometimes dogs are used because of their greater susceptibility to a number of toxicants. Rhesus monkeys do not appear to be preferable to dogs because they are less susceptible and are more variable in their response (Gray, 1976).

Route of Administration

The chemical to be tested should be administered to the animals by the same route as the expected human exposure. However, in view of the relative difficulty in carrying out inhalation studies, it is interesting to note that the relative rankings of a number of halogenated hydrocarbons administered by parenteral route were similar to those obtained after administration by inhalation (Gehring, 1968).

Examinations

Gross Pathology The color and appearance can often indicate the nature of toxicity, such as fatty liver, or cirrhosis. The organ weight is usually a very sensitive indicator of effect on the liver. Although an effect does not necessarily indicate toxicity, an increase in liver weight has been shown in certain cases to be the most sensitive criterion of toxicity. For instance, DA 1627 [α-methyl-(α-morpholinoethyl)-1-naphthyl acetic acid] was found to significantly increase the absolute and relative liver weight at a dose level of 250 mg/kg/d without histologic changes. Fatty degeneration was observed in the animals dosed at a higher level, 1000 mg/kg (Bianchi et al., 1968).

Microscopic Examinations Light microscopy can detect a variety of histologic abnormalities, such as fatty change, necrosis, cirrhosis, hyperplastic nodules, and neoplasia. Korsrud et al. (1972) found that CCl_4 produced histopathologic changes in the liver of rats at doses lower than those that induced changes in serum enzymes. Grice (1972) confirmed this finding with CCl_4 as well as with mercuric chloride, thioacetamide, and diethanolamine.

Electron microscopy can detect changes in various subcellular structures. Observations of subcellular changes, along with biochemical findings, are often useful in delineating the mechanism of action of toxicants.

Biochemical Tests A number of serum enzymes have been used as indicators of hepatic injuries. These enzymes are released to the blood from the cytosol and subcellular organelles. The serum level of alanine aminotransferase (ALT) is increased in good correlation with the severity of hepatic necrosis as determined histologically. It is therefore the choice test in liver necrosis (Leonard et al., 1986). In addition, ornithine carbamoyl transferase (OCT) and sorbitol dehydrogenase (SDH) are more sensitive, but less specific, than ALT. They are therefore often used in conjunction with ALT when testing new toxicants. In cholestatic lesions, both ALT and alkaline phosphatase (AP) are greatly elevated. On the other hand, serum cholinesterase may be reduced in certain cases of liver diseases. For additional details see Plaa and Charbonneau (1994).

There are also other tests. The liver is involved in the metabolism of carbohydrate, fat, and protein, as well as in the formation of prothrombin and the excretion of bilirubin and certain foreign chemicals. It is also the major site of biotransformation of toxicants. Tests have thus been devised to determine these hepatic functions.

For example, bilirubin is excreted by the liver; hence its level in the blood is an index of liver function, but it is relatively insensitive. The rate of excretion of bromsulphalein is a more sensitive indicator of liver damage. Clinically, the prolongation of prothrombin time, after excluding vitamin K deficiency, has been used in detecting acute hepatic lesions. A chemical may either potentiate or inhibit the pharmacologic and toxicologic actions of another by stimulating the hepatic microsomal enzymes (see chap. 5). Measurements of barbiturate-induced sleeping time and the duration of zoxazolamine-induced paralysis have been used as indications of hepatic effects.

In addition, a number of biochemical tests can be performed on the liver tissue itself: (1) level of triglycerides, (2) activity of glucose 6-phosphatase, (3) level of microsomal conjugated dienes, resulting from peroxidation of microsomal lipids, (4) covalent binding of reactive metabolites to tissue macromolecules, (5) arylation or alkylation of purine and pyrimidine components of DNA and RNA (carcinogenicity), and (6) arylation or alkylation of other macromolecules (necrosis?).

Because of the importance of lipid peroxidation in liver lesions, the extent of this reaction is often determined, using thiobarbituric acid (TBA). It combines with malonaldehyde, a degradation product of the lipid, to form a colored complex, which can be measured quantitatively.

IN VITRO TESTS

Isolated Perfused Liver

The rat liver can be isolated and perfused in the study of a wide range of effects on a variety of hepatotoxicants. For example, the effects of CCl_4 on the transport and metabolism of triglycerides and fatty acids have been studied by Heimberg et al. (1962). Frazier and Kingsley (1976) reported on the transport of cadmium by the isolated liver to the bile.

Isolated Hepatocytes

Isolated rat and human hepatocytes, in suspension or in culture, have been used in a variety of biochemical studies. Freshly isolated hepatocytes are often used, but they can be maintained for only 26 h. However, they can survive 15 d if kept in culture media. Normal hepatocytes have little or no mitotic activity. To study the effects on dividing liver cells, hepatocytes from very young animals or from liver tumors are used. The techniques involved in isolating and incubating these cells and in testing their viability are given by Klaassen and Stacey (1982).

The isolated hepatocytes can be used to determine the nature of various toxic effects:

1 Membrane damages can be detected microscopically or biochemically. Biochemical procedures include measuring the ability of the cells to take up cofactors (e.g., NADPH), polar dyes (e.g., trypan blue), and substrates (e.g., succinate) and leakage of cytoplasmic enzymes.
2 There may be changes in cellular macromolecules such as inhibition of protein and RNA synthesis and increased synthesis of DNA.
3 Other effects include alterations of intermediary metabolism and changes in the activity and growth of the hepatocytes.

EVALUATION

Nature of Toxicity

The seriousness of various types of liver lesion differs markedly. Thus, certain effects on the liver, such as malignant neoplasm, are irreversible and serious. Necrosis may or may not be serious, depending on the extent of the effect. Local necrotic cells may be replaced by new cells through mitosis of adjacent hepatocytes. An accumulation of triglycerides per se is not necessarily indicative of damage. Under certain conditions the hepatocytes, with accumulated fat, function normally. The mortality rate in drug-induced cholestatic jaundice is less than 1%, whereas that in hepatocellular jaundice (viral-like hepatitis) ranges from 10 to 50%.

As noted earlier, changes in organ weight are often a very sensitive indicator of toxicity. However, it is important to bear in mind that some enzyme inducers such as phenobarbital may increase the liver weight associated with biological effects that are generally considered as adaptive rather than toxic. These effects generally include proliferation of the smooth endoplasmic reticulum, increased cytochrome P-450 content, increased drug-metabolizing activity, and increased amount of polyunsaturated acyl side chains. On the other hand, hepatotoxicants generally disturb the structure of the endoplasmic reticulum membranes, decrease the cytochrome P-450 content, decrease drug-metabolizing activity, and increase the amount of saturated acyl side chains (de la Iglesia et al., 1982).

Quantitative Assessment

In general, microscopic changes are difficult to quantify. However, pathologic lesions can be graded according to their nature and extent (Grice, 1972). Quantitative stereology can be applied to light and electron microscopy. The tissue composition can be characterized in terms of volume, surface, and population density (de la Iglesia et al., 1982).

Biochemical findings can be readily analyzed statistically. The biochemical effects, when plotted against log dose, usually show a linear dose-response relationship. This has been demonstrated, for example, in CCl_4-treated mice, with the following parameters: BSP retention, SGPT, bilirubinemia and triglycerides, glucose 6-phosphatase, and peroxidation (Plaa and Priestly, 1976).

These dose-response relations can be used in comparing the relative toxicity of different chemicals. They can also be used in the assessment of the relative sensitivity of different parameters. For example, with a 10-fold increase in the dose of CCl_4, there was a 4- to 5-fold increase in SGPT, but only a 50% decrease in liver glucose 6-phosphatase (Plaa and Priestly, 1976).

REFERENCES

Bailie, M. B., Pearson, J. M., Lappin, P. B., Killam, A. L., and Roth, R. A. 1994. Platelets and α-naphthylisothiocyanate-induced liver injury. *Toxicol. Appl. Pharmacol.* 129: 207–213.

Bianchi, C., Bonardo, G., and Marazzi-Uberti, E. 1968. Toxicology of α-methyl-α-(2-morpholinoethyl)-1-naphthyl-acetic acid hydrochloride. *Toxicol. Appl. Pharmacol.* 12: 331–336.

Bridges, J. W., Benford, D. J., and Hubbard S. A. 1983. Mechanisms of toxic injury. *Ann. NY Acad. Sci.* 407:42–63.

de la Iglesia, F., Sturgess, J. M., and Feuer, G. 1982. New approaches for assessment of hepatotoxicity by means of quantitative functional-morphological interrelationship. In *Toxicology of the liver*, eds. G. L. Plaa and W. R. Hewitt, pp. 47–102. New York: Raven Press.

Frazier, J. M., and Kingsley, B. S. 1976. Kinetics of cadmium transport in the isolated perfused rat liver. *Toxicol. Appl. Pharmacol.* 38:583–593.

Gehring, P. J. 1968. Hepatotoxic potency of various chlorinated hydrocarbon vapors relative to their narcotic and lethal potencies in mice. *Toxicol. Appl. Pharmacol.* 13:287–298.

Gray, J. E. 1976. Assessment of hepatotoxic potential. *Environ. Health Perspect.* 15:4754.

Grice, H. C. 1972. The changing role of pathology in modern safety evaluation. *CRC Crit. Rev. Toxicol.* 1:119–152.

Hartroft, W. S. 1975. On the etiology of alcoholic liver cirrhosis. In *Alcoholic liver pathology*, eds. J. M. Khanna, Y. Israel, and H. Kalant, pp. 189–197. Toronto: Addiction Research Foundation.

Heimberg, M., Weinstein, I., Dishmon, G., and Dunkerly, A. 1962. The action of carbon tetrachloride on the transport and metabolism of triglycerides and fatty acids by the isolated perfused rat liver and its relationship to the etiology of fatty liver. *J. Biol. Chem.* 237:3623–3627.

Hubbard, A. K., Gandolfi, A. J., and Brown, R. R. 1988. Immunological basis of anesthetic-induced hepatotoxicity. *Anesthesiology* 69:814–817.

Kamiyama, T., Sato, C., Liu, J., Tajiri, K., Miyakawa, H., and Marumo, F. 1993. Role of peroxidation in acetaminophen-induced hepatotoxicity: Comparison with carbon tetrachloride. *Toxicol. Lett.* 66:7–12.

Klaassen, C. D., and Stacey, N. H. 1982. Use of isolated hepatocytes in toxicity assessment. In *Toxicology of the liver*, eds. G. L. Plaa and W. R. Hewitt, pp. 147–179. New York: Raven Press.

Klaassen, C. D., and Watkins, J. B. 1984. Mechanisms of bile formation, hepatic uptake and biliary excretion. *Pharmacol. Rev.* 36:1–67.

Korsrud, G. O., Grice, H. C., and McLaughlan, J. M. 1972. Sensitivity of several serum enzymes in detecting carbon tetrachloride-induced liver damage in rats. *Toxicol. Appl. Pharmacol.* 22:474–483.

Kulkarni, A. P., and Byczkowski, J. Z. 1994. Hepatoxicity. In *Introduction to biochemical toxicology*, eds. E. Hodgson and P. E. Levi. Norwalk, CT: Appleton & Lange.

Leonard, T. B., Hewitt, W. R., Dent, J. G., and Morgan, D. G. 1986. Serum alanine aminotransferase (ALT) as a quantitative indicator to hepatic necrosis. *Toxicologist* 6:184.

Levi, P. E. 1987. Types of liver injury. In *A textbook of modern toxicology*, eds. E. Hodgson and P. E. Levi, p. 169. New York: Elsevier.

Lewis, J. H., and Zimmerman, H. J. 1989. Drug-induced liver disease. *Med. Clin. North Am.* 73:775–792.

Lieber, C. S., and DiCarli, L. M. 1976. Animal models of ethanol dependence of liver injury in rats and baboons. *Fed. Proc.* 35:1232–1236.

Mitchell, J. R., Snodgrass, W. R., and Gillette, J. R. 1976. The role of biotransformation in chemical-induced liver injury. *Environ. Health Perspect.* 15:27–38.

Newberne, P. M. 1982. Assessment of the hepatocarcinogenic potential of chemicals: Response of the liver. In *Toxicology of the liver*, eds. G. L. Plaa and W. R. Hewitt, pp. 243–290. New York: Raven Press.

Plaa, G. L. 1993. Toxic responses of the liver. In *Casarett and Doull's toxicology*, 4th ed, eds. M. O. Amdur, J. Doull, and C. D. Klaassen, pp. 334–353. New York: McGraw Hill.

Plaa, G. L., and Charbonneau, M. 1994. Detection and evaluation of chemically induced liver injury. In *Principles and methods of toxicology*, ed. A. W. Hayes, pp. 839–870. New York: Raven Press.

Plaa, G. L., and Priestly, B. G. 1976. Intrahepatic cholestasis induced by drugs and chemicals. *Pharmacol. Rev.* 28:207–273.

Recknagel, R. O., and Glende, E. A., Jr. 1973. Carbon tetrachloride hepatotoxicity: An example of lethal cleavage. *CRC Crit. Rev. Toxicol.* 2:263–297.

Recknagel, R. O., Glende, E. A., Waller, R. L., and Lowrey, K. 1982. Lipid peroxidation: Biochemistry, measurement, and significance in liver cell injury. In *Toxicology of the liver*, eds. G. L. Plaa and W. R. Hewitt, pp. 213–241. New York: Raven Press.

Shah, H., Martman, S. P., and Weinhouse, S. 1979. Formation of carbonyl chloride in carbon tetrachloride metabolism by rat liver in vitro. *Cancer Res.* 39:3942–3947.

Smith, M. L., Loveridge, N., Wills, E. D., and Chayen, J. 1979. The distribution of glutathione in rat liver lobule. *Biochem. J.* 182:103–108.

Stott, W. T. 1988. Chemically induced proliferation of peroxisomes: Implications for risk assessment. *Regul. Toxicol. Pharmacol.* 8:125–159.

Thomas, C. E., and Reed, D. J. 1989. Current status of calcium in hepatocellular injury. *Hepatology* 10: 375–384.

Wogan, C. N. 1976. The induction of liver cell cancer by chemicals. In *Liver cell cancer*, eds. H. M. Cameron, D. A. Linsell, and G. P. Warwick, pp. 121–152. Amsterdam: Elsevier.

Appendix 12-1 Examples of Hepatotoxic Agents and Associated Liver Injury

Necrosis and fatty liver

Acetaminophen[a]	Ethionine[b]
Aflatoxin	Furosemide[a]
Allyl alcohol[a]	Galactosamine
Azaserine	Phosphorus
Beryllium[a]	Puromycin[b]
Bromobenzene[a]	Pyrrolizidine alkaloids
Carbon tetrachloride	Tannic acid[a]
Chloroform	Tetrachloroethane
Cycloheximide[b]	Tetracycline[b]
Dimethylnitrosamine	Thioacetamide[a]
Ethanol[b]	Trichloroethylene
	Valproic acid[b]

Cholestasis (drug-induced)

p-Aminosalicylic acid[c]	Imipramine[c]
Amitriptyline	Mepazine
Carbamazepine[c]	Mestranol
Carbarsone	Methandrolone
Chlorpromazine[c]	Methimazole
Chlorthiazide	Oxyphenisatin[c]
Diazepam	Perphenazine
Erythromycin estolate[c]	Phenindione[c]
Estradiol	Promazine
Ethacrynic acid[c]	Sulfanilamide
	Thioridazine

Viral-like hepatitis (drug-induced)

Colchicine	6-Mercaptopurine
Halothane	Methoxyflurane
Imipramine	α-Methyldopa
Indomethacin	Papaverine
Iproniazid	Phenylbutazone
Isoniazid	Zoxazolamine

Carcinogenesis (in experimental animals)

Acetylaminofluorene	Polychlorinated biphenyls
Aflatoxin B$_1$	Pyrrolizidine alkaloids
Cycasin	Safrole
Dialkyl nitrosamines	Urethane
Dimethylbenzanthracene	Vinyl chloride

Source: Adapted from Levi (1987) and Plaa (1993).
[a]Primary effect is necrosis.
[b]Primary effect is fatty liver.
[c]Also induces viral-like hepatitis.

Toxicology of the Kidney

CHAPTER 13 CONTENTS

INTRODUCTION

As noted in chap. 2, urine is the principal route by which most toxicants are excreted. As a result, the kidney has a high volume of blood flow, concentrates toxicants in the filtrate, transports toxicants across the tubular cells, and bioactivates certain toxicants. It is therefore a major target organ of toxic effects. To facilitate discussions on these effects, the renal structure and functions are briefly reviewed.

Structure

The predominant structures in the kidney are the nephrons, numbering approximately 1.3×10^6. Each nephron consists of a glomerulus and a series of tubules (see Fig. 13-1). The glomerulus is supplied with a high-pressure capillary system that produces an ultrafiltrate from the plasma. The filtrate collected in the Bowman's capsule flows through the proximal convoluted tubule, the loop of Henle, and the distal convoluted tubule and then drains through a collecting tubule into the renal pelvis for excretion as urine.

The proximal tubule is divided into three sections (S^1, S^2, and S^3). S^1 and S^3 consist of major portions of the convoluted tubule and the straight portion, respectively. S^2 consists of the end of the convoluted portion and the beginning of the straight portion.

The major functions of the kidney are to eliminate wastes resulting from normal metabolism and to excrete xenobiotics and their metabolites. These are effected through the production of urine, a process that also contributes to the maintenance of the homeostatic status of the body. In addition, the kidney has several nonexcretory functions.

Production of Urine

The production of urine is a complex process. It begins with filtration in the glomeruli. In humans, approximately 180 L of filtrate is formed per day. Since only 500–2500 ml of urine is excreted, some 99% of the filtered water is reabsorbed.

The reabsorption of water, through diffusion, takes place first at the proximal tubules, where Na^+ is actively reabsorbed. Further diffusion of water takes place at the descending limb of the loop of Henle to the hyperosmolar interstitium. The hyperosmolarity is produced by the active reabsorption of Cl^- (along with Na^+) at the ascending limb of the loop (Berndt, 1976). The spatial arrangement of the loops and the vasa recta provides an effective countercurrent multiplier mechanism.

Additional water is removed from the filtrate in the distal and the collecting tubules as Na^+ is actively reabsorbed. The extent of the removal

Figure 13-1 Schematic presentation of a cortical (short-looped) and a juxtamedallary (long-looped) nephron together with the collecting system: (1) glomerulus with Bowman's capsule, (2) proximal tubule, convoluted portion, (3) proximal tubule, straight portion, (4) descending thin limb (loop of Henle), (5) ascending limb (loop of Henle), (6) thick ascending limb, (7) distal convoluted tubule, (8) connecting tubule, (9) collecting tubule (adapted from Kriz and Bankir, 1988).

of water from these tubules depends on the activity of antidiuretic hormone (ADH). ADH reduces the urine volume by increasing the permeability of these structures to water.

Tubular Resorption and Secretion

As the glomerular capillaries have large pores (70 nm), substances with molecular weights under 60,000 are filtered into Bowman's capsules. Some of the filtered substances such as glucose and amino acids, which are vital to the body, are reabsorbed by the tubules. On the other hand, ammonia (NH_3), a metabolic waste of amino acids, diffuses through the cells to the filtrate, where it reacts with H^+ to form NH_4^+, which is nondiffusible and hence excreted.

To facilitate the passive reabsorption of water and to maintain the homeostasis, various electrolytes in the glomerular filtrate are reabsorbed nearly completely or to a great extent. The reabsorption of Na^+ at the distal and collecting tubules is regulated by the mineralocorticoids, that of phosphorus by the parathyroid hormone, and that of bicarbonate (HCO_3^-) by the acid–base balance. In addition, K^+ and H^+ are secreted by the tubules.

Nonexcretory Functions

The kidney possesses other functions, such as the regulation of blood pressure and volume. This is mediated through the renin–angiotensin–aldosterone system. Renin, a proteolytic enzyme, is formed in the cells of the juxtaglomerular apparatus and catalyzes the conversion of a plasma angiotensin prohormone to angiotensin I. The latter, a decapeptide, is converted in the lung to angiotensin II by an enzyme that removes a dipeptide from the C-terminal end.

A renal erythropoietic factor (REF) also acts on a plasma protein to form erythropoietin, which increases the production of normoblasts and the synthesis of hemoglobin. Renal prostaglandins are produced in the interstitial cells in the medulla and appear to have the capability of regulating renal blood flow and the excretion of Na^+ and urine. The kidney is also involved in the conversion of the relatively inactive 25-hydroxy-vitamin D_3 to the active 1,25-dihydroxy-vitamin D_3.

NEPHROTOXICANTS: MECHANISM AND SITE OF ACTION

The major groups of nephrotoxicants are heavy metals, antibiotics, analgesics, and certain halogenated hydrocarbons (Table 13-1). All parts of the nephron are potentially subject to the detrimental effects of toxicants. However, most toxicants preferentially affect specific parts of the kidney. The

Table 13-1   Nephrotoxicants

Toxicant	Site of action
Heavy metals	
Cadmium	Proximal tubules
Chromium	Proximal tubules
Gold	Glomeruli
Lead	Proximal tubules and blood vessels
Mercury, inorganic	Proximal tubules and glomeruli
Antibiotics	
Aminoglycosides	Glomeruli and proximal tubules
Amphotericin-B	Glomerular blood vessels and distal tubules
Cephaloridine	Proximal tubules
Puromycin	Glomeruli
Tetracycline	Interstitial tissues in medulla
Halogenated hydrocarbons	
Bromobenzene	Proximal tubules
Carbon tetrachloride	Proximal tubules
Chloroform	Proximal tubules
Hexachlorobutadiene	Pars recta
Analgesics/anesthetics	
Acetaminophen	Various parts of nephron and blood vessels
Methoxyflurane	Various parts of nephron
Antineoplastics	
Cisplatin	Pars recta and other parts of nephron
Immunosuppressants	
Cyclosporin	Blood vessels and interstitial tissue
Miscellaneous	
Glycol	Tubular blockade
Sulfapyridine	Tubular blockade

mechanisms of action of nephrotoxicants include interaction with receptors, inhibition of oxidative phosphorylation, disturbance of Ca^{2+} homeostasis, and adverse effects in plasma and subcellular membranes. Details of these are provided in a review article (Commandeur and Vermeulen, 1990).

Glomeruli

The antibiotic puromycin can increase the permeability of the glomerulus to proteins such as albumin. This has been attributed to an alteration in the electrical charge of glomerular basement membrane (Brenner et al., 1977). On the other hand, the aminoglycoside antibiotics, such as genta-mycin and kanamycin, decrease the glomerular filtration, in addition to their effects on renal tubules (Humes and O'Connor, 1988). Certain toxi-cants, such as gold, mercury, and penicillamine, may induce membranous glomerulonephritis by the deposition of antigen antibody conjugates in the glomerular basement membrane.

Proximal Tubules

Because of their active absorptive and secretory activities, the proximal tubules often have higher concentrations of toxicants. Furthermore, they have a higher level of cytochrome P-450 to detoxify or activate toxicants. They are thus often the site of toxic effects. Heavy metals, such as mercury, chromium, cadmium, and lead, can alter the functions of the tubules, characterized by glycosuria, aminoaciduria, and polyuria. After higher doses, they cause tubular cell death, elevated blood urea nitrogen (BUN), and anuria. The straight portion (pars recta) of the proximal tubules appears more susceptible than the convoluted portion to the toxicity of mercury (Phillips et al., 1977). The nephrotoxicity may result from a combination of direct cellular toxicity and ischemia secondary to vasoconstriction. Additional information on renal toxicity of metals is given in chap. 20.

As noted earlier, certain antibiotics affect the glomerular filtration. In addition, many antibiotics are also secreted by the proximal tubules and can induce alterations in the tubular functions. Various aminoglycoside antibiotics (streptomycin, neomycin, kanamycin, gentomycin, and amphotericin-B) have been reported to affect the proximal tubules. These drugs alter membrane phospholipid compositions, permeability, Na^+- K^+-ATPase activity, adenylate cyclase activity, and transport of K^+, Ca^{2+}, and Mg^{2+} (Kaloyanides, 1984; Mingeot-Leclercq et al., 1995). Cephaloridine, unlike the antibiotics just named, is not secreted from the proximal tubules but is accumulated in these cells, thereby causing damage.

Halogenated hydrocarbons such as carbon tetrachloride and chloroform are mainly hepatotoxic, but in certain animal species they may also exert toxic effects on the kidney, especially on the proximal tubules, as reflected in functional changes. At higher doses, however, morphologic changes may be produced in other parts of the nephron. Hexachlorobutadiene damages mainly the pars recta of the proximal tubules, resulting in decreased urinary concentrating ability. Bromobenzene, like hexachlorobutadiene, is also nephrotoxic, acting on the proximal tubules. While the former is bioactivated in the liver, the latter is bioactivated in the kidney, via a renal enzyme (C-S lyase) after biotransformation in the liver (Hewitt et al., 1993).

Other Sites

Tetracycline, especially outdated products, may affect the renal medulla and induce interstitial nephritis. Amphotericin-B induces renal toxicity in a majority of the patients, affecting various renal structures.

Methoxyflurane, an anesthetic, is known to be nephrotoxic in humans and certain animals, causing high-output renal failure. This chemical has been shown to be biotransformed to inorganic fluoride and oxalate. Experimental data suggest that the F^- acts on several parts of the nephron to reduce the reabsorption of water. First, it interferes with the capability of the proximal tubules to reabsorb water. Second, it inhibits the enzymes involved in the transport of ions at the ascending limb of the loop of Henle, thus reducing the interstitial osmolarity, thereby decreasing water reabsorption. It also damages the collecting tubules, rendering them insensitive to the antidiuretic hormone (ADH) (Mazze, 1976).

Analgesic mixtures containing aspirin and phenacetin, a derivative of acetaminophen, can cause chronic renal failure, with the toxic effects located predominantly in the medulla, that is, the loop of Henle, vasa recta, interstitial cells, and collecting tubules. The effects might be a result of a vasoconstriction of the vasa recta (the blood vessels surrounding the loop of Henle) due to an inhibition of the synthesis of vasodilator prostaglandin (Nanra, 1974). Cisplatin affects many parts of the tubules in patients taking this chemotherapeutic agent (Tanaka et al., 1986). Cyclosporin causes acute thrombotic microangiopathy and chronic nephropathy with interstitial fibrosis (Racusen and Solez, 1988).

Other types of toxicity include renal carcinogenicity of DMN (dimethylnitrosamine), and tubular blockade induced by the metabolites of sulfapyridine (acetylsulfapyridine) and glycols (oxalic acid). Penicillins and sulfonamides have been reported to cause inflammatory interstitial nephritis in humans. An immunologic mechanism has been suggested as responsible for this toxicity (Appel and Neu, 1977).

TESTING PROCEDURE

Functional and morphologic examinations of the kidney are routinely carried out as an integral part of short-term and long-term toxicity studies. The types of examinations involved are described in chap. 6 and are further elaborated in this section.

In studies designed specifically for nephrotoxicity, dogs, rabbits, and rats are the commonly used animals. Examinations of the kidney functions may be done in a number of ways.

Urinalysis

Proteinuria   Because of the size of their molecules, only a very small amount of proteins of low molecular weight pass through the glomerular filter. The low-molecular-weight proteins are readily reabsorbed by the proximal tubules. The occurrence of large amounts of such protein in the urine is thus an indication of a loss of tubular reabsorptive function, as in cadmium poisoning. On the other hand, excretion of high-molecular-weight protein indicates a loss of integrity of glomeruli. It is to be noted that normal rat urine may contain some protein. A critical comparison of the treated animals with the controls is therefore important.

Glycosuria   Glucose in the glomerular filtrate is completely reabsorbed in the tubules, provided the amount of glucose to be reabsorbed does not exceed the *transport maximum* (Tm). Glycosuria in the absence of hyperglycemia thus indicates tubular dysfunction.

Urine Volume and Osmolarity   These two values are usually inversely related and are useful indicators of renal function in a *concentration test*, wherein water is withheld from the animal, and also in a *dilution test*, wherein a large amount of water is given to the animal. The osmolarity can be estimated from the specific gravity, but the freezing point of urine provides a more accurate measurement. A toxicant may cause high-output renal failure as noted earlier. On the other hand, it may cause oliguria or even anuria, resulting from tubular injury, with concomitant interstitial edema and intraluminal sediment or debris, which blocks urine flow.

Acidifying Capacity   This can be assessed from urine pH, titratable acids, and NH_4^+. This capacity is reduced when there is distal tubular dysfunction.

Enzymes   Enzymes such as maltase and acid phosphatase in urine may indicate destruction of proximal tubules. Urine alkaline phosphatase, on the other hand, may be renal or hepatic in origin. Plummer (1981) suggests that the urinary enzymes not only are useful indicators of renal damage but also indicate the subcellular site of origin. For example, alkaline phosphatase is located in endoplasmic reticulum, glutamate dehydrogenase in mitochondria, and lactate dehydrogenase in cytoplasm. In general, urinary enzymes are more useful in acute nephrotoxic conditions.

Blood Analysis

Blood Urea Nitrogen   Blood urea nitrogen (BUN) is derived from normal metabolism of protein and is excreted in the urine. Elevated BUN usually indicates glomerular damage. However, its level can also be affected by poor nutrition and hepatotoxicity, which are common effects of many toxicants.

Creatinine   Creatinine is a metabolite of creatine and is excreted completely in the urine via glomerular filtration. An elevation of its level in the blood is thus an indication of impaired kidney function. Furthermore, data on its level in blood and its amounts in urine can be used to estimate the glomerular filtration rate. One drawback with this procedure is the fact that some creatinine is secreted by the tubules.

Special Tests

Glomerular Filtration Rate   The glomerular filtration rate (GFR) can be more accurately determined by the clearance of inulin, a polysaccharide. It is diffused into the glomerular filtrate and is neither reabsorbed nor secreted by the tubules. Reduced GFR indicates impairment of glomerular filtration.

Renal Clearance   This is the volume of plasma that is completely cleared of a substance in a unit of time. The renal clearance of *p*-aminohippuric acid (PAH) exceeds that of inulin because it is not only filtered through the glomeruli but also secreted by the tubules. A reduction of PAH elimination without a concomitant decrease of GFR indicates tubular dysfunction. PAH is nearly completely (up to 90%) removed from the blood in one passage. The rate of its clearance is therefore useful in determining the effective renal plasma flow (ERPF). The renal blood flow can also be determined by the use of radiolabeled microspheres or an electromagnetic flowmeter.

PSP Excretion Test   The rate of excretion of phenolsulfonphthalein is related to renal blood flow. It is, therefore, often used in the assessment of renal function. However, a reduced secretion rate can also result from cardiovascular diseases.

Morphologic Examinations

Gross Examination   The organ weight of the kidney per se or in terms of body weight of the animal, as a rule, is routinely determined at the end of short-term and long-term toxicity studies. Alterations in the organ weight, when compared to the controls, often suggest kidney lesions. A number of other pathologic lesions can also be detected on gross examination.

Microscopic Examination   Light microscopy can reveal the site, extent, and morphologic nature of renal lesions. Electron microscopy is useful in assessing ultrastructural changes in the cells. For example, prolonged exposure to methylmercury increased the volume density of mitochondria and lysosomes. Concomitantly, there were changes in various enzyme activities, the most notable of which was the marked increase in the specific activity of o-aminolevulinic acid synthetase (Fowler, 1980).

IN VITRO STUDIES

Kidney Slices Tissue slices provide a useful tool for the study of renal tubular function. In spite of the relatively artificial conditions imposed by in vitro studies, Berndt (1976) compiled data demonstrating that the in vitro uptakes of various organic acids, bases, sugars, amino acids, and inorganic electrolytes were essentially identical to those under in vivo conditions.

A toxicant to be studied can be added to the medium in which the slices are immersed, or it can be administered to the animal prior to the removal of the kidney for the preparation of the slices. For example, Koschier and Berndt (1976) reported that renal slices from animals pretreated with 2,4,5-trichlorophenoxyacetic acid (2,4,5-T) showed impaired renal transport of 2,4,5-T, 2,4-dichlorophenoxyacetic acid (2,4-D), and triethanolamine (TEA) in the absence of morphologic changes. A description of the method used in studying nephrotoxicants on kidney slices and the results obtained thereof as well as extensive literature citations are provided by Kacew and Hirsch (1982).

Perfused Renal Tubules Various sections of the renal tubules of the rabbit have been isolated and their transport functions studied. In addition, other species of animals have been used; these include the mouse, rat, hamster, snake, flounder, frog, salamander, and humans. Schafer (1981) described the technique and outlined the pros and cons of this procedure.

Isolated Nephrons Endou et al. (1983) isolated nephrons from rat kidney after perfusing it with 0.1% collagenase to facilitate the dissection. They found cytochrome P-450 existent only in the proximal tubules, with the straight portion containing more than the convoluted portion. Furthermore, the enzymes in these two portions of the tubule differ in their responses to 3-methylcholanthrene and starvation.

EVALUATION

Nature of Toxicity

The kidney has a remarkable compensatory capability. Even after appreciable changes in renal functions and morphology, the kidney may compensate and regain normal functions. Therefore, it is important to perform tests at repeated and appropriate time intervals.

Nephrotoxicants can exert adverse effects on various parts of the kidney, resulting in alterations of different functions. A variety of tests should therefore be performed. The most sensitive and reliable tests appear to vary depending on the nature of the nephrotoxicants as well as the experimental conditions (e.g., animal species, duration of exposure). In an article, Kluwe (1981) concluded from his studies that in vitro accumulation of organic ions (e.g., PAH, TEA), urinary concentrating ability, and kidney weight were the most sensitive and consistent indicators of nephrotoxicity. Standard urinalysis, serum analyses, qualitative enzymuria, and histopathologic changes were less sensitive and less consistent. Goldstein et al. (1981) observed that urine osmolarity was the most sensitive indicator of the nephrotoxicity of a platinum complex, whereas GFR and ERPF were affected only later and at higher doses.

In assessing the renal effects of a toxicant, extrarenal factors that might affect the blood volume or blood pressure should be taken into account, since they may indirectly impair renal functions. Furthermore, kidney diseases, such as those associated with aging, may be prevalent and should also be considered.

Quantitative Assessment

In general, morphologic changes are difficult to quantify. However, criteria for grading the microscopic changes have been suggested by Zbinden (1976). On the other hand, biochemical and functional tests usually yield data that can be statistically analyzed readily. Since nephrotoxicants may affect several renal functions differently, quantitative comparison of relative toxicity should be done with caution.

REFERENCES

Appel, G. B., and Neu, H. C. 1977. The nephrotoxicity of antimicrobial agents (parts 1 and 2). *N. Engl. J. Med.* 296:663–670, 722–728.

Berndt, W. O. 1976. Use of tissue slice technique for evaluation of renal transport processes. *Environ. Health Perspect.* 15:73–88.

Brenner, B. M., Bohrer, M. P., Baglis, C., and Deen, W. M. 1977. Determinants of glomerular permselectivity: Insights derived from observations in vivo. *Kidney Int.* 12:229–257.

Commandeur, J. N. M., and Vermeulan, N. P. E. 1990. Molecular and biochemical mechanisms of chemically induced nephrotoxicity: A review. *Chem. Res. Toxicol.* 3:171–194.

Endou, H., Koseki, C., and Sakai, F. 1983. Effects of 3-methylcholanthrene and starvation on intranephron distribution of cytochrome P-450. *Toxicol. Lett.* 18(suppl. 1):1–10.

Fowler, B. A. 1980. Ultrastructural morphometric/biochemical assessment of cellular toxicity. In *The scientific basis of toxicity assessment*, ed. P. R. Witschi, pp. 211–218. Amsterdam: Elsevier/North Holland.

Goldstein, R. S., Noordwier, B., Bond, J. T., Hook, J. B., and Mayor, G. H. 1981. *cis*-Dichlorodiammineplatinum nephrotoxicity: Time course and dose response of renal functional impairment. *Toxicol. Appl. Pharmacol.* 60:163–175.

Hewitt, W. R., Goldstein, R. S., and Hook, J. B. 1993. Toxic response of the kidney. In *Casarett and Doull's toxicology*, 4th ed., eds. M. O. Amdur, J. Doull, and C. D. Klaassen, pp. 354–382. New York: McGraw-Hill.

Humes, H. D., and O'Connor, R. P. 1988. Aminoglycoside nephrotoxicity. In *Diseases of the Kidney*, 4th ed, eds. R. W. Shrier and C. W. Gottschalk, vol. 2, pp. 1228–1273. Boston: Little, Brown.

Kacew, S., and Hirsch, G. H. 1982. Evaluation of nephrotoxicity of various compounds by means of in vitro techniques and comparison to in vivo methods. In *Toxicology of the kidney*, ed. J. B. Hook, pp. 77–98. New York: Raven Press.

Kaloyanides, G. J. 1984. Aminoglycoside-induced functional and biochemical defects in the renal cortex. *Fundam. Appl. Toxicol.* 4:930–943.

Kluwe, W. M. 1981. Renal function tests as indicators of kidney injury in subacute toxicity studies. *Toxicol. Appl. Pharmacol.* 57:414–424.

Koschier, E. F., and Berndt, W. O. 1976. In vitro uptake of organic ions by renal cortical tissue of rats treated acutely with 2,4,5-trichlorophenoxyacetic acids. *Toxicol. Appl. Pharmacol.* 35:355–364.

Kriz, W., and Bankir, L. 1988. A standard nomenclature for structures of the kidney. *Am. J. Physiol.* 254:F1–F8.

Mazze, R. I. 1976. Methoxyflurane nephropathy. *Environ. Health Perspect.* 15:111–120.

Mingeot-Leclercq, M.-P., Brasseur, R., and Schank, A. 1995. Molecular parameters involved in aminoglycoside nephrotoxicity. *J. Toxicol. Environ. Health* 44:263–300.

Nanra, R. S. 1974. Pathology, etiology and pathogenesis of analgesic nephropathy. *Aust. N. Z. J. Med.* 4:602–603.

Phillips, R., Yamaguchi, M., Cote, M. G., and Plaa, G. L. 1977. Assessment of mercuric chloride-induced nephrotoxicity by *p*-aminohippuric acid uptake and the activity of four gluconeogenic enzymes in rat renal cortex. *Toxicol. Appl. Pharmacol.* 41:407–422.

Plummer, D. T. 1981. Urinary enzyme in drug toxicity. In *Testing for toxicity*, ed. J. W. Gorrod, pp. 157–171. London: Taylor & Francis.

Racusen, L. C., and Solez, K. 1988. Cyclosporine nephrotoxicity. *Int. Rev. Exp. Pathol.* 30: 107–157.

Schafer, J. A. 1981. Transport studies in isolated perfused renal tubules. *Fed. Proc.* 40: 2450–2459.

Tanaka, H., Ishikawa, E. Teshima, S., and Shimizu, E. 1986. Histopathological study of human cisplatin nephrotoxicity. *Toxicol. Pathol.* 14:247–257.

Zbinden, G. 1976. *Progress in toxicology*, Vol. 2, pp. 44–49. New York: Springer-Verlag.

ADDITIONAL READING

World Health Organization. 1991. Principles and Methods for the Assessment of Nephrotoxicity Associated with Exposure to Chemicals. Environmental Health Criteria 119. Geneva: WHO.

Toxicology of the Skin

CHAPTER 14 CONTENTS

GENERAL CONSIDERATIONS

The body of humans, as well as that of animals, is almost entirely covered by skin. As a result, it is exposed to a variety of chemicals such as cosmetics, household products, topical medication, and industrial pollutants, especially in certain workplaces. Dermal exposure to chemicals can result in various types of lesions. Furthermore, skin lesions may follow systematic exposure to chemicals.

The skin consists of the epidermis and the dermis, which rests over the subcutaneous tissue (Fig. 14-1). The epidermis is relatively thin, averaging 0.1–0.2 mm in thickness, whereas the dermis is about 2 mm thick. These two layers are separated by a basement membrane.

The living layer of epidermis in turn consists of a basal cell layer (stratum germinativum), which provides the other layers with new cells.

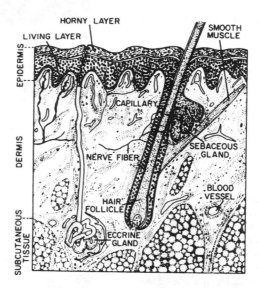

Figure 14-1 Cross section of the skin showing the two major layers of epidermis and dermis, and the various structures in the dermis (from Montagna, 1965, copyright © 1965 by Scientific American, Inc., all rights reserved).

These new cells become prickle cells (stratum spinosum) and, later, the granular cells (stratum granulosum). The nuclei in these cells disintegrate and dissolve. In addition, these cells produce keratohydrin, which later becomes keratin in the outermost stratum corneum, the horny layer. This layer is gradually shed. This development process takes about 4 wk. The epidermis also contains melanocytes, which produce pigments, and the Langerhans cells, which act as macrophages; and lymphocytes. The latter two types of cells are involved in immune responses. The epidermis thus forms an important protective cover of the body.

The dermis is mainly composed of collagen and elastin, which are important structures for the support of the skin. In this layer there are several types of cells, the most abundant being the fibroblasts, which are involved in the biosynthesis of the fibrous proteins and ground substances such as hyaluronic acid, chondroitin sulfates, and mucopolysaccharides. The other types of cells include fat cells, macrophages, histiocytes, and mast cells. Underneath the dermis is the subcutaneous tissue.

There are, in addition, a number of other structures, such as the hair follicles, sweat glands (the ecrine glands), sebaceous glands, small blood vessels, and neural elements.

The possibility of systemic toxicity following dermal exposure to toxicants is discussed in chap. 2. In addition, dermal reactions may appear following systemic administration of toxicants. The toxicities of pesticides, industrial chemicals, and metals from dermal exposure are discussed in chaps. 19–21.

TYPES OF TOXIC EFFECTS
AND DERMATOTOXICANTS

A variety of effects can result from dermal exposure to toxicants. Most of the effects involve the skin itself, but some of them affect its appendages—hair, sebaceous glands, and sweat glands.

Primary Irritation

Irritation is a reaction of the skin to chemicals such as strong alkalis, acids, solvents, and detergents. It ranges in severity from hyperemia, edema, and vesiculation to ulceration (corrosion). Primary irritations occur at the site of contact and, in general, on the first contact. It is thus different from sensitization.

Sensitization Reaction

The skin may show little or no reaction on the first contact with a chemical. However, a reaction or a more severe reaction occurs after a subsequent exposure to the chemical. The induction period ranges from a few days to years. A subsequent exposure to the specific toxicant will elicit a reaction after a delay of 12–48 h. It is therefore known as "delayed hypersensitivity." A complex immune mechanism is involved in this reaction. Briefly, the toxicant, upon entering the skin, becomes bonded to the surface of certain cells, which will process it for reaction with T lymphocytes. After such reaction, the sensitized T lymphocytes may release a variety of substances upon reexposure to the same toxicant and result in hyperemia and edema (see also chaps. 4 and 10).

A variety of chemicals, including topical medicaments, can induce sensitization reaction. Table 14-1 lists a number of them. They show positive response in human patch test with a frequency of 5–11% (Rudner, 1973).

Table 14-1   Selected Dermal Sensitizers

Antibiotics—neomycin
Hair dye ingredient—*p*-Phenylenediamine
Local anesthetics—benzocaine
Metals—nickel and nickel salts, beryllium, chromium salts,
    organomercurials (thimerosol)
Pesticides—captan, ethylenediamine
Poisonous plants—poison ivy, poison oak

Table 14-2   Comparison of Phototoxic and Photoallergic Reactions

Reaction	Phototoxic	Photoallergic
Reaction possible on first exposure	Yes	No
Incubation period necessary after first exposure	No	Yes
Chemical alteration of photosensitizer	No	Yes
Covalent binding with carrier	No	Yes
Clinical changes	Usually like sunburn	Varied morphology
Flares at distant previously involved sites possible	No	Yes
Persistent light reaction can develop	No	Yes
Cross-reactions to structurally related agents	Infrequent	Frequent
Broadening of cross-reactions following repeated photopatch testing	No	Possible
Concentration of drug necessary for reaction	High	Low
Incidence	Usually relatively high	Usually very low
Passive transfer	No	Possible
Lymphocyte stimulation test	No	Possible
Macrophage migration inhibition test	No	Possible

Source: Adapted from Harber and Baer (1972).

Phototoxicity and Photoallergy

These two types of skin reaction are similar in that both are light induced and may follow either systemic administration or topical application of the offending chemical. However, photoallergy involves immune reactions, whereas phototoxicity does not. This and other differences have been summarized by Harber and Baer (1972) (Table 14-2).

Phototoxicity is more common than photoallergy. The commonly reported phototoxic chemicals in humans, according to Harber et al. (1987), are aminobenzoic acid derivatives, anthraquinone dyes, chlorpromazine, chlorothiazides, phenothiazines, sulfanilamide, and coal tar derivatives

Table 14-3   Examples of Phototoxic and Photoallergic Chemicals

Chemicals	Phototoxicity	Photoallergy
Aminobenzoic acid derivatives	+	+
Chlorpromazine	+	+
Chlorothiazide	+	+
Methoxypsoralens	+	−
Psoralens	+	−
Sulfonamides	+	+
Tetracyclines	+	−
Coal tar derivatives	+	−
Nonsteroidal anti-inflammatory drugs	+	−

(e.g., anthracene, pyridine, acridine, and phenanthrene). The skin reaction consists of a delayed erythema, followed by hyperpigmentation and desquamation.

The commonly reported photoallergic chemicals include aminobenzoic acids, chlorpromazine, chlorpropamide, 2,2-thiobis(4-chlorophenol) (Fentichlor), halogenated salicylanilides, promethazine, sulfanilamide, and thiazides (Harber et al., 1987). Many compounds are therefore both phototoxic and photoallergic. Clinically, photoallergy usually manifests as delayed papules and eczema, but it may also appear as immediate urticarial reaction. Histologically it is characterized by a dense perivascular round-cell infiltrate in the dermis. The delayed reactions are type IV T-cell-mediated immune response, whereas the immediate reaction is probably antibody mediated (chap. 10).

The most biologically active rays that cause erythema and pigmentation are in the shorter ultraviolet (UV) range, that is, wavelengths below 320 nm. The sunlight ranges from 290 nm upward, but the UV rays emitted by artificial light sources may be shorter. However, the longer UV rays (320–400 nm) per se are less erythrogenic, but are responsible for both phototoxic and photoallergic reactions to chemicals (see Testing Procedures).

Contact Urticaria / Urticarial Reactions

These skin reactions, in the form of urticaria or eczema, appear within minutes to an hour after contact with the offending substance. Hence they are different from the sensitization reaction described earlier. The mechanism may be nonimmunologic, such as the case with aspirin and methyl nicotinate. In other cases, such as latex rubber and penicillin, an immunologic mechanism is involved. However, unlike the sensitization reaction described earlier, an antibody (immunoglobulin E, IgE), rather than T cell, is involved. In both immunologic and nonimmunologic cases, the dermal reactions are elicited by vasoactive substances, such as histamine along with prostaglandins, leukotrienes, and kinins. A great variety of substances have been reported to induce these reactions, including metals (copper, platinum), medicaments (antibiotics, local anesthetics), and biogenic polymers (released from arthropods, jellyfish). Amin et al. (1995) have provided extensive lists of agents that induce immunologic and nonimmunologic immediate contact reactions. Urticarial actions may also follow ingested or parenterally administered agents.

Cutaneous Cancer

It has been known for over two centuries that soots can cause skin cancer. More recent studies confirm that soots and related substances, such as coal tars, creosote oils, shale oils, and cutting oil, cause cancers of the skin and other sites in animals and humans. In addition, arsenic and certain arsenic compounds have been reported to be associated with skin cancer in humans (chap. 20).

A number of polycyclic aromatic hydrocarbons (e.g., benzo[a]pyrene) and heterocyclic compounds (e.g., benz[c]acridine) are known to induce skin cancer after topical applications on animals (IARC, 1973). UV radiation is an important cause of skin cancer in humans, and a number of chemicals can influence the effect of UV light and vice versa (Forbes, 1995).

Effects on Epidermal Adnexa

Hair   Loss of hair may result from various antimitotic agents used in cancer chemotherapy. These agents affect the anagen phase of hair growth. The affected hair starts to shed after about 2 wk of therapy, but hair growth resumes about 2 mo after the suspension of therapy.

A number of other medications are known to cause hair loss by converting hair follicles in anagen phase to telogen phase. In such cases, hair shedding generally starts 24 mo after therapy. The medications involved in this type of hair loss include oral contraceptives, anticoagulants, propranolol, and triparanol (Emmett, 1993).

Sebaceous Glands   These glands secrete lipid through expulsion of their lipid-laden cells and are therefore known as *holocrine*. Their activity is hormone dependent. For example, androgens stimulate and estrogens inhibit the excretion. Adrenocortical steroids and thyroid hormones also have some stimulatory activity. Acne may be formed as a result of proliferation of the follicular epithelium of the sebaceous gland. Topically applied substances such as greases and oils and systemically administered substances such as iodides and bromides may increase the formation of acnes.

A number of chlorinated aromatic hydrocarbons can cause various skin lesions, including *chloracne*, which is characterized by small straw-colored cysts and comedones, and in which the sebaceous gland is replaced by a keratinous cyst. The severity of chloracne varies, but it has been noted among occupational workers. However, it was more notable in the outbreaks in Japan among individuals after their consumption of a batch of rice oil contaminated with polychlorinated biphenyls (PCB) (WHO, 1976), and in Seveso, Italy, among residents near a factory that accidentally released a large amount of TCDD (2,3,7,8-tetrachlorodibenzo-*p*-dioxin) (Pocchiari, 1980). For other chloracne-inducing agents, see Emmett (1993).

Sweat Glands   Sweating serves useful physiologic functions such as regulation of body temperature. Blockage of the sweat ducts, a disorder known as miliaria, may occur after topical application of 95% phenol and chloroform (Shelley and Horvath, 1950).

TESTING PROCEDURES

For most effects on skin, the test animal of choice is the albino rabbit, although albino guinea pigs, white mice, and others are also used.

Primary Irritation

This effect is in general measured by a patch test on the skin of rabbits (Draize, 1959). A small amount (0.5 g or 0.5 ml) of the chemical to be tested is introduced under a 1-in^2 gauze pad that is placed over a shaved part of the skin. The pad is suitably fastened over the animal for 24 h. At the end of this period, the pad is removed and the skin reaction is graded according to the extent of (1) erythema and eschar formation and (2) edema formation. The skin reaction is read again at the end of 72 h. The same test is done on other rabbits, except that the skin has been abraded. The 24- and 72-h readings from both groups are added to obtain the *primary irritation index*. The test procedure, grading of skin reaction, and interpretation of the grading are given in Appendix 14-1.

There are a number of modified skin irritation tests based on the Draize procedure. The modifications involve the animal species and the number of animals used, amount of test material applied, repetitive applications, and types of examinations. For details see Henry (1992).

Sensitization Reaction

The procedure described by Draize (1959) calls for the use of guinea pigs that are given the chemical by 10 repeated intradermal injections on one flank and a challenging dose on the other flank after a 10- to 14-d resting period. A greater reaction after the challenging dose, in comparison with that after the sensitizing doses, indicates sensitization.

The *Draize test* is generally considered insufficiently sensitive to identify allergic potential. Magnusson and Kligman (1969) therefore recommended the use of the *maximization test*, in which the guinea pigs are given intradermally on d 0 the test substance with and without Freund's complete adjuvant. On d 7 the substance is applied at the same site occlusively. Two weeks later, the test substance is applied topically over the pretreated areas in these animals. Different concentrations of the agent are used in the challenge. Recently, OECD (1992) has adopted this and the

Buehler test, which requires the application of the chemical under closed patches.

Human experience is obtained either in patch tests or in a controlled population. In the latter case, the substance is widely distributed to the target population for use as directed. Their skin reactions are examined and evaluated. A patch test usually involves 100 males and 100 females, covering a wide age range. The test material (0.5 ml or 0.5 g) is applied by patch to an area on the arm or back. The skin reaction is examined on the following day after the removal of the patch.

Phototoxicity and Photoallergy

Phototoxicity appears to be more readily demonstrable in the hairless mouse, the rabbit, and the guinea pig. The substance to be tested may be administered topically or by a systemic route. The reaction of the skin to nonerythrogenic light (wavelength greater than 320 nm) is then determined. Significant erythema, compared to controls, indicates phototoxicity.

For the detection of photoallergy, albino guinea pigs are especially useful. The procedure involves, in principle, an induction of photosensitization by repeatedly applying a small amount of the chemical on a shaved and depilated area of the skin and exposing that area to appropriate UV rays. After a 3-wk interval, the guinea pigs are exposed to the chemical and the UV rays to elicit photoallergy. Details of the procedure are given by Harber et al. (1987).

Contact Urticaria

A number of animal models have been proposed based on the procedure devised by Jacobs (1940). These generally involve a patch test on the flank and nipples of guinea pigs. Recently, a test using guinea pig ears has been found satisfactory in screening human contact urticarigenic substances (Lahti and Maibach, 1984).

The open patch test can be applied to human volunteers or to patients suspected of being susceptible to the chemical. In the latter case, all necessary resuscitation equipment and qualified personnel should be available to respond to anaphylactoid reaction.

Any immunologic involvement can be demonstrated by the passive transfer test, in which 0.1 ml fresh serum from the patient is injected intradermally into the forearm of a volunteer and challenged 24 h later by applying the suspect chemical to the injection site.

Cutaneous Cancer

The procedure involves topical application of the substance on a shaved area of the skin. The substance per se, if a liquid, is applied directly. Otherwise, it is dissolved or suspended in a suitable vehicle. The skin painting is usually done once a week or more frequently. The commonly used animal is the mouse. It is advisable to include a vehicle control group as well as a positive control group, which is treated with a known skin carcinogen such as benzo[a]pyrene.

EVALUATION

Although various tests for primary irritation and sensitization reaction have been in use for many years, their reliability and reproducibility have been questioned. For example, Nixon et al. (1975) and Griffith and Buehler (1977) found the rabbit to be generally more susceptible than the guinea pig and humans, and the use of these two species is more reliable in predicting human reactions. Furthermore, the use of abraded skin did not enhance the value of the animal tests.

The various sensitization tests in guinea pigs and the human patch test yielded comparable results to a variety of chemicals. However, these tests appear to be more likely to yield false-positive results than false-negatives, compared to use experience in humans. There is less information comparing results from the various tests in animals and human experience with respect to the other types of dermal effects. However, the available information indicates that they are useful as screening procedures.

IN VITRO TESTS

In order to reduce the use of intact animals in dermal irritancy tests, several in vitro procedures have been developed. One of them involves the determination of the uptake of neutral red by normal human keratinocytes. Chemicals that damage these isolated cells will reduce the uptake of the dye (Borenfreund and Puerner, 1984; Shopsis et al., 1987). A method using cultured rat epidermal keratinocytes to measure toxic effects in terms of plasma membrane integrity and lysosomal and mitochondrial functions has been described (Hsieh and Acosta, 1991).

REFERENCES

Amin, S., Lahti, A., and Maibach, H. I. 1995. Immediate contact reactions: Contact urticaria and the contact urticaria syndrome. In *Dermatotoxicology*, eds. F. N. Marzulli and H. I. Maibach. Washington, DC: Taylor & Francis.

Borenfreund, E., and Puerner, J. 1984. A simple quantitative procedure using monolayer cultures for cytotoxicity assays. *J. Tissue Culture Methods* 9:7–9.

Draize, J. H. 1959. Dermal toxicity. In *U.S. appraisal of the safety of chemicals in foods, drugs and cosmetics*, ed. Editorial Committee of the Association of Food and Drug Officials of the United States. Austin, TX: Texas State Department of Health.

Emmett, E. A. 1993. Toxic responses of the skin. In *Casarett and Doull's toxicology*, eds. M. O. Amdur, J. Doull, and C. D. Klaassen, pp. 463–483. New York: McGraw-Hill.

Forbes, P. D. 1995. Carcinogenesis and photocarcinogenesis test methods. In *Dermatotoxicology*, eds. F. N. Marzulli and H. I. Maibach. Washington, DC: Taylor & Francis.

Griffith, J. F., and Buehler, E. V. 1977. Prediction of skin irritancy and sensitizing potential by testing with animals and man. In *Cutaneous toxicity*, eds. V. A. Drill and P. Lazar, pp. 155–174. New York: Academic Press.

Harber, L. C., and Baer, R. L. 1972. Pathogenic mechanisms of drug-induced photosensitivity. *J. Invest. Dermatol.* 58:327–342.

Harber, L. S., Shalita, A. R., and Armstrong, R. B. 1987. Immunologically mediated contact photosensitivity in guinea pigs. In *Dermatotoxicology*, eds. F. N. Marzulli and H. I. Maibach, pp. 413–430. Washington, DC: Hemisphere.

Henry, M. C. 1992. USEPA efforts in harmonization of acute toxicity test guidelines with OECD. *J. Am. College Toxicol.* 11:285–291.

Hsieh, G. C., and Acosta, D. 1991. Dithral-induced cytotoxicity in primary cultures of rat epidermal keratinocytes. *Toxicol. Appl. Pharmacol.* 107:16–26.

International Agency for Research on Cancer. 1973. Certain Polycyclic Aromatic Hydrocarbons and Heterocyclic Compounds. IARC Monographs on the Evaluation of Carcinogenic Risk of the Chemical to Man, vol. 3. Lyon, France: IARC.

Jacobs, J. L. 1940. Immediate generalized skin reactions in hypersensitive guinea pigs. *Proc. Soc. Exp. Biol. Med.* 43:641–643.

Lahti, A., and Maibach, H. I. 1984. An animal model for nonimmunologic contact urticaria. *Toxicol. Appl. Pharmacol.* 76:219–224.

Magnusson, B., and Kligman, A. M. 1969. The identification of contact allergens by animal assay. The guinea pig maximization test. *J. Invest. Dermatol.* 52:268–276.

Montagna, W. 1965. The skin. *Sci. Am.* (Feb.):60.

Nixon, G. A., Tyson, C. A., and Werz, W. C. 1975. Interspecies comparisons of skin irritancy. *Toxicol. Appl. Pharmacol.* 31:481–490.

Organization for Economic Cooperation and Development. 1992. OECD Guidelines for Testing Chemicals. Paris: OECD.

Pocchiari, F. 1980. Accidental release of 2,3,7,8-tetrachlorodibenzo-*p*-dioxin (TCDD) at Seveso, Italy. *Ecotoxicol. Environ. Safety* 4:282.

Rudner, E. F. 1973. Epidemiology of contact dermatitis in North America. *Arch. Dermatol.* 108:537–540.

Shelley, W. B., and Horvath, P. N. 1950. Experimental miliaria in man. II. Production of sweat retention anhidrosis and miliaria crystallina by various kinds of injury. *J. Invest. Dermatol.* 1:9–30.

Shopsis, C., Borenfreund, E., and Stark, D. M. 1987. Validation studies on a battery of potential in vitro alternatives to the Draize test. In *Alternative methods in toxicology*, vol. 5, ed. A. M. Goldberg, pp. 31–44. New York: Mary Ann Liebert.

World Health Organization. 1976. Polychlorinated Biphenyls and Terphenyls. Environmental Health Criteria 2. Geneva: WHO.

APPENDIX 14-1   PRIMARY IRRITATION*

Primary irritation of the skin is measured by a patch-test technique on the abraded and intact skin of the albino rabbit clipped free of hair. A minimum of six subjects is used per preparation tested. The method consists in introducing under a 1-in^2 patch 0.5 ml (in case of liquids) or 0.5 g (in cases of solids and semisolids) of the test substance. It is also desirable in the case of solids to attempt solubilizing in an appropriate solvent (discussed earlier) and to apply the solution as for liquids. The animals are immobilized in an animal holder with patches secured in place by adhesive tape. The entire trunk of the animal is then wrapped with rubberized cloth for the entire 24-h period of exposure. This latter procedure aids in maintaining the test patches in position, and, in addition, retards the evaporation of volatile substances. After the 24 h of exposure the patches are removed and the resulting reactions are evaluated on the basis of scores in Table A-1. Readings are made also after 72 h, and the final score represents an average of 24- and 72-h readings. An equal number of exposures are made on areas of skin that have been previously abraded. The abrasions are minor incisions through the stratum corneum, but not sufficiently deep to disturb the derma (that is, not sufficiently deep to produce bleeding).

The total erythema and edema scores are added in both the 24- and 72-h readings, and the averages of the scores for intact and abraded skin are combined; this combined average is referred to as the primary irritation index. It is useful for placing compounds in general groups with reference to irritant properties.

Compounds producing combined averages (primary irritation indexes) of 2 or less are only mildly irritating; those with indexes from 2 to 5 are moderate irritants, and those with scores above 6 are considered severe irritants.

*From Draize, 1959.

Table A-1   Evaluation of Skin Reactions

Erythema and eschar formation	
No erythema	0
Very slight erythema (barely perceptible)	1
Well-defined erythema	2
Moderate to severe erythema	3
Severe erythema (beet redness) to slight eschar formation (injuries in depth)	4
Total possible erythema score	4
Edema formation	
No edema	0
Very slight edema (barely perceptible)	1
Slight edema (edges of area well defined by definite raising)	2
Moderate edema (raised approximately 1 mm)	3
Severe edema (raised more than 1 mm and extending beyond area of exposure)	4
Total possible edema score	4

Toxicology of the Eye

CHAPTER 15 CONTENTS

GENERAL CONSIDERATIONS

Although the eyes are relatively small, they are important to one's well-being and they are complex in structure.

The eye is a spherical body that is covered mainly by three coats of tissues: the sclera, choroids, and retina. These coats mainly consist of, respectively, fibrous tissues, pigments and blood vessels, and nerve fibers, cells, and special receptors. They are nontransparent. However, light is admitted through the front of the eye, where the three coats are replaced by a number of tissues, notably the cornea and the lens (Fig. 15-1a).

The cornea is a continuum of the sclera. It consists of a relatively thick stroma and is covered, in front, by an epithelium, consisting of several layers of cells and Bowman's membranes, and, behind, by Descemet's membrane and an endothelium. The cornea and the front portion of the sclera as well as the inside of the eyelids are covered by a thin layer of conjunctiva.

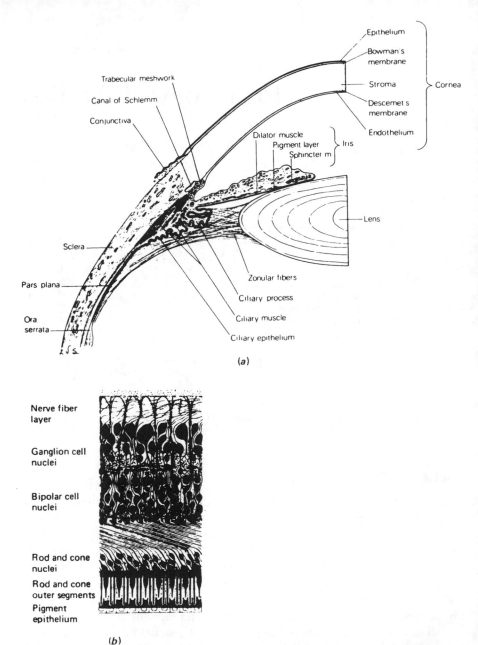

Figure 15-1 (*a*) Cross section of the anterior chamber angle and surrounding structures (from Vaughan and Asbury, 1983; copyright © 1983 by Lange Medical Publications). (*b*) Cross section of the retina (from Polyak, 1940, copyright © 1940 by University of Chicago Press).

The lens consists of transparent fibers enclosed in the lens capsule. It is suspended by the ciliary zonule to the ciliary body and its curvature is adjustable by the contraction and relaxation of the ciliary muscle.

The space between the lens and the cornea is filled with the aqueous humor. Also in this space and immediately in front of the lens is the iris. It is rich in blood vessels and heavily pigmented. The iris has a central opening, the pupil. Filling the space between the lens and retina is the vitreous humor.

The retina is the ocular structure that responds to light stimuli. It consists of several layers (Fig. 15-1b). The outermost is a pigmented epithelium. Next to it are the retinal rods and cones, which are the light-responsive neural structures. They are connected via the bipolar cells to the ganglion cells. The axons from the latter cells converge and exit from the eye at the optic papilla as the optic nerve.

Because of their diverse physiologic nature and spatial relations, these various ocular structures may exhibit a variety of effects as a result of exposure to toxicants.

TOXICANTS AND SITES OF THEIR EFFECTS

Cornea

The cornea is a delicate structure and is subject to toxic effects of chemicals, mainly from external exposure. Chemicals that affect the cornea include acids and alkalies, detergents, organic solvents, and smog. Acids and alkalies can readily damage the cornea. The extent of damage ranges from minor, superficial destruction of the tissue, which heals completely, to opacity of the cornea or even perforation. Acid burns are related to the low pH as well as the affinity of the anion for the corneal tissue. The effects of alkalies usually have slower onset than those caused by acids and are essentially pH dependent. However, ammonium ion, which is present in many household products, penetrates the cornea more readily and can thereby affect the iris (Potts, 1993).

Detergents are useful household and industrial products. In general, the nonionic detergents are less damaging than the ionic agents, and the cationics are more damaging than the anionics (Draize and Kelley, 1952). Organic solvents, such as acetone, hexane, and toluene, may enter the eye as a result of industrial or laboratory accidents. These substances can dissolve fat and damage the corneal epithelial cells.

Smog is a mixture of industrial smoke and fog. However, it now refers more often to the photochemical reaction products of automobile exhaust (see chap. 21). These products accumulate under certain meteorologic conditions. They affect mainly the respiratory tract, but even at low concentrations they irritate the corneal sensory nerve endings and cause reflex lacrimation.

Other chemicals can affect the cornea following systemic administration. These include quinacrine, chloroquine, and chlorpromazine. Potts (1993) reviewed the corneal effects of these drugs and other chemicals. They affect the cornea likely via tears and/or after passing through the blood–aqueous barrier. However, they affect humans only rarely and only after large doses.

Iris, Aqueous Humor, and Ciliary Body

Because of its proximity to the cornea, the iris is susceptible to physical trauma and chemical irritation. The effects of such irritation consists of leakage of serum proteins and fibrin as well as leukocytes from the blood vessels. These may be followed by fibroblast metaplasia. Severe damages to the iris cause liberation of melanin granules from the posterior epithelium of the iris.

The *iris* is innervated by sympathetic nerves (for the dilator muscles) and parasympathetic nerves (for the constrictor muscles). Therefore, the pupil can be dilated by chemicals that are sympathomimetic or parasympatholytic, and it can be constricted by parasympathomimetic and sympatholytic chemicals. Furthermore, the size of the pupil can be altered via the central nervous system by chemicals such as morphine and general anesthetics.

The *aqueous humor* is secreted by the epithelium of the ciliary body into the posterior chamber. It flows through the pupil into the anterior chamber and drains through the canal of Schlemm at the angle of the anterior chamber. Inflammatory changes of the iris can block the drainage of the fluid through the canal of Schlemm and raise the intraocular pressure, thereby inducing glaucoma. Atropine and other mydriatics may also precipitate glaucoma by dilating the pupil, thus blocking the drainage. Corticosteroids, applied topically or systematically, can also increase the intraocular pressure and cause glaucoma.

In the *ciliary body* is the ciliary muscle, the contraction of which allows relaxation of the ciliary zonule, which in turn allows the lens capsule to assume a more spherical form. This muscle is parasympathetically innervated; therefore, cholinesterase inhibitors and parasympatholytic agents such as atropine can cause the lens to be fixed in different states of visual accommodation.

Lens

A number of chemicals are known to alter the lenticular transparency, resulting in the formation of cataract. Examples are 2,4-dinitrophenol, corticosteroids, busulfan, triparanol, and thallium. Their cataractogenic property has been noted in humans as well as animals, such as the rabbit, rat, and young fowl. The effects generally follow systemic exposure, but with certain chemicals (e.g., corticosteroids, anticholinesterases), they may occur after topical application (Woods et al., 1967; Axelsson, 1968).

Diabetic patients are more likely to have cataracts, which can also be produced in rats and rabbits rendered diabetic with alloxan or streptozotocin (Heywood, 1982).

In addition, rats fed large amounts of galactose develop cataract (Sippel, 1966). This condition may be comparable to the cataract observed in infants with galactosemia. Such galactosemia results from a metabolic inability, inherited as an autosomal recessive trait, to convert galactose to glucose because of absence of the enzyme galactose-1-phosphate uridylyl transferase (Kinosita, 1965).

On the other hand, deficiencies of certain nutrients may also induce cataract. These nutrients include tryptophan, proteins, vitamin E, riboflavin, and folic acid (Gehring, 1971).

The mechanism underlying the formation of cataract is not fully understood. It is likely that it varies with the nature of the toxicant. For example, corticosteroid cataract may be mediated through an inhibition of protein synthesis in the lens (Ono, 1972). Busulfan may act through an interference of mitosis of the lenticular epithelial cells (Grimes and von Sallmann, 1966). Triparanol may interfere with the Na^+ pump, resulting in an increase of Na^+ and water in the lens (Harris and Gruber, 1972). The effect of dinitrophenol is likely to be mediated through the uncoupling of oxidative phosphorylation (see also chap. 4).

An extensive review of cataractogenic chemicals has been prepared by Gehring (1971). These chemicals are listed in Appendix 15-1.

Apart from cataractogenic effects, transient lens opacity has been noted in young beagle dogs following administration of some tranquilizers, some diuretics, and diisophenol. In addition, the transparency and refraction of the lens may also be altered by dimethyl sulfoxide and p-chlorophenylalanine (Heywood, 1982).

Retina

Certain polycyclic compounds, such as chloroquine, hydroxychloroquine, and thioridazine, can induce retinopathy in humans and animals. They affect the visual acuity, dark adaptation, and retinal pigment pattern. Hyperoxia and iodate also may induce retinal changes. Meier-Ruge (1972) reviewed the literature on various retinopathic chemicals.

Different mechanisms are involved in these retinal effects. Inhibition of protein metabolism in the pigment epithelium has been suggested as the primary toxic effect of chloroquine and hydroxychloroquine, which have strong affinity for melanin (Meier-Ruge, 1972). Increased oxygen supply to the retina induces vasoconstriction, which is associated with a decrease in the supply of nutrients. The latter effect is probably responsible for the hyperoxia-induced retinal changes. Iodate apparently affects the pigment epithelium, the derangement of which results in degeneration of the rod layer. A recent review of the various modes of action has been provided by Heywood (1982). These include the early formation of membranous cytoplasmic bodies (myeloid bodies), degenerative changes in the cell body of the rods and cones, derangement of the intracytoplasmic rods, and the appearing of vacuoles around these rods in the tapetum.

More recently, Leong et al. (1987) reported that an important chemical intermediate, 4,4-methylenedianiline, a well-known hepatotoxicant, induces degeneration of the inner and outer segments of the photoreceptor cells in albino and pigmented guinea pigs. Other retinal effects include hemorrhage from rupture of blood vessels or disturbance of blood clotting mechanism and exudates, which may cause partial detachment of retina.

Optic Nerve

As noted earlier, the retina contains, among other structures, the ganglion cells, the axons of which form the optic nerve. Toxicants can affect either the ganglion cells or the optic nerve. Damage to one of them often results in the degeneration of the other.

Some toxicants affect mainly the central vision. The most notable example is methanol. Others include carbon disulfide, disulfuram, ethambutol, and thallium. On the other hand, quinine, chloroquine, pentavalent arsenic, and carbon monoxide cause constriction of visual fields by damaging the structures responsible for peripheral vision. Interestingly, nitrobenzol affects both the central and peripheral vision (Harrington, 1976).

While methylmercury also causes constriction of visual field, its toxic effect is on the visual cortex instead of the optic nerve (chap. 20).

These toxicants can also be classified according to their effects on other peripheral nerves. For example, quinine, ethambutol, and methanol generally do not affect other peripheral nerves, while carbon disulfide, disulfiram, and thallium cause both optic and peripheral neuropathies. It is worthy of note that certain organic solvents can induce peripheral neuropathy but spare the visual system. These include tri-o-cresyl phosphate, acrylamide, n-hexane, and methyl n-butyl ketone (Grant, 1980).

Clioquinol (also known as Vioform and Entero-Vioform) was widely used for the prevention and treatment of "traveler's diarrhea." It has reportedly caused more than 10,000 cases of SMON (subacute myelo-opticoneuropathy), a disease affecting the optic nerves, spinal tracts, and peripheral nerves (Potts, 1993).

TESTING PROCEDURES

Effects on the eye can be examined after topical application of the toxicants. In addition, systemic administration can also result in ocular alterations. Several types of examinations are available.

Albino rabbits are commonly used to determine the ocular irritancy of ophthalmic medications and other chemicals that might come in contact with the eye. Dogs and nonhuman primates (rhesus monkeys) have also been used. For effects on the lens, retina, and optical nerve, many species of animals are used, such as rat, rabbit, cat, dog, monkey, and pig.

Gross Examination

The test described by Draize and Kelley (1952) has been a standard procedure for testing ocular irritancy. It specifies the use of nine rabbits. Into one eye of each rabbit is instilled 0.1 ml of the test material. In three of the nine rabbits, the test material is washed with 20 ml of lukewarm water 2 s after the instillation, and in three others, the washing is done with a 4-s delay. In the three remaining rabbits, the material is left in the eye. The ocular reactions are read with the unaided eye or with the aid of a slit-lamp at 24, 48, and 72 h and at 4 and 7 d after treatment. The reactions of the conjunctiva (redness, chemosis, and discharge), cornea (the degree and extent of opacity), and iris (congestion, swelling, and circumcorneal injection) are scored according to a specified scale. A series of colored pictures, originally provided by the U.S. Food and Drug Administration in 1965 as a guide for grading eye irritation, are available from the U.S. Consumer Product Safety Commission, Washington, DC 20207. Samples were reproduced in Hackett and McDonald (1995).

Several modified versions of the Draize and Kelley test have been proposed. Griffith et al. (1980) reported on their results of assessing eye irritancy of a large number of substances. The irritancy ranged from nil to corrosive. The authors recommend that the following points be taken into account in conducting eye irritation tests:

1 A 0.01-ml dose, or its weight equivalent for solids and powders, should be applied directly to the central corneal surface of at least six eyes without subsequent rinsing or manipulation of the eyelids.

2 Evaluation of the irritancy should be based on the median duration for the eyes to return to normal, instead of using a scoring system based on the type and extent of the effects.

The latest U.S. federal agency regulation (Consumer Product Safety Commission, 1988) requires the use of six albino rabbits for each test substance. For test liquids 0.1 ml is used, and for solids and pastes, 100 mg. The test material is instilled into one eye of each rabbit without washing. Ocular examinations are done after 24, 48, and 72 h. A rabbit is considered as having a positive reaction if the eye shows, on any examination, ulceration or opacity of the cornea, inflammation of the iris, or swelling of the conjunctiva with partial eversion of the eyelids.

Another variation of the Draize procedure calls for the use of three rabbits whose eyes are examined at 1, 24, 48, and 72 h. However, only one albino rabbit should be used first, if marked effects are expected. Furthermore, if it is thought that the substance could cause unreasonable pain, a local anesthetic should be used. The grading of the eye irritation is shown in Appendix 15-2.

Instrumental Examinations

Ophthalmoscopy The ophthalmoscope is used in assessing effects of toxicants on various parts of the retina. The examination is generally intended to discover the existence of edema, hyperemia or pallor, atrophy of the optic disk, pigmentation, or the state of the blood vessels. Changes in the vitreous humor, lens, aqueous humor, iris, and cornea can also be revealed.

Visual Perimetry Effect on the visual field can be readily determined in humans, but not in laboratory animals, except the nonhuman primates. Merigan (1979) described a procedure using macaque monkeys to demonstrate the loss of peripheral vision resulting from exposure to methylmercury.

Other Procedures Visual acuity and color vision are sensitive and useful indicators of effects on the visual system in humans. Procedures involving instrumentation, such as electro-oculography, and visual-evoked responses are also useful and can be incorporated in animal experimentation (Grant, 1980).

Histologic and Biochemical Examinations

Light microscopy can usually pinpoint the site of action of toxicants, electron microscopy can demonstrate ultrastructural changes, and biochemical studies can reveal the mechanism of toxic effects. For example, with light microscopy chloroquine has been observed to cause a thickening of the pigment epithelium, followed by migration of the pigment to the outer nuclear layer, and finally total atrophy of the photoreceptors (Meier-Ruge, 1968). Electron microscopy showed mitochondrial swelling and disorganization of the endoplasmic reticulum in the photoreceptor inner segment (Solze and McConnell, 1970). Biochemical studies revealed inhibition of many enzymatic reactions, especially those related to protein metabolism of the pigment epithelium.

In Vitro Tests   Because of humane concerns about the use of animals in eye irritation tests, a number of in vitro tests have been developed. They involve the use of cells from isolated cornea and chorioallantoic membrane and measuring their uptake of dyes, such as neutral red, as an indicator of toxicity. A number of other procedures have been proposed (see Frazier et al., 1987). However, these tests apparently require much refinement and extensive validation.

EVALUATION

Eye irritation tests are widely used to assess the ocular irritancy of chemicals. In general, the albino rabbit is the animal of choice. Some intralaboratory and interlaboratory variations in the scores were noted in a collaborative study (Marzulli and Ruggles, 1973). Nevertheless, periodic collaborative studies tend to improve the reliability of the scores. The various modifications made on the Draize test also tend to reduce the variability of the results.

A large number of animal experimentations and clinical studies indicate that there is a fair correlation between humans and animals in their reactions to toxicants with respect to cataract formation and retinopathy (Grant, 1980; Potts, 1993).

REFERENCES

Axelsson, U. 1968. Glaucoma, miotic therapy and cataract. III. Visual loss due to lens changes in glaucoma eyes treated with paraoxon (Mintacol), echothiophate or pilocarpine. *Acta Ophthalmol.* 46:831.

Consumer Product Safety Commission. 1988. Test for Eye Irritants. Code of Federal Regulations, Title 16. Federal Hazardous Substances Act Regulation, Part 1500.42.

Draize, J. H., and Kelley, E. A. 1952. Toxicity to eye mucosa of certain cosmetic preparations containing surface-active agents. *Proc. Sci. Sect. Toilet Goods Assoc.* 17:1–4.

Frazier, J. M., Gad, S. C., Goldberg, A. M., and McCalley, J. P. 1987. *A critical evaluation of alternatives to acute irritation testing.* New York: Mary Ann Liebert.

Gehring, P. J. 1971. The cataractogenic activity of chemical agents. *CRC Crit. Rev. Toxicol.* 1:93–118.

Grant, W. M. 1980. The peripheral visual system as a target. In *Experimental and clinical neurotoxicology,* eds. B. S. Spencer and H. H. Schaumburg. Baltimore: Williams & Wilkins.

Griffith, J. F., Nixon, G. A., Bruce, R. D., Reer, P. J., and Bannan, E. A. 1980. Dose-response studies with chemical irritants in the albino rabbit eye as a basis for selecting optimum testing conditions for predicting hazard to the human eye. *Toxicol. Appl. Pharmacol.* 55: 501–513.

Grimes, P., and Von Sallmann, L. 1966. Interference with cell proliferation and induction of polyploidy in rat lens epithelium during prolonged Myleran treatment. *Exp. Cell Res.* 62: 265–273.

Hackett, R. B., and McDonald, T. O. 1995. Assessing ocular irritation. In *Dermatotoxicology*, eds. F. N. Marzulli and H. I. Maibach. Washington, DC: Taylor & Francis.

Harrington, D. O. 1976. *The visual fields.* St. Louis, MO: Mosby.

Harris, J. E., and Gruber, L. 1972. Reversal of triparanol-induced cataracts in the rat. II. Exchange of ^{22}NA, ^{42}K, ^{86}Rb in cataractous and clearing lenses. *Invest. Ophthalmol. Visual Sci.* 11:608–616.

Heywood, R. 1982. Histopathological and laboratory assessment of visual dysfunction. *Environ. Health Perspect.* 44:35–45.

Kinosita, J. H. 1965. Cataracts in galactosemia. *Invest. Ophthalmol. Visual Sci.* 4:786–799.

Leong, B. K. J., Lund, J. E., Groehn, J. A., Coombs, J. K., Sabaitis, C. P., Weaver, R. J., and Griffin, R. L. 1987. Retinopathy from inhaling 4,4-methylenedianiline aerosols. *Fundam. Appl. Toxicol.* 9:645–658.

Marzulli, F. N., and Ruggles, D. I. 1973. Rabbit eye irritation test: Collaborative study. *J. Am. Assoc. Anal. Chem.* 56:905–914.

Meier-Ruge, M. 1968. The pathophysiological morphology of the pigment epithelium and its importance for retinal structure and function. *Med. Prob. Ophthalmol.* 8:32–48.

Meier-Ruge, W. 1972. Drug induced retinopathy. *CRC Crit. Rev. Toxicol.* 1:325–360.

Merigan, W. H. 1979. Effects of toxicants on visual systems. *Neurobehav. Toxicol.* 1(suppl. 1):1522.

Organization for Economic Cooperation and Development. 1987. *OECD guidelines for testing of chemicals.* Paris: OECD.

Ono, S. 1972. Presence of corticol-binding protein in the lens. *Ophthal. Res.* 3:233–240.

Potts, A. M. 1993. Toxic responses of the eye. In *Casarett and Doull's toxicology*, eds. M. O. Amdur, J. Doull, and C. D. Klaassen. New York: McGraw-Hill.

Polyak, S. 1940. *The retina.* Chicago: University of Chicago Press.

Sippel, T. O. 1966. Changes in water, protein and glutathione contents of the lens in the course of galactose cataract development in rats. *Invest. Ophthalmol. Visual Sci.* 5:568–575.

Solze, D. A., and McConnell, D. G. 1970. Ultrastructural changes in the rat photoreceptor inner segment during experimental chloroquine retinopathy. *Ophthal. Res.* 1:140–148.

Vaughan, D., and Ashbury, T. 1983. *General ophthalmology*, 10th ed. Los Altos, CA: Lange.

Woods, D. C., Contaxis, I., Sweet, D., Smith, J. C. II, and Van Dolah, J. 1967. Response of rabbits to corticosteroids. I. Influence on growth, intraocular pressure and lens transparency. *Am. J. Ophthalmol.* 63:841–849.

Appendix 15-1   Cataractogenic Chemicals

Sugars (glucose, galactose, xylose)
Streptozotocin
Corticosteroids
Naphthalene
Tyrosine
2,4-Dinitrophenol (DNP) and related
   compounds
Alkylating agents
Mimosine (leucenol)
Methoxsalen
Methionine sulfoximine
Polyriboinosinic acid polyribocytidylic acid
Quietidine [1,4-bis (phenylisopropyl)-
   piperazine . 2HCl]
N-Phenyl-β-hydrazinopropionitriles and
   related compounds
4-[3(7-Chloro-5,11-dihydrodibenz[b,e]
   [1,4]-oxyazepin-5-YL) propyl]-1-
   piperazineethanol dichloride

Anticholinesterases
Chlorpromazine
Triparanol
Dimethyl sulfoxide (DMSO)
2,4,6-Trinitrotoluene (TNT)
Sympathomimetic drugs and morphine-
   like drugs
2,6-Dichloro-4-nitroaniline
Iodoacetic acid
Mephenytoin
Diquat
Oral contraceptives
Sulfaethoxypyridazine
Thallium
Heptachlor

Desferal
Thioacetamide

Source: Gehring (1971).

Appendix 15-2   Grading of Eye Irritation

Description	Grade
Cornea	
No ulceration or opacity	0
Scattered or diffuse areas of opacity (other than slight dulling of normal lustre), details of iris clearly visible	1
Easily discernible translucent area, details of iris slightly obscured	2
Nacrous area, no details of iris visible, size of pupil barely discernible	3
Opaque cornea, iris not discernible through the opacity	4
Iris	
Normal	0
Markedly deepened rugae, congestion, swelling, moderate circumcorneal hyperaemia, or injection, any of these or combination of any thereof, iris still reacting to light (sluggish reaction is positive)	1
No reaction to light, haemorrhage, gross destruction (any or all of these)	2
Conjunctivae	
Redness (refers to palpebral and bulbar conjunctivae, cornea, and iris)	0
Blood vessels normal	
Some blood vessels definitely hyperemic (injected)	1
Diffuse, crimson color, individual vessels not easily discernible	2
Diffuse beefy red	3
Chemosis: lids and/or nictating membranes	0
No swelling	
Any swelling above normal (includes nictitating membranes)	1
Obvious swelling with partial eversion of lids	2
Swelling with lids about half closed	3
Swelling with lids more than half closed	4

Source: OECD (1987).

Toxicology of the Nervous System

CHAPTER 16 CONTENTS

INTRODUCTION

As a vital part of the body, the nervous system is shielded from toxicants in the blood by a unique protective mechanism, namely, the blood–brain and blood–nerve barriers. Nonetheless, it is susceptible to a variety of toxicants. For example, methylmercury affects mainly the nervous system, although its concentration in the brain is comparable to that in most other tissues, and in fact it is much lower than that in the liver and kidneys.

The greater susceptibility may be attributed partly to the fact that neurons have a high metabolic rate, with little capacity for anaerobic metabolism. Furthermore, being electrically excitable, neurons tend to lose cell membrane integrity more readily. The great length of the axons is another reason why the nervous system is especially susceptible to toxic effects, since the cell body must supply its axon structurally and metabolically.

To facilitate the description of the various types of toxic effects and the procedures for their testing, the various parts of the nervous system are presented.

Central and Peripheral Nervous Systems

The system consists of two major parts: the central nervous system (CNS) and the peripheral nervous system (PNS). The CNS is made up of the brain and the spinal cord, and the PNS includes the cranial and spinal nerves, which are either motor or sensory. The neurons of the sensory spinal nerves are located in the ganglia in the dorsal roots. In addition, the PNS also includes the sympathetic nerve system, which arises from neurons in the thoracic and lumbar region of the spinal cord, and the parasympathetic system, which stems from nerve fibers leaving the CNS via the cranial nerves and the sacral spinal roots.

Cells and Appendages

The principal cells in the nervous system are neurons, composed of perikarya, along with their dendrites and axons. These structures are responsible for the conduction of nerve impulses. The main supporting structure consists of various types of glial cells. Apart from a lack of conductivity, the glial cells differ from neurons in that the former, as most other types of cells, do reproduce whereas the latter do not.

In the CNS the glial cells include astrocytes, oligodendrocytes (oligodendroglia), and microglia. Astrocytes help maintain a proper microenvironment around the neurons and support the blood–brain barrier. Oligodendroglia surround the axons in the CNS with a lipid-rich material, the myelin sheath, which provides electrical insulation. Microglia are basically macrophages that are located in the CNS. In the PNS the Schwann cells provide the myelin sheath that wraps around the axon. The myelin sheath is interrupted by the nodes of Ranvier.

Neurotransmitters

Neurons are connected, via their axons, to other neurons at their dendrites or to the receptors in the glands or muscles. At nerve terminals, on excitation by an action potential, chemical neurotransmitters are released. The most common transmitters are acetylcholine and norepinephrine. However, there are several amine neurotransmitters in addition to norepinephrine, dopamine, serotonin, and histamine. Furthermore, the following amino acids also act as neurotransmitters: γ-aminobutyric acid (GABA), glycine, glutamate, and aspartate. These transmitters are small molecules and act rapidly. They are synthesized in the presynaptic terminals. These neurotransmitters are presynthesized, stored in synaptic vesicles, and released upon excitation. Nitric oxide (NO), a recently discovered neurotransmitter, is different from the others in that, as a labile free radical, it is not presynthesized for storage in synaptic vesicles. It is synthesized, on demand, from L-arginine by NO synthase (Zhang and Snyder, 1995).

In addition to these small molecule neurotransmitters, a large number of neuropeptides are slow-acting neurotransmitters/modulators. Some are released by the pituitary gland: ACTH, β-endorphin, growth hormone, thyrotropin, oxytocin, and vasopressin. A number of peptide transmitters act on gut and brain, such as leucine enkephalin and methionine enkephalin.

Blood–Brain and Blood–Nerve Barriers

These barriers protect the nervous system from certain neurotoxicants. Difference in neurotoxicity sometimes can be explained on the basis of these barriers.

Blood–Brain Barrier (BBB)   The endothelium in the brain is impermeable to substances of medium molecular weight, such as horseradish perioxidase (mol. wt. 40,000; diameter 5–6 nm), because the adjacent cells are tightly joined. Further, these cells have few micropinocytotic vesicles, which in capillaries of other tissues serve as an important transport mechanism across endothelial cells. However, highly lipid-soluble substances and the nonionized fraction of a chemical are more permeable across the BBB. It is, therefore, similar to intact cell membranes in permeability.

The BBB is absent where the cells produce hormones or act as hormonal or chemoreceptors. Glutamate and a number of related compounds, such as aspartate, have been shown to affect areas in the brain not protected by the BBB, such as the arcuate nucleus of the hypothalamus and the area postrema in various laboratory animals. These effects, while not observed in humans, are of interest because they may be used as tools in the study of such clinical conditions as Huntington's disease, drug-induced parkinsonism, tardive dyskinesia, and sulfur amino acidopathies.

The BBB is effective in excluding many neurotoxicants, such as diphtheria, staphylococcus, and tetanus toxins. This is also true with doxorubicin, which affects the dorsal root ganglia but not the CNS. Mercury chloride has a small molecule but is hydrophilic and mainly in ionic form. Its concentration in the brain is minimal and so are its CNS effects. On the other hand, methylmercury is lipophilic and thus readily crosses the BBB, thereby damaging the brain.

Blood–Nerve Barrier (BNB)   Peripheral nerves are covered by two connective tissue sheaths, the perineurium and epineurium, and interlaced with the endoneurium. The BNB is provided by the blood vessels in the endoneurium and supplemented by the lamellated cells of the perineural sheath. It is not as effective as the BBB; therefore, the dorsal root glanglia are generally more susceptible than the neurons in the CNS to neurotoxicants. For example, doxorubicin affects neurons in the dorsal root ganglia but not those in the brain.

NEUROTOXIC EFFECTS AND NEUROTOXICANTS

The effects may be classified according to the site of action. These include the neurons, the axons, the glial cells, and the vascular system. A toxicant, however, may affect more than one site. The following is a brief description of certain neurotoxic effects, along with the putative mode of action, grouped according to the site of action.

Figure 16-1 depicts damages to neurons, axons and myelin sheath. *Neuronopathy* is represented by the damage to a second-order sensory neuron (4), which innervates corpuscle A, and a neuron in the dorsal root ganglion (3), which innervates corpuscle B. *Axonopathy* is represented by the damaged central axonal process of a sensory neuron that innervates corpuscle C, and the axons of the lower motor neurons (2) that innervate muscle fibers D and E. *Myelinopathy* is shown along the axons of upper (1) and lower (2) motor neurons that innervate muscle fiber F.

Figure 16-1 Cellular target sites of some neurotoxic chemicals illustrated by upper (1) and lower (2) motor neurons, dorsal root ganglion cells (3), and second-order sensory neurons (4) in the gracile nucleus of the medulla oblongata. The central nervous system (CNS) is represented above the sloping horizontal line, the peripheral nervous system (PNS) below. The peripheral receptors on fibers A–C are pacinian corpuscles. Fibers D–F innervate extrafusal muscle fibers. (a), Axonal degeneration; (d), demyelination; (r), remyelinatiion of ventral root and medulla oblongata. Adapted from Spencer et al. (1980).

Some neurotoxicants that induce these and other damages are described next.

Neuronopathy

Neurons, being dependent mainly on glucose as an energy source, are susceptible to anoxic and hypoglycemic conditions. A number of chemicals are well known for their anoxigenic effects in the brain. Barbiturates induce anoxia in the brain, especially in certain areas of the cerebral cortex: hippocampus and cerebellum. Permanent CNS damage even after barbiturate coma, however, is rare, possibly because of the reduced cell metabolism. On the other hand, prolonged exposure to carbon monoxide may induce permanent effects in the brain, arising from the development of a diffuse sclerosis of the white matter (leukoencephalopathy). Cyanide and azide inhibit cytochrome oxidase, thereby producing cytotoxic anoxia.

The cell body of neurons may be affected directly by toxicants. Methylmercury first causes focal loss of ribosomes and then disintegration and disappearance of the Nissl substances, especially in the small cells. These are followed by nuclear and perinuclear changes and finally by the loss of the entire neuron including its axon (Jacobs et al., 1977). Doxorubicin (Adriamycin) affects neurons by intercalating with DNA, leading to a breakdown of the helical structures (Cho et al., 1980). This derangement inhibits the synthesis of RNA and neuronal protein. Since this drug does not cross the blood–brain barrier, it can affect the neurons in the dorsal root ganglia (Fig. 16-1, B) and autonomic ganglia, but not those in the CNS. On the other hand, methylmercury does penetrate the blood–brain barrier and thus damages the neurons in the dorsal root ganglia as well as those in the CNS.

Organotins are used as pesticides and as plasticizers. Upon entering the nervous system, they accumulate in the Golgi-like structures in the cell body. The cells then undergo swelling and necrosis (Bouldin et al., 1981).

Aluminum also penetrates the BBB and induces encephalopathy with neurofibrillar degeneration in cat and rabbit and might be responsible for certain cases of Alzheimer's disease (DeBoni et al., 1976). A number of references to aluminum toxicity have been cited by Liu and Stemmer (1990).

Glutamate, alanosine, and related chemicals, in very large doses, are known to affect areas of the CNS devoid of BBB (see Blood–Brain Barrier subsection) and are considered as having neuroexcitatory and neurotoxic effects. The dendrites are the primary site of action. The perikarya are then affected, but the axons are spared (Fig. 16-1, A). The toxicity may be mediated through NO (Dawson et al., 1991). Kainic acid is derived from a particular seaweed and it has been used in ascariasis; it is similar to glutamate but much more potent (Olney et al., 1974).

Alcohol in pregnant women may induce in their offspring abnormalities in the nervous system including abnormal neuronal migration and abnormal development of dendritic spines (Abel et al., 1983).

Axonopathy

Some axons are very long (up to 1 m), and the elements in the axons, such as neurofibrils, are synthesized not locally but in the cell body and are transported along the axon. The axon may therefore be attacked either directly by toxicants or indirectly through damages to the cell body.

Lesions may occur either in the proximal or in the distal sections of axons.

Proximal Axonopathy β,β-Iminodiproprionitrile (IDPN) produces typical lesions of this type. It has therefore been used as a model to study motor neuron diseases such as amyotrophic lateral sclerosis. The primary effect of IDPN is the impairment of slow axonal transport of neurofilaments, probably through aberrant phosphorylation of neurofilaments (Gold and Austin, 1991), while their synthesis is continued in the cell body. The accumulation of neurofilaments in the proximal axon causes it to enlarge and the distal axon to atrophy (Fig. 16-1, E). The enlarged proximal axon in turn elicits local proliferation of the subpial astrocytic processes and extension of the processes filled with glial filaments along the proximal ventral root. The proximal swelling also stimulates splitting of myelin at the intraperiod line, formation of intramyelinic vacuoles, and ultimate demyelination. The Schwann cells in the demyelinated segment divide and remyelinate, and the repeated demyelination and remyelination give rise to "onion-bulb" formation (Griffin and Price, 1980). Abou-Donia (1995) found an increased aberrant phosphorylation of cytoskeletal proteins resulting in axonal swelling and decreased transport of neurofilament down the axon.

Distal Axonopathy Axons contain three types of neurofibrillary structures, namely, neurotubules, neurofilaments, and microfilaments. In addition, they contain mitochondria and smooth endoplasmic reticulum. These structures are especially susceptible to a variety of neurotoxicants. For example, thallium induces mitochondrial swelling and degeneration, and certain organophosphates and organic solvents cause derangement of the neurofibrillary structures, resulting in distal axonopathy.

An important type of distal axonopathy is produced by certain organophosphorus compounds such as TOCP (tri-o-cresyl phosphate), EPN, and leptophos. These compounds, besides inhibiting cholinesterase, cause *delayed neuropathy*, which manifests mainly as paralysis of muscles. It affects especially long and large nerve fibers; hence the hindlimbs are paralyzed before the forelimbs. Although a number of other animals may also be affected, especially after repeated exposures, this toxicity can be readily reproduced in hens, usually with a delay of 8–10 d after exposure. Because of the severity of delayed neurotoxicity, new organophosphorus chemicals are routinely tested for this potential hazard. The Organization for Economic Cooperation and Development (OECD, 1995) and U.S. Environmental Protection Agency (U.S. EPA, 1994) have published guidelines for such tests both after a single dose and after repeated administrations, using domestic hens. The condition is unrelated to cholinesterase inhibition because such potent inhibitors as malathion, parathion, and carbaryl do not possess this toxic property. It is apparently associated with phosphorylation of the enzyme neuropathy target esterase (NTE; formerly known as neurotoxic esterase) (Abou-Donia, 1981; Johnson, 1990). More recent studies indicate an increased aberrant phosphorylation of cytoskeletal proteins resulting in axonal swelling and decreased transport of neurofilament down the axon (Abou-Donia, 1995).

A different type of distal axonopathy is known to be caused by hexacarbons such as n-hexane and methyl n-butyl ketone. These solvents have caused toxic polyneuropathy among industrial workers, as has acrylamide. Both cause marked neurofilament proliferation in axons, probably as a result of altered phosphorylation of certain proteins (Berti-Mattera et al., 1990). However, giant axonal swellings are common with hexacarbons (Fig. 16-1, D), but rare with acrylamide. Furthermore, sensory nerves are involved early with acrylamide but late with hexacarbons, which affect certain motor nerves first. Vincristine may cause accumulation of neurofibrils in the perikarya and axons. It disrupts the axonal neurotubules and neurofilaments and blocks axoplasmic transport of these ultrastructures.

Clioquinol, a popular remedy and preventive for "travelers' diarrhea" in the 1960s and 1970s, induced disorders of the nervous system known as subacute myelo-opticoneuropathy (SMON) in thousands of individuals (Appendix 1-2). In humans and experimental animals, it causes central axonal degeneration of the dorsal root ganglion (Fig. 16-1, C), as well as the optic nerves (Worden et al., 1978).

Distal axonopathy has also been hypothesized as resulting from impairment of glycolytic enzyme activities in the axon (Spencer et al., 1979). These enzymes are responsible for the transport of neurofilaments, which are synthesized in the perikaryon and transported along the axon. Impairment of the activities of these enzymes would thus first affect the distal portion of the axon as well as the large, long nerve fibers, which have a greater energy demand on the perikarya. A second hypothesis postulates that the neurofilaments are directly affected by toxicants such as hexacarbons and acrylamide (Savolainen, 1977). Neurofilaments exposed to the toxicant for the longest period, namely, those located distally in long fibers, would be affected first.

Interference with Impulse Conduction   A number of toxicants act mainly on nerve membranes. These membranes normally maintain a negative resting potential. When stimulated, an action potential is generated. The resting and action potentials result from differences in the Na^+ and K^+ concentrations across the membrane, and their concentrations are maintained by the Na^+ channels. Tetrodotoxin, the toxic principle of puffer fish, has been shown to block the action potential by blocking the Na^+ channels. Saxitoxin, the toxic principle produced by the dinoflagellate *Gonyaulax* and taken up by the clam *Saxidomas giganteus*, also acts by blocking the sodium channels. Consumption of improperly cleaned puffer fish or contaminated clam can cause death by respiratory failure. The binding with saxitoxin, however, is more readily reversible. These toxins have been useful tools in investigating the mode of action of neurotoxins (Narahashi, 1974).

Interference with Synaptic Transmission   Botulinum toxin, the most potent biologic toxin, is produced by *Clostridium botulinum*. It causes paralysis of muscles by impairing the release of acetylcholine from motor nerve endings. Black widow spider venom, on the other hand, causes a massive release of acetylcholine and results in cramps and paralysis.

Tetanoplasmin, from the microbe *Clostridium tetani*, causes tetanus through its effect on the CNS. It blocks release of the inhibitory amino acid transmitters GABA and glycine, thereby causing spastic paralysis. The molecular weight of this proteinaceous dimer is about 150,000; therefore it is too large to cross the blood–brain barrier. However, it reaches the CNS by retrograde axonal transport (Schield et al., 1977).

DDT and pyrethroids are markedly different in chemical structure. However, their effects on the nervous systems are similar. They prolong the opening of the sodium channel, thereby initiating repetitive activity at the synapses and neuromuscular junctions (Narahashi, 1992).

Glial Cells and Myelin

Myelinating Cells   Demyelination can result from injuries to myelinating cells (oligodendrocytes and Schwann cells). Neurotoxins of this type include lead, which affects Schwann cells possibly by interfering with their $Ca2+$ transport. Hypocholesterolemic agents such as triparanol, as expected, disrupt myelin sheath because of the high (70%) lipid content of myelin. However, they produce ultrastructural changes in oligodendrocytes before demyelination occurs. Diphtheria toxin demyelinates, possibly by affecting both the myelin and the myelinating cells. Triethyltin, ethidium bromide, and actinomycin are other examples of demyelinating toxins that act on the myelinating cells.

Myelin Sheath   Demyelination can also result from effects on the myelin sheath. This type of effect generally involves a disruption of the membrane structure. Other modes of action include (1) inhibition of carbonic anhydrase or other enzymes involved in ion and water transport, (2) inhibition of enzymes involved in oxidative phosphorylation, and (3) chelation of metals. Neurotoxicants that act directly on the myelin sheath include triethyltin, lysolecithin, isoniazid, cyanate, hexachlorophene, and lead. Acetyl ethyl tetramethyl tetralin (AETT) also causes myelinopathy through a complex mechanism (Fig. 16-1, F).

Lead has been known for centuries as a serious neurotoxicant. It affects various parts of the nervous system, including myelin sheath. The PNS is affected before the CNS, while the reverse is true with the toxicants mentioned in the previous paragraph. In addition, lead affects motor nerves before the sensory, resulting in "wrist-drop" and "foot-drop." Its effects on the blood vessels are discussed next.

Blood Vessels and Edema

The permeability of the vascular system in the CNS and PNS may be increased by higher blood pressure or lower plasma osmolarity. It may also result from exposure to certain toxins. The greater permeability generally leads to an accumulation of fluids in the extracellular space. In addition, a number of neurotoxicants are known to induce cellular edema.

Extracellular Edema   Lead can damage the endothelial cells and cause extravasation of plasma in the brain, especially in the white matter, which has a greater compliance than the gray matter. That suckling rats are more susceptible to lead has been attributed to the immaturity of the vascular system (Press, 1977). Lead has similar effects in the endoneurium, leading to increased endoneural fluid pressure and demyelination. Organic lead, such as tetraethyllead, more readily penetrates the barriers and is therefore more toxic in this respect.

Mercury compounds can damage the endothelial cells and increase their permeability. Organic arsenicals cause edema and focal hemorrhages in the brain. Tellurium causes edema in the endoneurium. Chronic alcoholism is associated with endoneural edema.

Endoneural edema can also result from intramyelinic edema in hexachlorophene intoxication. It may also be associated with wallerian degeneration due to mechanical injury.

Cellular Edema   Various parts of neurons may become edematous following exposure to toxicants. For example, υ-aminonicotinamide affects the perikaryon, cyanide and carbon monoxide affect the axon, and ouabain and methylsulfoxime affect the presynaptic nerve endings.

Edema of astrocytes and oligodendrocytes may be caused by 6-aminonicotinamide. Ouabain can also affect astrocytes. Edema of Schwann cells may be induced by lead, which, as noted earlier, also may cause extracellular edema.

Triethyltin and isoniazid also cause edema of the myelin sheaths in the CNS. Hexachlorophene induces edema of the myelin sheaths both in the white matter of the brain and in the peripheral nerves.

TESTING PROCEDURES

Functional Observational Battery (FOB)

A battery of observations has been devised to assess the neurotoxic effects (U.S. EPA, 1994; Kallman and Fowler, 1994). These are done in intact animals, usually rats or mice, and can be incorporated in other tests (chap. 6). These animals are exposed to the toxicant at two or three doses by an appropriate route. The duration of treatment and observation period vary from days to months according to the nature of the toxicant.

The animals are observed for the following abnormalities:

1   Unusual body position, activity level, gait, etc.
2   Unusual behavior such as compulsive biting, self-mutilation, circling, and walking backward.
3   The presence of convulsions, tremors, lacrimation, red-colored tears, salivation, diarrhea, vocalization, etc.
4   Changes in sensory and motor functions (for details, see the following sections).

Neurologic Examinations

These examinations often provide an indication of the site of neurotoxicity; therefore they play a preliminary but important part. Most of these examinations can be performed in humans as well as in animals. The exceptions relate to the determination of mental state and many sensory functions, which can be more readily assessed in humans. However, appropriate behavioral tests are available for examining animals.

Cranial nerves I through XII have different functions, and their tests therefore vary. For example, tests of the acoustic and optic nerves involve the evaluation of responses to sound and light stimuli.

Motor examination includes inspection of muscles for weakness, atrophy, and fasciculation, which indicate dysfunction of the lower motor neuron, that is, the anterior horn cells, motor roots, and peripheral nerves. Spasticity is a sign of dysfunction of the upper motor neurons in the brain and their axons down to the spinal cord. Resting tremor is often associated with lesions in the basal ganglia or cerebellum. Intention tremor occurs during voluntary movement and is a manifestation of cerebellar disease.

Reflex examination includes deep tendon reflexes, the functioning of which involves the intrafusal receptors, dorsal root ganglia, anterior horn cells and their axons, neuromuscular junction, and muscle. Damages to any of these structures will cause these reflexes to be absent or hypoactive. On the other hand, when there is upper motor neuron dysfunction, these reflexes will be exaggerated. The Babinski reflex is the most important superficial cutaneous reflex. Abnormal response is an indication of cortico-spinal dysfunction.

Gait abnormalities may also aid in locating the site of toxicity. For example, lower motor neuron disease causes high-stepping gait. A scis-soring, or stiff, gait indicates upper motor neuron lesion. Cerebellar dys-function results in an ataxic or reeling gait.

Neurologic signs usually develop rapidly with neuronopathy and mye-linopathy but slowly with axonopathy. Axonopathy generally affects both the sensory and motor fibers. On the other hand, neuronopathy affects predominantly the sensory fibers and myelinopathy the motor fibers (Dewar, 1981).

Morphologic Examinations

As described in the section Categories of Neurotoxic Effects and depicted in Fig. 16-1, neurotoxicants may act on the CNS, the PNS, or both. They may induce lesions in the neuronal perikaryon or its axon, either proxi-mally or distally, the myelinating cells or the myelin sheath itself, the astrocytes, or the endothelial cells. Morphologic examinations are therefore important in establishing the precise site of toxic lesions on an anatomic level. Examinations on cellular and ultrastructural levels often facilitate the differential diagnosis of the neuropathy.

Some of the commonly used techniques, along with a list of references, have been provided by Spencer et al. (1980). It is worth noting, however, that damages to endothelial cells can be demonstrated not only by signs of edema (fewer cells and nerve fiber per unit area) but also by increases of the pressure of the intracranial and endoneural fluids as well as by the penetration of tracer substances, such as horseradish peroxidase, through the endothelium.

Electrophysiologic Examinations

Peripheral Nerves   A frequently used examination involves the mea-surement of *motor nerve* conduction velocity. This can be done on intact animals subjected to short-term or chronic exposure to neurotoxicants or on exposed nerves after local application of the toxicants. *Sensory nerve* conduction velocity and action potentials have also been measured in the study of neurotoxicity. deJesus et al. (1978) described a procedure using the sural nerve in rats and observed that hexachlorophene decreased the sensory nerve conduction velocity but had no effect on the amplitude of the action potential. On the other hand, zinc pyridinethione reduced the amplitude of the action potential but had no effect on the conduction velocity. Another useful procedure is the measurement of conduction velocity of *slow fibers* (Seppalainen and Hernberg, 1972).

Electromyography   This procedure calls for the examination of the electrical activities of a muscle, at rest and when contracted, recorded with the aid of a needle electrode inserted into the muscle. Neurotoxicities may manifest as (1) abnormal insertional activity, (2) occurrence of spontaneous electrical activity of a resting muscle, and (3) interference pattern of electrical activity of motor units during voluntary muscle contraction (Goodgold and Eberstein, 1977).

Biochemical Examinations

As noted earlier, the nervous system depends almost entirely on glucose metabolism for its energy. Since the enzyme systems involved in glucose metabolism are often the target of toxicants, their activities merit investigation, as do the systems involved in ion transport, which is vital to nerve impulse conduction. Protein synthesis is impaired by a number of neurotoxicants. The compositions of various subcellular structures and myelin sheath are also fruitful subjects of biochemical examination. The migration of radiolabeled materials along axons and transneurally is another useful procedure. Other biochemical parameters include the levels of neurotransmitters at specific sites in the nervous system and the binding of neurotransmitter receptors by the use of agonists and antagonists (Dewar, 1981). For certain organophosphorus esters, determination of NTE with a method described by, for example, Caroldi and Lotti (1982) is useful in assessing the potential for delayed neurotoxicity.

Nerve Cell Cultures

Apart from the various testing procedures described already, cells from fetal brain, the spinal cord, and dorsal root ganglia can be mechanically or enzymatically segregated and grown in suitable culture media. The cells grow and differentiate in the media. They can be subjected to electrophysiologic, morphologic, and biochemical examinations to assess the effects of neurotoxicants (Nelson, 1978).

BEHAVIORAL STUDIES

There is a large body of information on behavioral toxicology, resulting from a widespread feeling that behavior is a subtle and sensitive indicator of toxicity. However, this view has been questioned, for example, by Norton (1980), who stated: "Scientific data supporting this view are not only

scanty but the available evidence often flatly contradicts this assumption."
In the hope that improved testing procedures would increase the sensitivity
and utility of this approach in neurotoxicology, this branch of neurotoxicology will undoubtedly grow. A few highlights of this subject are presented next.

The tests involve two types of responses: (1) unconditioned responses,
which are either emitted (spontaneous) or elicited (reflex), and (2) condi-
tioned responses, which may be considered as either "classic conditioning"
(Pavlov) or operant conditioning (Skinner). The extent of training of the
experimental animals required and the neurobehavioral function to be assessed are also useful criteria for classification of the tests.

The U.S. EPA (1994) has provided some guidelines on schedule-
controlled operant behavior.

Simple Tests

Tilson et al. (1980) listed tests that require little or no prior training of the
experimental animals (rats and mice) (see Table 16-1).

Table 16-1 Examples of Primary Level Neurobehavioral Tests for Rats or Mice

Neurobehavioral function	Behavioral test
Sensory	
Visual, olfactory, somatosensory, auditory	Localization
Pain	Tail flick
Orientation in space	Negative geotaxis
Motor	
Spontaneous activity	Activity in Automex
Muscular weakness	Forelimb grip; hindlimb extensor
Fatigability	Swim endurance
Tremor	Frequency of occurrence
Cognitive-associative	
Learning and retention	One-way avoidance; step-through passive avoidance
Affective-emotional	
Responsiveness	Startle to air puff; emergence in a novel environment
Physiologic-consummatory	
Thermoregulation	Body weight; food and water ingestion; core temperature

Source: From Tilson et al. (1980). Reproduced with permission of Peter S. Spencer, editor.

More Involved Tests

The tests listed in Table 16-2 require extended or special training, frequent evaluation, and/or manipulation of motivational factors.

Procedures to Enhance Sensitivity

Because of the large functional reserve of the brain, focal damages may not result in any overt brain dysfunction. Such damages, however, may be demonstrated clinically with the use of *provocative* tests. These involve administering sodium amobarbital, raising body temperature, or lowering blood pH with the intravenous infusion of ammonium chloride (Lehrer, 1974).

Animals

Apart from rats and mice, other animals such as pigeons, cats, dogs, and monkeys are also commonly used, with testing procedures similar to those already listed.

Table 16-2 Examples of Secondary Level Neurobehavioral Tests for Rats or Mice

Neurobehavioral function	Behavioral test
Sensory	
Visual, auditory, olfactory	Operant psychophysics
Gustatory	Taste discrimination
Somatosensory	T-maze discrimination
Orientation in space	T-maze discrimination
Pain	Operant titration
Motor	
Spontaneous activity	Diurnal cyclicity; patterning
Muscular strength	Operant response force
Tremor	Spectral analysis
Cognitive-associative	
Learning and retention	Autoshaping; temporal discriminating; repeated acquisition
Affective-emotional	
CNS excitability	Brain self-stimulation; aversion thresholds
Physiologic–consummatory	
Thermoregulation	Diurnal patterning; cyclicity; preference

Source: From Tilson et al. (1980). Reproduced with permission of Peter S. Spencer, editor.

EVALUATION

In view of the wide range of toxic effects on the nervous system, as outlined earlier, there is clearly need for a battery of tests for the evaluation of neurotoxicants. It is also worth noting that the choice of animal species is critical in eliciting certain types of toxicity, such as delayed neurotoxicity. Furthermore, the nature of the toxicity on the nervous system, as on other organs, can vary according to the duration of exposure. For example, n-hexane and TOCP produce, after acute exposure, narcosis, a CNS effect, but they induce axonopathy after repeated exposures.

The significance of a neurotoxic effect depends on its reversibility. In general, irreversible effects are more serious than reversible ones. The site of the effect also plays an important role. There are areas in the nervous system more critical to physiologic function than others. In addition, focal damages in areas with abundant functional reserve are likely to be less serious.

The behavioral effects are especially susceptible to endogenous and environmental variations. For example, Norton (1980) reported data to indicate a large variability of results both between animals of the same species and within the same animal at different times. It is therefore important to adhere to proper experimental procedures, such as sufficiently large number of animals, rigorously controlled experimental environment, and statistical analysis of results.

REFERENCES

Abel, E. J., Jacobson, S., and Sherwin, B. J. 1983. *In utero* ethanol exposure: Functional and structural brain damage. *Neurobehav. Toxicol. Teratol.* 5:139–146.

Abou-Donia, M. B. 1981. Organophosphorus ester-induced delayed neurotoxicity. *Annu. Rev. Pharmacol. Toxicol.* 21:511–548.

Abou-Donia, M. B. 1995. Involvement of cytoskeletal proteins in the mechanisms of organophosphorus ester-induced delayed neurotoxicity. *Clin. Exper. Pharmacol. Physiol.* 22: 358–359.

Berti-Mattera, L.N., Eichberg, J., Schrama, L., and LoPachin, R.M. 1990. Acrylamide administration alters protein phosphorylation and phospholipid metabolism in rat sciatic nerve. *Toxicol. Appl. Pharmacol.* 103:502–511.

Bouldin, T. W., Gaines, N. D., Bagvell, C. R., and Krigman, M. R. 1981. Pathogenesis of trimethyltin neuronal toxicity. *Am. J. Pathol.* 104:237–249.

Caroldi, S., and Lotti, M. 1982. Neurotoxic esterase in peripheral nerve: Assay, inhibition, and rate of resynthesis. *Toxicol. Appl. Pharmacol.* 62:498–501.

Cho, E. S., Spencer, P. S., and Jortner, B. S. 1980. Doxorubicin. In *Experimental and clinical neurotoxicology*, eds. P. S. Spencer and H. H. Schaumberg, pp. 440–455. Baltimore: Williams & Wilkins.

Dawson, V. L., Dawson, T. M., London, E. D., Bredt, D. S., and Snyder, S. H. 1991. Nitric oxide mediates glutamate neurotoxicity in primary cortical culture. *Proc. Natl. Acad. Sci. USA* 88:6368–6371.

DeBoni, U., Otros, A., Scott, J. W., and Crapper, D. B. 1976. Neurofibrillary degeneration induced by systemic aluminum. *Acta Neuropathol.* 35:285–294.

deJesus, C. P. V., Towfighi, J., and Snyder, J. R. 1978. Sural nerve conduction study in the rat: A new technique for studying experimental neuropathies. *Muscle Nerve* 1:162–167.

Dewar, A. J. 1981. Neurotoxicity testing with particular reference to biochemical methods. In *Testing for toxicity*, ed. J. W. Gorrod, pp. 199–217. London: Taylor & Francis.

Gold, G. B., and Austin, D. R. 1991. Regulation of aberrant neurofilament phosphorylation in neuronal perikarya. *Brain. Res.* 563:151–162.

Goodgold, J., and Eberstein, A. 1977. *Electrodiagnosis of neuromuscular diseases*. Baltimore: Williams & Wilkins.

Griffin, J. W., and Price, D. L. 1980. Proximal axonopathies induced by toxic chemicals. In *Experimental and clinical neurotoxicology*, eds. P. S. Spencer and H. H. Schaumberg, pp. 161–178. Baltimore: Williams & Wilkins.

Jacobs, J. M., Carmichael, N., and Cavanagh, J. B. 1977. Ultrastructural studies in the nervous system of rabbits poisoned with methyl mercury. *Toxicol. Appl. Pharmacol.* 39:249–261.

Johnson, M. K. 1990. Contemporary issues in toxicology. Organophosphates and delayed neuropathy—Is NTE alive and well? *Toxicol. Appl. Pharmacol.* 103:385–399.

Kallman, M. J., and Fowler, S. C. 1994. Assessment of chemically induced alterations in motor functions. In *Principles of neurotoxicology*, ed. L. W. Chang, pp. 373–396. New York: Marcel Dekker.

Lehrer, G. M. 1974. Measurement of minimal brain dysfunction. In *Behavior toxicology*, eds. C. Xintaras, B. L. Johnson, and I. de Groot. Washington, DC: National Institute for Occupational Safety and Health.

Liu, J. Y., and Stemmer, K. L. 1990. Interaction of aluminum with zinc and copper and its effects on pituitary-testicular axis: A histological study. *Biomed. Environ. Sci.* 3:1–19.

Narahashi, T. 1974. Chemicals as tools in the study of excitable membranes. *Physiol. Rev.* 54: 813–889.

Narahashi, T. 1992. Nerve membrane Na^+ channels as targets of insecticides. *Trends Pharmacol. Sci.* 13:236–241.

Nelson, P. G. 1978. Neuronal cell cultures as toxicologic test systems. *Environ. Health Perspect.* 13:236–241.

Norton, S. 1980. Behavioral toxicology: A critical appraisal. In *The scientific basis of toxicity assessment*, ed. H. R. Witschi, pp. 91–107. Amsterdam: Elsevier/North Holland.

Olney, J. W., Rhee, V., and Ho, O. L. 1974. Kainic acid: A powerful neurotoxic analogue of glutamate. *Brain Res.* 77:507–512.

Organization for Economic Cooperation and Development. 1995. Delayed neurotoxicity of organophosphorus substances. In *Guidelines for testing chemicals*. Paris: OECD.

Press, M. F. 1977. Lead encephalopathy in neonatal Long-Evans rats: Morphologic studies. *J. Neuropathol. Exp. Neurol.* 36:169–193.

Savolainen, J. 1977. Some aspects of the mechanism by which industrial solvents produce neurotoxic effects. *Chem. Biol. Interact.* 18:1–10.

Schield, L. K., Griffin, J. W., Drachman, D. B., and Price, D. L. 1977. Retrograde axonal transport: A direct method for measurement of rate. *Neurology* 27:393.

Seppalainen, A. M., and Hernberg, S. 1972. Sensitive technique for detecting subclinical lead neuropathy. *Br. J. Ind. Med.* 29:443–449.

Spencer, P. S., Sabri, M. I., Schaumberg, H. H., and Moore, C. 1979. Does a defect in energy metabolism in the nerve fiber cause axonal degeneration in polyneuropathies? *Ann. Neurol.* 5:501–507.

Spencer, P. S., Bischoff, M. C., and Schaumberg, H. H. 1980. Neuropathological methods for the detection of neurotoxic disease. In *Experimental and clinical neurotoxicology*, eds. P. S. Spencer and H. H. Schaumberg, pp. 743–757. Baltimore: Williams & Wilkins.

Tilson, H. A., Cabe, P. A., and Burne, T. A. 1980. Behavioral procedures for the assessment of neurotoxicity. In *Experimental and clinical neurotoxicology*, eds. P. C. Spencer and H. H. Schaumberg, pp. 758–766. Baltimore: Williams & Wilkins.

U.S. Environmental Protection Agency. 1994. Health Effects Testing Guidelines. Code of Federal Regulations, Title 40, Part 798.

Worden, A. N., Heywood, R., Prentice, D. E., Chesterman, H., Skerrett, K., and Thomann, P. E. 1978. Clioquinol toxicity in the dog. *Toxicology* 9:227.

Zhang, J., and Snyder, S. H. 1995. Nitric oxide in the nervous system. *Am. Rev. Pharmacol. Toxicol.* 35:213–233.

ADDITIONAL READING

Weiss, B., and Cory-Slechta, D. A. 1994. Assessment of behavioral toxicity. In *Principles and methods of toxicology*, 3rd ed., ed. A. W. Hayes. New York: Raven Press.

Appendix 16-1 Select Neurotoxicants Whose Neurotoxicity Is Briefly Described in Text

Acrylamide-A	n-Hexane-A
Actinomycin-M	IDPN-A
Alcohol-N, T	Kainic acid-N
Alanosine-N	Lead-MS
Aluminum-N	Leptophos-A
6-Aminonicotinamide BV	Methyl n-butyl ketone-A
Arsenic-BV	Methylmercury-N, BV
Azide-N	Nicotine-C
Barbiturate-N	Organic solvents-A
Botulinum toxin-C	Pyrethroids-C
Carbon monoxide-N	Saxitoxin-C
Clioquinol-A	Tellurium-BV
Cyanide-N, BV	Tetanoplasmin-C
DDT-C	Tetrodotoxin-C
Diphtheria toxin-M	Thallium-A
Doxorubicin-N	Triethyltin-M
EPN-A	Triparanol-M
Ethidium bromide-M	TOCP-A
Glutamate-N	Vincristine-A
Hexachlorophene-M, BV	

Note: A, axonopathy; N, neuropathy; M, myelinopathy; C, conduction and transmission; T, teratogenicity; BV, blood vessel and edema; MS, multiple sites.

Chapter 17

Reproductive and Cardiovascular Systems

CHAPTER 17 CONTENTS

REPRODUCTIVE SYSTEM

INTRODUCTION

Reproductive Process and Organs

The reproductive process starts with gametogenesis. In the female animal, oogenesis involves the formation of primary oocytes from the primordial germ cells (oogonia) through mitosis. This development takes place during the fetal period and ceases at birth. Primary oocytes divide by meiosis to form secondary oocytes just before they are ovulated.

On the other hand, spermatogenesis starts with gonocytes during the fetal period, and these cells are transformed to spermatogonia after birth. Spermatogonia remain dormant until puberty, when proliferative activity begins again. Some of the spermatogonia multiply to form additional spermatogonia, while others mature to spermatozoa. There are three intermediate stages. Spermatogonia divide by mitosis to form primary spermatocytes, which divide by meiosis to form secondary spermatocytes. These in turn divide to form spermatids. Finally spermatids become spermatozoa by metamorphosis. The entire process is continuous, and the time required for spermatogonia to become spermatozoa is about 60 d (Fig. 17-1).

Fertilization requires not only functional ovum and spermatozoa but also effective delivery of the sperm and proper milieu. The conceptus, the fertilized ovum, is then implanted in the uterus and develops through embryonic and fetal stages. At the end of the gestational period, parturition takes place. The pups are suckled until weaning. They then grow and mature to start the reproductive process again, thus completing a reproductive cycle.

Other Cells and Organs   While gametocytes are the essential elements of the reproductive process, other cells and organs also play important roles. In the male reproductive system, spermatogenesis takes place in the seminiferous tubules in the testis. In these tubules are the Sertoli cells, which extend from the basement membrane to the lumen of the seminiferous tubules and contain androgen-binding proteins (ABP). The ABP facilitate the movement of androgen to the spermatocytes for their development.

In addition, there are the Leydig cells, which are located in the interstitial tissue surrounding the seminiferous tubules. These cells are the main

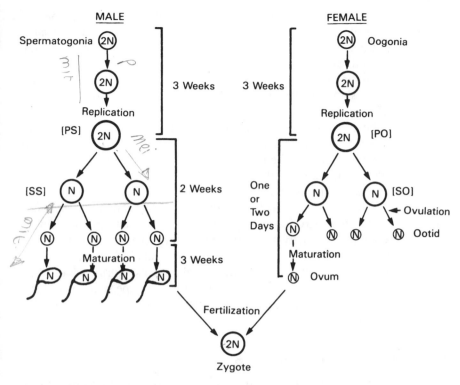

Figure 17-1 Gametogenesis and fertilization. 2N, diploid; N, haploid; PS, primary spermatocyte; SS, secondary spermatocyte; PO, primary oocyte; SO, secondary oocyte (from
Brusick, 1987, by permission).

site of synthesis of testosterone, which is essential not only for the development of the reproductive system but also for its proper functioning.

After leaving the testis, spermatozoa are stored in the epididymis to
undergo changes in order to gain fertility capacity and for later delivery to
the female reproductive system. In addition, the accessory organs prostate
and seminal vesicle provide special nutrients and proper milieu for the
sperm. These organs respond to the effect of testosterone, and hence their
weights are indicators of the blood level of this hormone.

In the female reproductive system the ova can be affected while they
are in the ovaries. However, more often the fertilized ova are affected either
directly or indirectly through damages to the uterus.

Pharmacokinetics

Throughout the reproductive cycle, toxicants can interfere with the various
events and processes just enumerated. They may act directly on the repro-

ductive system or the conceptus or indirectly via certain endocrine organs. Before chemicals act directly, they must reach the target organs in sufficiently high concentration. This concentration may be higher or lower than that in the blood. For example, with DDT, the concentration is almost 80 times higher in the ovary than in the plasma. A number of other substances have also been shown to penetrate the oocyte, oviduct, uterine fluid, and blastocyst (Fabro, 1978).

Unlike the ovaries, the testis is protected by the blood–testis barrier (BTB) (Lee and Dixon, 1978). The BTB is a complex multicellular system composed of capillary endothelial cells, myoid cells, and membranes surrounding the seminiferous tubules and the tightly joined Sertoli cells in the tubules. This barrier, however, is less effective than the blood–brain barrier. The penetration rate of chemicals into the testis is governed by their molecular weights, their partition coefficients, and ionic characteristics.

Testis contains both activating and detoxicating enzyme systems. These two enzyme systems, as noted in chap. 3, are capable of, respectively, increasing and decreasing the toxicities of chemicals. Furthermore, there is an efficient DNA repair system in the premeiotic spermatogenic cells, but there is none in spermatids nor in spermatozoa. Mutations can therefore be induced by electrophilic substances.

TOXICANTS AND THEIR EFFECTS

The reproductive functions may be affected by toxicants through their effects on the reproductive system of either sex. In the male, the formation, development, storage, and delivery of spermatozoa may be adversely affected. The oocytes, in the females, are also susceptible to certain toxicants. In addition, the implantation of the fertilized ova as well as the growth and development of the conceptus may be affected. In both sexes, some of the toxic effects are mediated through hormonal or nervous system activities.

Male Reproductive System

Many cells adversely affect spermatogenesis and cause testicular atrophy. These include food colors (e.g., Oil Yellow AB and Oil Yellow OB) (Allmark et al., 1955), pesticides (e.g., DBCP), metals (e.g., lead and cadmium), and organic solvents. Various other chemicals affect the testis, such as steroid hormones, alkylating agents, cyclohexylamine, and hexachlorophene.

In addition to reduced sperm count resulting from adverse effects on spermatogenesis, a toxicant may render spermatozoa defective, less mobile, or even dead. For example, methylmethane sulfonate (MMS) and busulfan both cause lethal mutation, but MMS affects spermatids and spermatozoa whereas busulfan affects the prespermiogenic cells. These alkylating agents apparently attack the DNA of these cells with different repair mechanisms (Lee, 1983).

Spermatozoa may also be affected while being stored in epididymis. For example, the male antifertility agent α-chlorohydrin inhibits the fertilizing capacity of spermatozoa. Gossypol, another such agent that was extensively tried in China (Quain and Wang, 1984), probably acts through a similar mechanism.

The testis is hormonally regulated by the hypothalamus–pituitary–testis axis: Follicle-stimulating hormone (FSH) is required in the initiation of spermatogenesis through the production of ABP in the Sertoli cells, whereas luteinizing hormone (LH) acts on Leydig cells to synthesize testosterone. A toxicant may thus affect the reproductive function via these endocrines. An example is DBCP (dibromochloropropane), a fumigant used in agriculture. It has been observed among occupational workers to induce azoospermia and oligospermia, along with an elevated serum concentration of LH and FSH (Miller et al., 1987).

In addition, reproductive functions are under the influence of the autonomic nervous system. Therefore, the hypotensive drug losulazine, which acts by depleting norepinephrine, causes reversible infertility in male rats, probably through altered sexual behavior and ejaculatory disturbances (Mesfin et al., 1989). Guanethidine, another hypotensive drug, can induce nonpregnancy by interfering with seminal emission (Palmer, 1976).

Tumors may develop in the testis. For example, the herbicide linuron may induce Leydig-cell tumors. The tumorigenesis is mediated through a sustained hypersecretion of luteinizing hormone (Cook et al., 1993). Furthermore, the calcium channel blocker SDZ 200-110 has been reported to induce Leydig-cell tumors in rats through elevated levels of serum gonadotropins (Roberts ct al., 1989). In contrast to rats, which are likely to develop Leydig-cell tumors, testicular tumors in men are more likely to arise from germ cells. Certain occupational workers, such as aircraft repairmen, seem at greater risk (Thomas and Barsano, 1995). Cadmium has been reported to induce prostate caner in men (Waalkes and Rehm, 1994).

Female Reproductive System

Oocytes may be damaged by chemotherapeutic agents such as nitrogen mustard and vinblastine and polycyclic aromatic hydrocarbons (PAH) such as 3-methylcholanthrene and benzo[a]pyrene. Prostaglandin synthetase inhibitors, such as aspirin-like drugs, may block the release of ovulation. Oocytes before puberty are more resistant to the toxic effects of chemicals, evidently because they are dormant.

Certain organochlorine pesticides such as methoxychlor, similar to estradiol, may increase the weight of uterus (Eroschenko and Rourke, 1992).

Other reproductive functions may also be affected. Haloperidol prevents implantation. DDT and nicotine may affect the development and growth of the conceptus and thus lower the fetal weight (Fabro, 1978). Spironolactone may interfere with ovulation and implantation of the fertilized ovum; it may also retard the development of the sex organs of the offspring (Nagi and Virgo, 1982). Gossypol is also toxic in the female. It suppresses ovarian steroid hormone secretion, interrupts regular cyclicity, and inhibits embryo implantation (Lin et al., 1994).

PAH are ubiquitous in the environment, including cigarette smoke. There is a relationship between the extent of cigarette smoking and the onset of menopause; menopause is an indication of oocyte depletion (Miller et al., 1987).

The toxic effects that are specifically related to the production of congenital anomalies are dealt with in chap. 9, Teratogenesis.

Somewhat more comprehensive lists of toxicants that affect the male and female reproductive capacity are provided by Thomas (1993).

ROUTINE TESTING: MULTIGENERATION REPRODUCTION STUDIES

Procedure

In general, rats are the animal of choice. A minimum of 20 females and 10 males is placed in each of three dose groups and a control group. OECD (1995), however, recommends 10 animals of each sex. The doses are so selected that the high dose will produce some minimal toxic signs but will not result in a mortality greater than 10%. The low dose will not induce any observable effect.

Prior to breeding, the animals are dosed for 10 wk. However, because of the difference in the time required for maturation of the gametes, according to certain recommended protocols the males are dosed for 70 d, the period of spermatogenesis, and the females are dosed for 14 d, the length of the development of the ova. Dosing of the females is continued through the gestation and lactation periods. The test chemical should be administered by a route that most closely resembles the human exposure condition.

To determine the potential effect of the chemical on the reproductive function of the offspring (F_1), a second generation offspring (F_2) is bred and reared to reproductive maturity.

Observations and Examinations

The adult animals are observed for body weight, food consumption, general appearance, estrus cycle, and mating behavior. In addition, the fertility and nesting and nursing behaviors are also noted. Half of the maternal rats are killed on d 13 of gestation for examination of corpora lutea, implantations, and resorptions.

The other half of the maternal rats are allowed to deliver their pups. The pups are examined for litter size, number stillborn, sex distribution, and congenital anomalies. In addition, the viability and pup weight are recorded at birth, on d 4, and at weaning, and preferably also on d 12 or 14. Auditory and visual functions and behavior are also examined for subtle congenital defects.

An appropriate number of males and females are randomly selected from all generations and examined by gross necropsy and histopathology, especially with respect to the reproductive organs. In the males, weights and histopathology of the testes, epididymides, seminal vesicles, prostate, and pituitary often provide useful information on the site of action of the toxicant under test. Other indicators of the mode of action are the sperm count and its motility and morphology, as well as the levels of certain hormones, especially testosterone, and luteinizing and follicle-stimulating hormones. In the females, weights and histopathology of the vagina, uterus, oviduct, ovaries, and pituitary should be assessed, along with the levels of the relevant hormones.

Additional details and references to the reproduction and fertility studies are provided in the U.S. Environmental Protection Agency (U.S. EPA) test guidelines (1994).

Evaluation

From the data described, a number of disturbances of reproductive function can be deduced from the following indices:

1   Fertility index: the percentage of matings resulting in pregnancy.
2   Gestation index: the percentage of pregnancies resulting in the birth of live litters.
3   Viability index: the percentage of live pups that survive 4 d or longer.
4   Lactation index: the percentage of pups alive on d 4 that survive 21 d or longer.

Other indicators of effects include (1) mating index (the percentage of estrus cycles that had matings), (2) male fertility index (the percentage of males exposed to fertile nonpregnant females that resulted in pregnancies), (3) female fertility index (the percentage of females exposed to fertile males that resulted in pregnancies), and (4) 12- or 14-d survival indices.

Multigeneration reproductive study can reveal a variety of toxic effects on the reproductive function as well as on the conceptus. Examples are indices of gestation, viability, and survival. However, nonspecific response (e.g., nonpregnancy) is common. It may follow unusual routes of administering the chemical, such as inhalation, topical application to the eye or nose, and parenteral administration. Excessive handling may also disturb the normal reproductive function. A number of other interfering factors are discussed by Palmer (1976).

The pathologic examination may reveal suppression of spermatogenesis, advanced rates of follicle atresia, and ovulatory or meiotic failure.

Adjunct Tests

To save time and expense, the males of the parent generation (F_0) used in the multigeneration study may be used in a *dominant lethal* test (see chap. 8), and a second litter of the first generation offspring (F_{1b}) may be bred for a *teratogenicity* study (see chap. 9).

Perinatal and postnatal studies are often conducted to determine effects on late development of the offspring. The procedure is essentially the same as that of the multigeneration study, except that only the females are treated and their treatment covers only the last third of gestation and throughout lactation. The litter data, as described earlier, are recorded and evaluated (Palmer, 1976).

OTHER TESTS

The effects revealed in multigeneration reproduction studies outlined earlier may result from paternal, maternal, or fetal exposure. Thus, additional tests are often conducted to establish the cause of the effect. A few such tests are outlined next.

Pathological examinations are useful in identifying a variety of toxic effects. The weight of testis is a simple but sensitive index of testicular damages. The extent and nature of such damages can often be assessed microscopically. The weights of prostate and seminal vesicle are often correlated with levels of testosterone. Similarly, gross and microscopic analysis of *semen* is useful in epidemiologic and animal studies. The sperm count and the motility, survival, and morphology of the spermatozoa often provide information on toxic effects on the testis (Eliasson, 1978).

As noted earlier, certain toxicants affect the reproductive function through disturbances of *hormones*, especially testosterone, estrogens, luteinizing hormone, and follicle-stimulating hormone. Assays of their levels will thus be useful in ascertaining the mode of action of the toxicant.

The *perfused male reproductive tracts* have been shown to be useful models in studying the effects of chemicals on the secretion and accumulation of androgens (Bardin et al., 1978).

Brackett (1978) described a procedure using *in vitro fertilized ova* in the study of toxic effects by observing development of the ova.

Certain *biomarkers* have been used in a variety of tests for disorders of the reproductive system. For example, DNA probes have been used to detect gene mutation and massive deletion and translocations in meiotic and postmeiotic germ cells as well as Sertoli and Leydig cells in the testis (Hecht, 1987).

CARDIOVASCULAR SYSTEM

GENERAL CONSIDERATIONS

The cardiovascular system is composed of two parts: the heart and the blood vessels. The heart is a vital organ in the body. Although it is not a common target organ, it can be damaged by a variety of chemicals. They act either directly on the myocardium or indirectly through the nervous system or blood vessels. A list of such chemicals, as compiled by Van Stee (1980), is reproduced in Table 17-1.

The heart is mainly composed of myocardial cells, each measuring about 15 × 80 θm. Unlike skeletal muscle cells, each of which is inner-

Table 17-1 Cardiotoxic Drugs and Chemicals

Cardiomyopathy	
Allylamine	Adrenergic agonists
Furazolidone	Methysergide
Ethanol	Vasodilators
Cobalt	

Interference with nucleic acid metabolism and protein synthesis	
Antineoplastic drugs	

Electrophysiologic mechanisms	
Cardiotonic drugs	Local anesthetics
Phenytoin (diphenylhydantoin)	Emetine
Tricyclic antidepressants	Chlordimeform
Clofibrate	Contrast media
Lithium	Antimalarial drugs
Propylene glycol	Calcium antagonists

Nonspecific myocardial depression	
Lipid-soluble organic compounds	Antimicrobial antibiotics
Myocardial depressant factor	Carbromide, carbromal

Involvement with lipid metabolism	
High-cholesterol diet	Brominated vegetable oils
Rapeseed oil	

Miscellaneous	
Phenothiazines	

Source: Van Stee (1980).

vated, only some of the heart muscle cells are innervated. However, these cells are joined, at their ends, to each other by the nexus. It has low resistance and thus allows rapid transmission of electrical stimulus from one cell to the next. These characteristics are essential to the programmed sequence of contraction of different parts of the heart.

The myocardium is different from skeletal muscles also in that there is less contractile material (50% vs. 80%) but much more mitochondrial material (35% vs. 2%). Mitochondria evidently play an important role in the cardiac contractility and are a common subcellular target of cardiotoxicity.

Myocardial contraction involves the liberation of energy from oxidative metabolism, conservation of the energy by adenosine triphosphate and creatine phosphate, and utilization of the energy by contractile proteins. The most vulnerable mechanisms probably include the utilization of energy and intracellular movement of calcium ion, which is involved in the contractility of myocardium as well as regulating enzyme activities, transduction of hormonal information, etc.

The vascular system consists of arteries, arterioles, capillaries, venules, and veins. A toxicant may affect any of these vessels; the seriousness of the effect depends on the vital role of the organ that is supplied by the affected blood vessel.

TOXIC EFFECTS ON THE HEART

Cardiomyopathy

The usual toxic effects of cobalt are polycythemia, goiter, and signs of gastrointestinal irritation such as vomiting and diarrhea. However, its inclusion in beer as a foam stabilizer caused a number of serious and fatal cases of cardiomyopathy. Subsequent studies showed that there is also intramitochondrial accumulation of calcium. The toxicity of cobalt on the heart was greatly enhanced by malnutrition, especially the deficiency of certain amino acids. Among heavy beer drinkers, this condition existed because of the large caloric intake of beer. It was also noted that cobalt ions depressed oxygen uptake and interfered with cardiac energy metabolism in the tricarboxylic acid cycle, as thiamine deficiency does (Grice, 1972). As noted earlier, Ca^{2+} plays a vital role in various functions of myocardium. Cobalt may reduce the available myocardial Ca^{2+} by complexing with macromolecules and may also be antagonistic to endogenous Ca^{2+}.

A number of adrenergic B-receptor agonists, notably isoproterenol, and vasodilating antihypertensive drugs, such as hydralazine and diazoxide, are capable of inducing myocardial necrosis. The former chemicals have direct adrenergic effects, whereas the antihypertensive drugs exert adrenergic effects via the induced hypotension. These effects produce an augmented transmembrane calcium influx, which in turn causes an increase in the rate and force of contraction. This, along with the concomitant hypotension, results in cardiac hypoxia. The hypoxia and the calcium deposits in the mitochondria cause disintegration of organelles and sarcolemma (Balazs et al., 1981).

Interference with Nucleic Acid Synthesis

The anthracycline antibiotics doxorubicin and daunorubicin are effective antineoplastic drugs. However, they produce hypotension, tachycardia, and arrhythmias acutely. More prolonged administration causes degeneration and atrophy of cardiac muscle cells and interstitial edema and fibrosis. The likely mode of action is the binding of these antibiotics to mitochondrial and nuclear DNA, which in turn interferes with synthesis of RNA and protein. This effect on the heart is important because the half-life of the contractile proteins is short (12 wk). Other possible mechanisms of action include (1) inhibition of Q enzymes, (2) peroxidation of membrane lipids, and (3) hypotension resulting from release of histamine (Van Stee, 1980).

Arrhythmias

A number of fluorocarbons are capable of producing cardiac arrhythmias. This effect is mediated by a sensitization of the heart to epinephrine, depression of contractility, reduction of coronary blood flow, and reflex increase in sympathetic and vagal impulses to the heart following irritation of mucosa in the respiratory tract (Aviado, 1978).

Tricyclic antidepressants also can cause cardiac arrhythmias. These effects are likely the result of imbalances within the autonomic regulatory system of the heart. Propylene glycol, a common solvent, can convert ventricular tachycardia induced by deslanoside into ventricular fibrillation (Van Stee, 1980).

Myocardial Depression

A number of lipid-soluble organic compounds, such as general anesthetics, depress cardiac contractility. The probable mechanism of action is a nonspecific expansion of various cellular membranes by the insertion of chemically indifferent molecules in the hydrophobic regions of integral proteins and membrane phospholipids.

The aminoglycoside antibiotics, such as neomycin and streptomycin, cause hypotension through depression of cardiac contractility. However, the mechanism of action appears to be related to an inhibition of a portion of Ca^{2+} bound to superficial membrane sites (Adams et al., 1978).

Miscellaneous

Rapeseed oil, a common cooking oil in many parts of the world, causes accumulation of lipid globules in heart muscles in rats. This effect was attributed to the high content of erucic acid in rapeseed oil. Brominated vegetable oils, used in adjusting the density of flavoring oils and in enhancing cloudy stability in beverages, induce biochemical and morphologic changes in cardiac myofibrils. The colorant Brown F.K. also produces severe morphologic changes in the heart muscles (Grice, 1972).

TOXIC EFFECTS ON BLOOD VESSELS

Increased Capillary Permeability   Lead, mercury, and several other toxicants damage endothelial cells of capillaries in the brain. This effect will result in brain edema and an impairment of the blood–brain barrier (chap. 16). Inhalation of irritating gas induces pulmonary edema (chap. 11).

Endothelial Damage   Monocrotaline, a plant toxin, may cause pulmonary vascular damage. This chemical, after ingestion, is bioactivated in the liver, but sufficient amounts of the active metabolite leave the liver and cause cross-linking of DNA in the endothelial cells of the pulmonary vasculature. This effect may damage the repair capability of the endothelial cells leading to thrombosis and progressive pulmonary hypertension (Boor et al., 1995). Arsenic has been suggested as the cause of the *black-foot* disease, a result of peripheral endarteritis (see chap. 20).

Vasoconstriction   Consumption of ergot alkaloids (fungal contaminants in certain foods) may cause gangrene resulting from vasoconstriction. A clinical syndrome known as black-foot disease is endemic in certain areas in South America and Taiwan. It has been attributed to vasoconstriction following consumption of drinking water with high levels of arsenic (chap. 20).

Exposure to pure oxygen over a prolonged period may result in blindness, especially among premature infants, evidently because of the associated vasoconstriction in the eye.

Occupational workers exposed to nitroglycerin on work days have been reported to have died suddenly of heart attack on weekends. Apparently the continued exposure to a coronary dilator has rendered the workers accustomed to a low level of coronary flow, and the sudden cessation of exposure to the coronary dilator precipitated coronary insufficiency.

Vasodilation　The musculature of the coronary artery may be damaged by large doses of certain hypotensive drugs, such as minoxidil and hydralazine. The lesion may be a result of exaggerated pharmacodynamic changes (Boor et al., 1995).

Degenerative Changes　Atherosclerosis is a complex degenerative disease affecting mainly large blood vessels such as the coronary and carotid arteries. Narrowing of these arteries may result in heart attacks and strokes, respectively. While the etiology of atherosclerosis is complex, certain toxicants may aggravate the pathological condition. CO may increase the permeability of capillaries surrounding these arteries and promote the degenerative process. So does CS2 by damaging their endothelium. Ramos et al. (1994) observed that certain allylamines and aromatic hydrocarbons may contribute to the development of atherosclerosis. These toxicants may act through nitric oxide and endothelin on the smooth muscle and endothelium of arteries and induce vascular lesions which may contribute to the development of atherosclerosis.

Fibrosis　Cadmium and lead may affect blood vessels in the kidney causing renal fibrosis. The impairment of blood supply may interfere with the "nonexcretory functions" of the kidney (chap. 13), and indirectly cause hypertension.

Hypersensitivity Reaction　Gold salts, penicillin, sulfonamides, and a number of other toxicants may induce vasculitis or exacerbate preexisting polyarteritis. The condition usually affects small vessels and is associated with infiltration of eosinophils and mononuclear cells, indicating involvement of the immune system.

Tumors　Tumors of blood vessels may result from certain toxicants. For example, vinyl chloride has been shown to cause hemangiosarcoma in the liver in humans and animals, and hemangioendothelioma has been reported to result from exposure to thorium dioxide.

TESTING PROCEDURES

Cardiovascular toxicity can be studied in intact normal animals, in animals with specific pathologic conditions, or in isolated hearts and blood vessels.

Normal Animals

A variety of examinations for cardiovascular toxicity can be performed on animals in conventional toxicity studies. These include blood pressure, heart rate, and electrocardiography. The rate of blood flow is a useful indicator of the functions of the cardiovascular systems, and can be measured using, among others, a pulsed Doppler flowmeter (Haywood et al., 1981). The status of the arteriole, capillaries, and venules can be studied either at a special site of the organism (e.g., conjunctiva and retina), or through a microvascular chamber that can be chronically placed on a laboratory animal (Smith et al., 1994). Functional tests, such as swimming until exhaustion, have been suggested. At necropsy, the organ weight is often determined. Gross, light, and, in particular, electron microscopic examinations are valuable. Biochemical studies of the myocardium and of the blood are also useful.

Animals with Pathologic Conditions

The hearts of rabbits fed a diet containing 2% cholesterol become atherosclerotic. These hearts are more susceptible to myocardial ischemia (Lee et al., 1978). Other models, such as infarcted myocardium, cardiomyopathic hamster, obesity, and drug interaction models, have been briefly described and referenced by Van Stee (1980).

Isolated Heart

The isolated, perfused heart is a common model for studying the effects of drugs on the strength and rate of heart contractions and the rate of coronary flow. It has also been used to detect the cardiac effects of toxicants. For example, Toy et al. (1976) have shown that certain halogenated alkanes depressed the peak left ventricular pressure as well as the rate of increase of that pressure. The isolated atrium and cultured heart cells have also been used in the study of cardiotoxicity (Adams et al., 1978; Sperelakis, 1978).

Evaluation

The cardiovascular toxicity of chemicals is not readily detected in conventional toxicity studies. For example, the toxic effects of cobalt and the anthracycline antibiotics on the heart were reproduced in animal experiments only after they were detected in humans first. Negative results therefore do not necessarily exclude potential cardiotoxicity.

To demonstrate such toxicity, specific testing procedures may be required. These procedures usually mimic the clinical conditions. For example, intermittent administration of the anthracycline antibiotics was necessary to elicit the cardiotoxicity; presumably continuous treatment caused the animals to die from other toxic effects before heart lesions developed. The toxicity of adrenergic -receptor agonists is best detected in acute studies; the effects of prolonged treatment may be masked by tolerance development. The effect of cobalt on the heart is more readily revealed when the animals are on a protein- and vitamin-deficient diet (Balazs and Ferrans, 1978).

REFERENCES

Adams, H. R., Parker, J. L., and Durrett, L. R. 1978. Cardiac toxicities of antibiotics. *Environ. Health Perspect.* 26:217–231.

Allmark, M. G., Grice, H. C., and Lu, F. C. 1955. Chronic toxicity studies on food colors: Observations on the toxicity of FD&C Yellow No. 3 (Oil Yellow AB) and FD&C Yellow No. 4 (Oil Yellow OB) in rats. *J. Pharm. Pharmacol.* 7:591–603.

Aviado, D. M. 1978. Effects of fluorocarbons, chlorinated solvents, and inosine on the cardiopulmonary system. *Environ. Health Perspect.* 26:207–216.

Balazs, T., and Ferrans, V. J. 1978. Cardiac lesions induced by chemicals. *Environ. Health Perspect.* 26: 181–191.

Balazs, T., Ferrans, V. J., et al. 1981. Study of the mechanism of hydralazine-induced myocardial necrosis in the rat. *Toxicol. Appl. Pharmacol.* 59:524–534.

Bardin, C. W., Baker, H. W. G., Jefferson, L. S., and Santen, R. J. 1978. Methods for perfusing male reproductive tract: Models for studying drugs and hormone metabolism. *Environ. Health Perspect.* 24:51–59.

Boor, P. J., Gotlieb, A. I., Joseph, E. C., Kerns, W. D., Roth, R. A., and Tomaszewski, K. E. 1995. Chemical-induced vasculature injury. *Toxicol. Appl. Pharmacol.* 132:177–195.

Brackett, B. G. 1978. In vitro fertilization: A potential means for toxicity testing. *Environ. Health Perspect.* 24:65–71.

Brusick, D. 1987. *Principles of genetic toxicology*, 2nd ed. New York: Plenum Press.

Cook, J. C., Mullin, L. S., Frame, S. R., and Biegel, L. B. 1993. Investigation of a mechanism for Leydig cell tumorigenesis by linuron. *Toxicol. Appl. Pharmacol.* 119:195–204.

Eliasson, R. 1978. Semen analysis. *Environ. Health Perspect.* 24:81–85.

Eroschenko, V. P., and Rourke, A. W. 1992. Stimulating influences of the technical grade methoxychlor and estradiol on protein synthesis in the uterus of the immature mouse. *J. Occup. Med. Toxicol.* 1:307–315.

Fabro, S. 1978. Penetration of chemicals into the oocyte, uterine fluid and preimplantation blastocyst. *Environ. Health Perspect.* 24:25–29.

Grice, H. C. 1972. The changing role of pathology in modern safety evaluation. *CRC Crit. Rev. Toxicol.* 1:119–152.

Haywood, J. R., Shaffer, R. A., Fink, G. D., and Brody, M. J. 1981. Regional blood flow measurements with pulsed Doppler flowmeter in conscious rat. *Am. J. Physiol.* 241: 14273–14278.

Hecht, N. B. 1987. Detecting the effects of toxic agents on spermatogenesis using DNA probes. *Environ. Health Perspect.* 74:31–40.

Lee, I. P. 1983. Adaptive biochemical repair response toward germ cell DNA damage. *Am. J. Ind. Med.* 4:135–147.

Lee, I. P., and Dixon, R. L. 1978. Factors influencing reproduction and genetic toxic effects on male gonads. *Environ. Health Perspect.* 24:117–127.

Lee, R. J., Zaidi, I. H., and Baky, S. H. 1978. Pathophysiology of the atherosclerotic rabbit. *Environ. Health Perspect.* 26:225–231.

Lin, Y. C., Coskun, S., and Sanbuissho, A. 1994. Effects of gossypol on in vitro bovine oocyte maturation and steroidogenesis in bovine granulosa cells. *Theriogenology* 41:1601–1611.

Mesfin, G. M., Morris, D. F., Seaman, W. J., and Marks, T. A. 1989. Testicular lesions in rats treated with a sympatholytic hypotensive agent (losulazine). *J. Am. Coll. Toxicol.* 8: 525–538.

Miller, R. K., Kellogg, C. K., and Saltzman, R. A. 1987. Reproductive and perinatal toxicology. In *Handbook of toxicology*, eds. T. J. Haley and W. O. Berndt, pp. 195–309. Washington, DC: Hemisphere.

Nagi, S., and Virgo, B. B. 1982. The effects of spironolactone on reproductive functions in female rats and mice. *Toxicol. Appl. Pharmacol.* 66:221–228.

OECD. 1995. OECD Guidelines for Testing of Chemicals: Reproduction/Developmental Toxicity Screening Test. Paris: OECD.

Palmer, A. K. 1976. Assessment of current test procedures. *Environ. Health Perspect.* 18: 97–104.

Quain, S., and Wang, Z. 1984. Gossypol: A potential antifertility agent for males. *Annu. Rev. Pharmacol. Toxicol.* 24:329–360.

Ramos, K. S., Bowes, R. C., Ou, X.-L., and Weber, T. J. 1994. Responses of vascular smooth cells to toxic insult: Cellular and molecular perspectives for environmental toxicants. *J. Toxicol. Environ. Health* 43:419–440.

Roberts, S. A., Nett, T. M., Hartman, H. A., Adams, T. E., and Stoll, R. E. 1989. SDZ 200-110 induces Leydig cell tumors by increasing gonadotropins in rats. *J. Am. Coll. Toxicol.* 8:487–505.

Smith, T. L., Koman, L. A., and Mosberg, A. T. 1994. Cardiovascular physiology and methods for toxicology. In *Principles and methods of toxicology*, ed. A. W. Hayes, pp. 917–935. New York: Raven Press.

Sperelakis, N. 1978. Cultured heart cell reaggregate model for studying cardiac toxicology. *Environ. Health Perspect.* 26:243–267.

Thomas, J. A. 1993. Toxic responses of the reproductive system. In *Casarett and Doull's toxicology*, eds. M. O. Amdur, J. Doull, and C. D. Klaassen, pp. 484–520. New York: McGraw-Hill.

Thomas, J. A., and Barsano, C. P. 1995. Occupational reproductive risks. In *Encyclopedia of environmental control technology*, vol. 7, *High-hazard pollutants*, ed. P. N. Cherimisinoff, pp. 195–215. Houston, TX: Gulf.

Toy, P. A., Van Stee, E. W., Harris, A. M., Horton, M. L., and Back, K. C. 1976. The effects of three halogenated alkanes on excitation and contraction in the isolated, perfused rabbit heart. *Toxicol. Appl. Pharmacol.* 38:7–17.

U.S. Environmental Protection Agency. 1994. *Health effects test guidelines.* Washington, DC: U.S. Environmental Protection Agency.

Van Stee, E. W. 1980. Myocardial toxicity. In *The scientific basis of toxicity assessment*, ed. H. R. Witschi, pp. 167–182. New York: Elsevier/North Holland.

Waalkes, M. P., and Rohm, S. 1994. Cadmium and prostate cancer. *J. Toxicol. Environ. Health* 43:251–269.

Part Four

Toxic Substances and Risk Assessment

Food Additives and Contaminants

CHAPTER 18 CONTENTS

INTRODUCTION

With the increasing world population, there has been a growing demand for more food. Various physical means and chemical substances have been developed and utilized to increase the food supply. However, the increased efficiency of farming reduced the number of farmers. In addition, with industrialization and urbanization, more and more people lived away from the farmland. These social changes have resulted in an ever-increasing demand for processed foods that can be transported from the farm to the city and that will retain their nutritive value and organoleptic properties.

These demands have been met largely by the addition of chemicals known as food additives. These chemicals serve a variety of technological functions as described in the subsection Functional Groups of Direct Food Additives.

Legal Definition of Food Additives

The following definition has been adopted by the Codex Alimentarius Commission, an intergovernmental agency consisting of more than 150 nations (FAO/WHO, 1994).

> *Food Additive* means any substance not normally consumed as a food by itself and not normally used as a typical ingredient of the food, whether or not it has nutritive value, the intentional addition of which to food for a technological (including organoleptic) purpose in the manufacture, processing, preparation, treatment, packing, packaging, transport or holding of such food results, or may be reasonably expected to result (directly or indirectly) in it or its by-products becoming a component of or otherwise affecting the characteristics of such foods. The term does not include "contaminants" or substances added to food for maintaining or improving nutritional qualities.

The U.S. legal definition appearing in the U.S. Federal Food, Drug and Cosmetic Act, as amended in October 1976 (1979), is different from the foregoing one in several aspects. The U.S. legislation excludes color additives and those substances that are to be added to food but are defined as "generally recognized as safe (GRAS)." On the other hand, the U.S. legislation considers nutritional supplements and irradiated foods as food additives.

There is another important difference between the U.S. legislation and that of many other nations. The U.S. Food Additive Amendment of 1958, also known as the Delaney Clause, stipulates "that no additive shall be deemed to be safe if it is found to induce cancer when ingested by man or animal, or if it is found, after tests which are appropriate for the evaluation of the safety of food additives, to induce cancer in man or animal." The protection of the consumers in other nations is provided for through the general safety clause, and its interpretation, especially with respect to questionable carcinogens, is left to the judgment of experts. On the other hand, the U.S. legislation provides little leeway for scientific judgment and has thus created much controversy among scientists and regulatory agencies (see Coulston, 1979; NRC/NAS, 1987).

Classification of Food Additives and Contaminants

Functional Groups of Direct Food Additives   A number of chemicals are added to food to increase its shelf life, to render it more amenable to mass production, or to enhance its consumer appeal with respect to color, flavor, texture, and convenience. These chemicals are grouped according to their technological functions. A detailed listing of various groups of food additives and their uses is given in a National Academy of Sciences (NAS) publication (1965) and a Codex document (FAO/WHO, 1994). The following are some examples.

1 Preservatives are added to prolong the shelf life of foods by preventing or inhibiting microbial growth. Examples are benzoic acid, propionic acid, and sorbic acid, their salts, nitrates and nitrites, and sulfur dioxide and related compounds.

2 Antioxidants are added to oils to prevent them from becoming rancid, which is a result of oxidative changes. Some are added to fruits and vegetables to prevent enzymatic browning. The commonly used ones include butylated hydroxyanisole (BHA), butylated hydroxytoluene (BHT), various gallates, ascorbic acid and its salts, and α-tocopherol.

3 Emulsifying, stabilizing, and thickening agents are added to improve the homogeneity, stability, and "body" of a variety of food products. These include mono- and diglycerides, sucrose esters of fatty acids, lecithin, salts of various types of phosphate, modified starches, calcium gluconate, calcium citrate, agar, alginic acid and its salts, various vegetable gums, and cellulose derivatives.

4 Colors are used to enhance visual appeal of food products. Some of these substances are derived from natural colors, such as carotene, chlorophyll, and cochineal. Others are synthetic, such as allura red, amaranth, azorubine, indigotine, and tartrazine.

5 Flavors and flavor enhancers. The flavors constitute the largest group of food additives. However, they are used, in general, at very low levels in foods. Some are synthetic (mainly esters, aldehydes, and ketones); others are derived from natural sources (such as oleoresins, plant extracts, and essential oils). Flavor enhancers, such as monosodium glutamate, enhance the flavor of the food to which they are added.

6 Artificial sweeteners have a strong sweet taste but little or no caloric value. They are therefore useful for diabetics and those who wish to enjoy the sweet taste without increasing the caloric intake. The notable ones are the cyclamates, saccharin, and aspartame.

7 Nutrients include vitamins, minerals, and essential amino acids. As noted earlier, national regulations in most countries, contrary to those of the United States, do not consider these as food additives. However, a food additive used for a technological reason may incidentally have certain nutritional values. For example, riboflavin may be used as a color but is also a vitamin.

8 Miscellaneous groups. These include (a) acidity regulators (acids and bases), which are used to adjust the pH of beverages and canned fruits and vegetables; (b) anticaking agents, which are added to salt, sugar, etc. to maintain their free-flowing property; (c) antifoaming agents, which are added to liquids to prevent foaming; (d) flour treatment agents, which are added to flour to improve its baking qualities; (e) glazing agents; (f) propellants; and (g) raising agents.

Indirect (Unintentional) Food Additives The substances just described are intentionally added to foods for specific technological purposes. Consequently they are considered "direct" or "intentional" food additives. However, a number of substances may become part of the foods as a result of their use during the production, processing, or storage of the foods. These include antibiotics and anabolic agents used during the raising of farm animals, residues from food processing machinery, and migrants from packaging materials.

Food Contaminants These substances are present in foods as a result of environmental pollution or faulty handling of the food. In other words, they serve no useful purpose either in the final food product or in its processing. Examples are mercury in fish harvested from contaminated waters, and mycotoxins found in improperly stored nuts and grains. Thus they differ from both the direct and indirect food additives.

TOXICOLOGICAL TESTING AND EVALUATION

Categories of Data Required

Because these chemicals are added to foods to be consumed by large numbers of people, they are in general extensively tested and strictly evaluated. Furthermore, because of their low toxicity, precise LD_{50}s are as a rule not required. The categories of studies include:

1 Biochemical studies—absorption, distribution, elimination (and storage), biotransformation, and effects on biochemical parameters.
2 Acute toxicity studies.
3 Short-term toxicity studies.
4 Long-term toxicity studies.
5 Reproductive function studies.
6 Short-term tests for carcinogenicity potential.
7 Carcinogenicity studies.
8 Teratogenicity studies.
9 Observation in humans.

Brief descriptions of these studies are given in chaps. 2, 3, 6, 7, 8, 9, and 17.

Extent of Testing

The Joint Food and Agriculture Organization/World Health Organization (FAO/WHO) Expert Committee on Food Additives considers, as a general rule, that the types of biological data just listed are required for proper evaluation of food additives. However, for certain groups of additives, depending on their chemical nature, source, and usage, much less data are required. These include (1) components of food and closely related chemicals, (2) certain enzymes used in food processing, (3) certain food colors, and (4) certain metals (e.g., copper, iron, and zinc). Detailed descriptions of the types of additives and the required data are given in several WHO reports (WHO, 1974, 1982a, 1986). These descriptions are summarized in a review article (Lu, 1988).

The U.S. Food and Drug Administration (FDA) established a set of criteria to determine the "level of concern," which in turn dictates the extent of testing required (FDA, 1982a). The level of concern is determined by the chemical structure of the additive and by its use level in food. Their relationship is shown in Table 18-1.

Additives are placed according to their chemical structure in three categories: A, B, and C. Additives of low probable toxicity are assigned to category A. This category comprises nine types of chemicals, such as simple aliphatic, noncyclic hydrocarbons with no unsaturation; sugars and polysaccharides; fats, fatty acids; and endogenous inorganic salts of alkali metals (Na, K) and alkaline earth metals (Mg, Ca). Additives with functional groups of high probable toxicity are assigned to category C. This category comprises 52 types of chemicals, such as those with an organic halogen (not salts), three-membered heterocyclic ring systems, and α,B-unsaturated lactones. Additives of intermediate or unknown probable toxicity are assigned to category B.

The testing required for a Concern Level I compound consists of (a) a battery of short-term carcinogenicity potential tests and (b) a short-term (28 d or longer) multiple-dose rodent study. If either or both tests yield positive results, a long-term carcinogenicity study in one rodent species and/or a chronic or subchronic rodent study, depending on the no-effect level observed, will be required. If the two initial studies (a and b) are negative, no further studies will be required, provided that the existing data from a multiple-dose nonrodent study and reproductive organ toxicity tests are negative. If they are positive, certain additional studies will be required.

For Concern Level II and III compounds, additional initial and more extensive followup studies are required. For example, both types of compounds require a two-generation reproduction study, subacute toxicity stud-

Table 18-1   Levels of Concern About Food Additives as Determined by Extent of Exposure (ppm in Foods) and Chemical Structure

Chemical structure	Level of concern		
	I	II	III
A	<0.05 ppm	<1.0 ppm	>1.0 ppm
B	<0.025 ppm	<0.5 ppm	>0.5 ppm
C	<0.0125 ppm	<0.25 ppm	>0.25 ppm

Source: FDA (1982a).

ies in a rodent and a nonrodent species, and short-term tests for carcinogenic potential. For a Concern Level III compound, chronic toxicity studies
in a rodent and a nonrodent species and long-term carcinogenicity studies
in two rodent species will be required when the short-term carcinogenicity
potential test is positive; even when it is negative, such carcinogenicity
studies will be required, although they will be assigned a low priority.

Evaluation

As described in chap. 22, toxicological evaluation of food additives follows
the procedure of determining the adequacy of data, establishing an appropriate no-effect level, and selecting a proper safety factor to obtain the
acceptable daily intake. This procedure is generally adopted by many national regulatory agencies including the U.S. Food and Drug Administration, as well as the international organizations WHO and FAO. The toxicological basis for drafting the provisions for food additives in the
International Food Standards is provided by the Joint FAO/WHO Expert
Committee on Food Additives. The interrelationship between the various
national and international bodies is described in a review article (Lu, 1988).

GRAS

As noted already, the U.S. legislation considers certain chemicals as "generally recognized as safe." This was done originally in 1958, and that list
included more than 600 direct additives with a variety of technological
functions and some 2000 indirect additives. Since then, the list of direct
additives has been expanded mainly by the addition of more than 1000
flavoring ingredients proposed by the Flavor and Extract Manufacturers'
Association (FEMA).

On the basis of new toxicological information, the safety of a number
of substances on the list has since been questioned. The most notable was
the suspected carcinogenicity of the artificial sweetener cyclamate. As a
result, FDA in 1970 asked the Life Sciences Research Office of the Fed-
eration of American Societies for Experimental Biology to evaluate the
safety of all the substances on the GRAS list. A Select Committee on
GRAS Substances was formed and issued 144 reports containing its con-
clusion and summaries of the available information on 468 substances. A
listing of these reports is included in two overview reports (Select Committee on GRAS Substances, 1977, 1982). A detailed account of the work
of the committee is given by Carr (1987).

ADDITIVES OF TOXICOLOGICAL CONCERN

Some 600 intentional food additives are being added to a variety of our
foods. The toxicity of most of these additives has been evaluated according

to prevailing procedure and found to be "safe." However, the use of some additives has been restricted, suspended, or requires label declaration because of toxicological concern.

Carcinogenicity

For example, the safety of *saccharin* has been questioned because of its reported carcinogenicity. In fact, the first study that revealed increased bladder tumors in rats involved the dosing of the animals with a combination of saccharin and cyclamate at the ratio of 1:9. Saccharin has been found to be excreted as such and nonmutagenic in most test systems. However, a large-scale experiment carried out in a Canadian government laboratory showed that rats fed saccharin at 7.5% in the diet developed bladder tumors (Arnold et al., 1977). The significance of this finding is somewhat doubtful because of the excessively high dosage and because the tumors occurred mainly among the male rats of the second generation.

Cyclamates were considered innocuous and were used widely in foods and beverages for many years. However, doubt was cast on their safety because of the discovery that they are metabolizable by intestinal flora in animals and humans to cyclohexylamine, which appears to be more toxic (Classen et al., 1968). Its use as a food additive was suspended in 1969 when it was discovered that a mixture of saccharin and cyclamate increased the incidence of bladder tumors in rats (Price et al., 1970). Subsequent studies on cyclamate showed no carcinogenicity and the short-term mutagenicity tests yielded no consistent results. This is also true with cyclohexylamine. Summaries of the reports are included in two publications (IARC, 1980; WHO, 1982b). Its use has been restored in a number of countries, although it is still not permitted for use as an additive in the United States.

Nitrates and nitrites are useful preservatives and they impart a special color and flavor to treated meat such as ham and corned beef. However, they can form, with certain amines, a variety of nitrosamines, many of which are potent carcinogens. Nitrates and nitrites are valuable in controlling toxin-forming microorganisms such as *Clostridium botulinum*. Furthermore, nitrites occur in the body, notably in the saliva, and it has been demonstrated that nitrosation of certain amines can occur in the stomach.

For these reasons, the use of these preservatives has not been suspended, but the use levels have been reduced. On the other hand, the preservative *diethylpyrocarbonate* (DEPC) presents a distinctly different picture. It had been used in a variety of beverages, but its use was suspended. This decision was based on the finding that DEPC may combine with ammonium ion in beverages to form urethane, a wide-spectrum carcinogen in all animal species tested, and on the fact that its use was not indispensable.

BHA (butylated hydroxyanisole) and *BHT* (butylated hydroxytoluene) are widely used antioxidants and have been investigated in several long-term studies without revealing any serious adverse effects. However, Ito et al. (1983) reported that BHA at very high dietary levels induced hyperplasia and tumors in the forestomach of rats. Since the tumors were only found in the forestomach, the relevance of this finding in terms of human health hazard was questioned. Additional studies using species without a forestomach were performed. The results were negative in the dog, and the increased mitotic rate in the esophagus of pigs was questionable (WHO, 1989). Olsen et al. (1983) reported an increase in the hepatocellular adenoma and carcinoma. However, several other studies yielded negative results. Furthermore, other studies on these antioxidants produced cancer-protective effects (Prochaska et al., 1985). In light of these conflicting results, BHA and BHT are still being used.

Hypersensitivity Reactions

A number of food additives are known to induce hypersensitivity reactions in susceptible individuals. Because they affect only a small proportion of the general population, and because their effects are usually mild and transitory, most regulatory agencies consider label declaration as sufficient to provide warning to these individuals. The following are the more commonly known ones:

Tartrazine, a widely used yellow color in a variety of processed foods, has been known to induce allergic reactions, especially among those who are allergic to aspirin (Juhlin, 1980).

Sulfur dioxide (SO2) and related chemicals, such as bisulfites and metabisulfites, are used as preservatives in processed foods as well as salads. In the latter case, these chemicals help to preserve the freshness of the vegetables. Since it is difficult to provide warning labels, such use has been discouraged.

Monosodium glutamate (MSG) has been used as a flavor enhancer for many decades in China and Japan. No untoward effects have been reported. However, a "Chinese restaurant syndrome" has been reported (Schaumberg et al., 1969). It usually appears after the individual has consumed a special Chinese soup, which contains relatively large amounts of MSG. The hypersensitivity reaction consists of a burning sensation, tingling in the face and neck, tightness in the chest, etc. Because of these findings, it is now possible, in many restaurants, to order soups and other dishes specifying "no MSG." For additional details, see Kenney (1986). The fact that adverse reactions to MSG have not been observed in the Far East is evidently related to the custom of consuming the soup as the last course, that is, on a full stomach, thereby delaying the absorption of this chemical and preventing a dramatic rise in blood level.

Other Adverse Effects

In addition to carcinogenicity and hypersensitivity reactions, the discovery of other adverse effects has prompted regulatory decisions or additional investigations. Examples are heart lesions in laboratory animals associated with brominated vegetable oils (BVO), a suspending agent in certain beverages, and liver lesions associated with Orange RN and Ponceau 2R, which were responsible for the suspension of their use. Other effects such as red blood cell damage (Orange RN), storage in tissues (BVO), and testicular atrophy (cyclohexylamine from cyclamate) were contributing factors to toxicological decisions on these additives (see Lu, 1979a).

INDIRECT FOOD ADDITIVES

Apart from direct food additives, there are a large number of indirect additives and some contaminants that pose toxicological problems and require different control measures. The problems are highlighted as follows.

The most important of these chemicals are (1) the constituents of packaging material, which may migrate into the food that is in contact with them, and (2) anabolic agents and antibiotics that are commonly used in raising food-producing animals.

Packaging Materials A number of substances may migrate from food containers, wrappers, etc. to the food that is packaged in them. Most of the chemicals that might migrate from the conventional types of packaging materials, such as paper and wood, had been considered safe and were included in FDA's GRAS list. More recently, however, the packaging items are generally made of polymeric materials. The polymers per se are generally inert, but the components—the monomers, which are present to some extent, residual reactants, intermediates, manufacturing aids, solvents, and plastic additives—as well as the products of side reaction and chemical degradation may migrate into the food that is in contact with them. Some of these chemicals have been shown to be toxic. For example, vinyl chloride has been shown to be a human carcinogen at high levels of exposure, and acrylonitrile is a probable human carcinogen. Both are carcinogenic in a number of animal species (chap. 7). However, because of the exceedingly low levels of exposure from migration to food, their continued use has been provisionally approved.

Animal Drug Residues in Human Food There are three types of drugs used in food-producing animals that may leave residues in human food such as meat, milk, and eggs. The drugs present not only a problem related to the parent chemicals. It is also necessary to consider their metabolites, which are produced as a result of the metabolic processes, including bioactivation, of the animals and which may possess different toxic properties (Hayes and Borzelleca, 1982).

Therapeutic drugs, such as the anthelmintic agents febantel, fenbendazole, and oxfendazole, are generally used in individual animals for specific disease and only over short periods of times. Therefore they do not pose a widespread health concern. On the other hand, tranquilizing agents such as chlorpromazine and propylpromazine are used shortly before slaughter and hence leave residues in the meat. Their use is therefore not allowed (WHO, 1995).

Antibiotics such as benzylpenicillin and oxytetracycline are usually incorporated in the animal feeds to prevent outbreaks of bacterial diseases and to promote growth. The residue levels are generally extremely low and not expected to induce toxic effects.

Anabolic agents are growth-promoting substances and are implanted subcutaneously in a part of the animal that is usually not eaten, such as the ear. Their residue levels in the meat are low enough to be essentially devoid of general toxic effects, except carcinogenicity. A carcinogen may be effective at extremely low dose levels. Diethylstilbestrol (DES) is no longer used as a growth promoter, because of the discovery that tumors of genital organs have developed in the offspring of mothers who had taken DES during the pregnancy in large doses for medical purposes.

The anabolic agents in use may be considered either "endogenous" or "exogenous." The former includes estradiol, progesterone, and testosterone. The latter includes trenbolone acetate and zeranol. The "endogenous" anabolic agents are considered indistinguishable from the endogenous hormones. Furthermore, the amount of the residues of such substance in meat is small in comparison with the amount normally present in the body. On the other hand, trenbolone acetate, a synthetic steroid, and zeranol, a nonsteroidal substance, are xenobiotics and have been evaluated as such. Temporary acceptable daily intakes of $0.01\mu g/kg$ and $0-0.5\mu g/kg$ have been allocated to trenbolone acetate and zeranol, respectively (WHO, 1988).

In compliance with the Delaney Clause, the U.S. Food and Drug Administration has regulated such agents, if shown to be carcinogenic, by stipulating that their use should leave "no residue" in the meat and other products. The condition of "no residue" is to be determined by a designated method of analysis (FDA, 1982b).

CONTAMINANTS

There are three main types of food contaminants: mycotoxins, heavy metals, and synthetic chemicals. They contaminate food because of growing or harvesting from contaminated soil or water, improper handling, and accidental release from industrial sources.

Mycotoxins *Aflatoxins*, produced by the mold *Aspergillus flavus*, occur in nuts and grains, especially when these commodities are stored in a humid and warm climate. These toxins exist as mixtures of aflatoxins B_1, B_2, G_1, and G_2. Among these aflatoxins, B_1 is the most potent carcinogen in most species of animals, especially the rat. In one experiment, rats fed a diet containing 1 ppb of aflatoxin B_1 had hyperplastic nodules and carcinoma of the liver (Wogan et al., 1974). Aflatoxins G_1 and M_1 (a metabolite of B_1 and occurring in milk) are also carcinogenic but much less potent. Positive correlation was noted between aflatoxin intake and liver cancer incidence in certain regions in Africa and Thailand (IARC, 1976). As noted in chap. 3, aflatoxin is bioactivated to aflatoxin- 8,9-epoxide, which may covalently bind to DNA, thus initiating carcinogenesis.

A number of other mycotoxins also occur in foods. Their characteristics are summarized in Table 18-2. Additional information on these and other mycotoxins may be found in a publication of NAS/NRC (1980).

Metals The toxic properties of a number of metals are described in chap. 20, but human exposure via food is highlighted in this section. Among the metals that have caused the most concern are mercury, lead, and cadmium.

A number of acute and chronic poisoning episodes have resulted from improper application or consumption of *alkylmercury* compounds used as fungicides to preserve seed grains. Others followed consumption of fish contaminated with methylmercury. The compound can be formed via bioactivation (aided by microorganisms in the mud) of mercury discharged from factories (e.g., in Minamata and Niigata, Japan; chap. 1, Appendix 1-2). Because of the biomagnification factor along the food chain, large carnivorous fishes generally contain much higher levels of methylmercury (WHO, 1976).

Lead has been used as a fuel additive, in lead batteries, in paints, etc. Humans are exposed to this metal from air, water, and food. According to

Table 18-2 Source, Occurrence, and Toxicity of Certain Mycotoxins

Mycotoxin	Source	Occurrence	Toxic effects
Trichothecenes	*Fusarium* *Trichoderma*	Grains	Vomiting, diarrhea, skin inflammation, multiple hemorrhage
Zearalenone	*Fusarium*	Grains	Estrogenic effects
Ochratoxins	*Aspergillus* *Penicillium*	Grains	Nephropathy
Ergot	*Claviceps* *purpura*	Grains, especially rye	Ergotism (spasm, cramps, dry gangrene)

Source: NAS/NRC (1980).

one analysis, daily intakes from these media amount to 15, 20, and 140 μg, respectively (NRC Canada, 1973). One unusual source of lead intake is improperly fired ceramic foodware, which may release large amounts of lead from the glaze and which has caused a number of poisonings. This fact has prompted the promulgation of limits in the extent of release of lead from various types of foodware (WHO, 1979). The estimated intake of lead from ceramic ware would be in the range of 30–80 μg per day if all the wares in use released this metal to the legal limit (Lu, 1979b). Among certain populations, ceramic foodware still constitutes an important source of lead (Rojas-Lopez et al., 1944).

Cadmium is used as a pigment and occurs in the environment, especially through the refining of zinc ores, which contain varying concentrations of cadmium. It enters the food chain through pollution of soil and water. Itai-itai disease in Japan has been attributed to chronic exposure to cadmium, through long-term ingestion of contaminated rice. It may also be leached from decorated ceramic foodware.

Certain Organic Compounds   Among these chemicals are *organochlorine insecticides*, which had been widely used. Their use has been discontinued because of their persistence in the environment. However, they are still present in foods in trace amounts. Others include *polychlorinated biphenyls* (PCB), which are used in electrical capacitors and transformers, as plasticizers and heat exchangers, and in paper manufacturing. Through leakage and discharge of waste, they enter the environment. Because of their persistence and biomagnification properties, they enter the food chain. These chemicals attracted much attention because of the epi-

Table 18-3   Action Levels for Certain Food Contaminants

Contaminants	Commodity	Action level
Aflatoxin	Nuts	20 ppb
	Foods and feeds	20 ppb
	Milk	0.5 ppb
Aldrin and dieldrin	Various foods	0.02–0.3 ppm
Cadmium, in	Flatware	0.5 fg/ml
leaching solution	Small hollowware	0.5 fg/ml
from ceramic ware	Large hollowware	0.25 fg/ml
Lead, in leaching	Flatware	3.0 fg/ml
solution from	Small hollowware	2.0 fg/ml
ceramic ware	Large hollowware	1.0 fg/ml
Mercury	Fish, shellfish, crustaceans	1.0 ppm
	Wheat	1.0 ppm
Polychlorinated biphenyls	Red meat (fat basis)	3 ppm

Source: FDA (1994).

sode of consumption of a batch of rice oil contaminated with PCB through a leak in a heat exchanger in 1968. Thousands of consumers in Japan were affected (chap. 1, Appendix 1-2). The main sign of toxicity was chloracne, although there were many other symptoms and signs (see chap. 21). Similarly, an inadvertent addition of *polybrominated biphenyls* (PBB) to cattle feed in Michigan resulted in the contamination of a large amount of beef and milk.

The "action levels" for these and other contaminants have been established by the FDA to control their levels in food and feed. Some of them are listed in Table 18-3.

REFERENCES

Arnold, D. L., Moodie, C. A., Stavric, D., Soltz, D.R., Grice, H. C., and Munro, I. C. 1977 Canadian saccharin study. *Science* 197:320.

Carr, C. J. 1987. Food additives: A benefit/risk dilemma. In *Handbook of toxicology*, eds. T J. Haley and W. O. Berndt, pp. 426–438. Washington, DC: Hemisphere.

Classen, H. G., Marquardt, P., and Spath, M. 1968. Sympathomimetic effects of cyclohexy lamine. *Arzneim. Forsch.* 18:590–594.

Coulston, F., ed. 1979. *Regulatory aspects of carcinogenesis and food additives: The Delane clause.* New York: Academic Press.

FAO/WHO. 1994. Food Additives. *Codex Alimentarius*, vol. XIV. Rome: Food and Agriculture Organization of the United Nations.

Food and Drug Administration. 1982a. Toxicological Principles for the Safety Assessment of Direct Additives and Color Additives Used in Food. Springfield, VA: National Technical Information Service, PB 83-170696.

Food and Drug Administration. 1982b. Chemical compounds in food-producing animals; availability of criteria for guideline. Fed. Reg. 42(22):4972–4977.

Food and Drug Administration. 1994. Action Levels for Poisonous or Deleterious Substances in Human Food and Animal Feed. Washington, DC: Food and Drug Administration.

Hayes, J. R., and Borzelleca, J. F. 1982. Biodisposition of xenobiotics in animals. In *Animal products in human nutrition*, eds. D. C. Beitz and R. Hanson, pp. 225–259. New York: Academic Press.

International Agency for Research on Cancer. 1976. *Evaluation of carcinogenic risk of chemicals to man*, vol. 10, *Some naturally occurring substances.* Lyon, France: IARC.

International Agency for Research on Cancer. 1980. *Evaluation of the carcinogenic risk of chemicals to humans*, vol. 22, *Some non-nutritive sweetening agents.* Lyon, France: IARC.

Ito, N., Fukushima, S., Hagiwara, A., Shibata, M., and Ogiso, T. 1983. Carcinogenicity of butylated hydroxyanisole in F344 rats. *JNCI* 70:343–352.

Juhlin, L. 1980. Incidence of intolerance to food additives. *Int. J. Dermatol.* 19:548–551.

Kenney, R. A. 1986. The Chinese restaurant syndrome: An anecdote revisited. *Food Chem. Toxicol.* 24:351–354.

Lu, F. C. 1979a. The safety of food additives: The dynamics of the issue. In *Toxicology and occupational medicine*, ed. W. B. Deichmann, pp. 175–189. New York: Elsevier/North Holland.

Lu, F. C. 1979b. Review of Total Intake of Lead from All Sources. HCS/CER/79.5. Geneva: World Health Organization.

Lu, F. C. 1988. Acceptable daily intake: Inception, evolution and application. *Regul. Toxicol. Pharmacol.* 8:45–60.

National Academy of Sciences-National Research Council. 1965. *Chemicals Used in Food Processing.* Washington, DC: NAS/NRC.

National Academy of Sciences-National Research Council. 1980. *Toxicants occurring naturally in food.* Washington, DC: NAS/NRC.

National Research Council/National Academy of Sciences. 1987. *Regulatory problems in foods: The Delaney paradox.* Washington, DC: National Academy Press.

National Research Council of Canada. 1973. Lead in the Canadian Environment. NRCC No. 13682. Ottawa: NRC of Canada.

Olsen, P., Bille, N., and Meyer, O. 1983. Hepatocellular neoplasms in rats induced by butylated hydroxytoluene (BHT). *Acta Pharmacol. Toxicol.* 54:433–434.

Price, J. M., Biava, C. G., Oser, B. L., Vogen, E. E., Steinfeld, J., and Ley, H. L. 1970. Bladder tumors in rats fed cyclohexylamine or high doses of a mixture of cyclamate and saccharin. *Science* 167:1131–1132.

Prochaska, H. J., DeLong, M. J., and Talalay, P. 1985. On the mechanisms of induction of cancer-protective enzymes: A unifying proposal. *Proc. Natl. Acad. Sci. USA* 82: 8232–8236.

Rojas-Lopez, M., Santos-Burgoa, C., Rios, C., Hernandez-Avila, M., and Romieu, I. 1994. Use of lead-glazed ceramics is the main factor associated to high lead in blood levels in two Mexican rural communities. *J. Toxicol. Environ. Health* 42:45–52.

Schaumberg, H. H., Byck, R., Gerstl, R., and Marshman, J. H. 1969. Monosodium glutamate: Its pharmacology and role in the Chinese restaurant syndrome. *Science* 163:826.

Select Committee on GRAS Substances. 1977. Evaluation of health aspects of GRAS food ingredients: Lessons learned and questions unanswered. *Fed. Proc.* 36:2519–2562.

Select Committee on GRAS Substances. 1982. Insights on Food Safety Evaluation. Bethesda, MD: Life Sciences Research Office, FASEB.

U.S. Federal Food, Drug, and Cosmetic Act, As Amended. 1979. Washington, DC: U.S. Government Printing Office.

Wogan, G. N., Paglialunga, S., and Newberne, P. M. 1974. Carcinogenic effects of low dietary levels of aflatoxin B in rats. *Food Cosmet. Toxicol.* 12:681–685.

World Health Organization. 1974. Toxicological Evaluation of Certain Food Additives with a Review of General Principles and of Specifirtain Food Additives and Contaminants (26th Report). Tech. Rep. Ser. 683. Geneva: WHO.

World Health Organization. 1976. Mercury. Environmental Health Criteria 1. Geneva: WHO.

World Health Organization. 1979. Ceramic Foodware Safety. Report of a Meeting of Experts. HCS/79.7. Geneva: WHO.

World Health Organization. 1982a. Evaluation of Certain Food Additives and Contaminants (26th Rep.). Tech. Rep. Ser. 683. Geneva: WHO.

World Health Organization. 1982b. Evaluation of Certain Food Additives. WHO Food Additives Series 17. Geneva: WHO.

World Health Organization. 1986. Evaluation of Certain Food Additives and Contaminants (29th Rep.). Tech. Rep. Ser. 733. Geneva: WHO.

World Health Organization. 1988. Evaluation of Certain Veterinary Drug Residues in Food (32nd Rep.). Tech. Rep. Ser. 763. Geneva: WHO.

World Health Organization. 1989. Evaluation of Certain Food Additives and Contaminants. WHO Food Additives Ser. 24. Geneva: WHO.

World Health Organization. 1995. Evaluation of Certain Veterinary Drug Residues in Food (38th Rep.). Tech. Rep. Ser. 815. Geneva: WHO.

ADDITIONAL READING

Davidek, J. 1995. *Natural toxic compounds of foods.* Boca Raton, FL: CRC Press.

Toxicity of Pesticides

CHAPTER 19 CONTENTS

INTRODUCTION

Value of Pesticides

Pesticides are substances that kill or control pests. There are various types of pests. The most common are insects. Some of them serve as vectors for diseases. The most important vector-borne diseases, malaria and onchocerciasis ("river blindness"), are transmitted to humans by mosquitoes and black flies. Both diseases are debilitating and affect millions of people in the tropical and subtropical regions. Other vector-borne diseases include filariasis, yellow fever, rickettsial pox, viral encephalitis, typhus, and bubonic plague. Insecticides have helped to control these diseases.

Insects are also detrimental to various plants and their products. Insecticides are therefore widely used to protect farmers' products. Although most of the insecticides currently in use are synthetic chemicals, a number of natural substances have been used by farmers for a long time. These substances include nicotine from tobacco, pyrethrum from flowers of a species of chrysanthemum, and various compounds of lead, copper, and arsenic.

Aside from insects, weeds constitute a very important nuisance to the farmer. Before the introduction of herbicides, farmers used to spend much time removing the weeds manually, a very time-consuming and backbreaking task. Other pesticides have also been developed to control other pests such as fungi, rodents, and others. The great variety of agricultural uses and chemical categories may be seen from a recent compilation of the 230 pesticides that have been evaluated and reevaluated by the World Health Organization (WHO) Expert Committee on Pesticide Residues since 1965 (Lu, 1995).

A number of household pesticide products are also available to control household nuisance pests, such as flies and mosquitoes.

Adverse Effects of Pesticides

These may involve human health and/or the environment. The most dramatic of such effects on humans are the accidental acute poisonings. Several major outbreaks of poisoning with methyl- and ethylmercury compounds and hexachlorobenzene as fungicides and with parathion, an organophosphorus insecticide, have occurred in several parts of the world involving thousands of individuals and hundreds of deaths. A few examples are listed in chap. 1, Appendix 1-2. Individual cases of acute poisoning have usually resulted from ingestion of large quantities of pesticides accidentally or with suicidal intent.

Occupational exposure to pesticides may involve workers engaged in the manufacturing, formulating, and application of pesticides. The pesticides enter the body generally through the respiratory tract and by dermal absorption, but small amounts may enter the gastrointestinal tract through the use of contaminated hands and utensils. This type of poisoning is more likely to happen with pesticides that are more toxic acutely. The major public health concern, however, is the ingestion of pesticide residues in foods, as this may involve large populations over long periods of time.

In addition to these human health hazards, pesticides may have serious impact on the environment. Apart from large-scale accidental release to the environment, only minimal levels are found in various environmental media. However, the levels are likely to be higher with pesticides that are persistent and/or have a propensity for biomagnification. In the latter case, the concentration of a pesticide increases as it moves through the trophic chain. The organism with a high concentration may be adversely affected. For example, the bald eagle was nearly extinct, resulting from its fragile egg shells as a toxic effect of high levels of DDT bioaccumulated through the contaminated food chain of the bird. Such environmental pollution may also affect human health by virtue of the contaminated soil and water, which then result in the production of contaminated human food and drinking water.

CATEGORIES OF PESTICIDES

Pesticides are usually grouped according to their uses and their chemical nature. The major groups are the following.

Insecticides

As noted earlier, this is the largest group of pesticides and consists of a number of different chemical subgroups.

Organophosphorus Insecticides These are esters of phosphoric acid or thiophosphoric acid, represented by dichlorvos and parathion, respectively. They act by inhibiting acetylcholinesterase (AChE), resulting in an accumulation of acetylcholine (ACh). The excess ACh induces a variety of symptoms and signs (see also Toxicological Properties section). The severity of the symptoms and signs is more or less correlated with the extent of the inhibition of cholinesterase in blood, but the precise relationship varies depending on the compound (Wills, 1972).

In addition to parathion and dichlorvos, other pesticides in this group include parathion-methyl, azinphos-methyl (Guthion), chlorfenvinphos, diazinon, dimethoate, disulfoton (Di-Syston), malathion, mevinphos, and trichlorfon (Dipterex). Their toxicities vary over a wide range (see Appendix 19-1).

Carbamate Insecticides These are esters of *N*-methylcarbamic acid. They also act by inhibiting AChE. However, their effects on the enzyme are much more readily reversible than those of the organophosphorus insecticides. Insecticides of this class include carbaryl (Sevin), aldicarb (Temik), carbofuran, methomyl, and propoxur (Baygon). In addition, with carbamates signs of toxicity appear more promptly, and for many of them there is a greater range from the doses that cause minor toxic effects and those that are lethal. For this reason, on an acute basis, the carbamates are safer than the organophosphorus insecticides. Appendix 19-1 also lists their toxicities.

Organochlorine Insecticides   These include the chlorinated ethane derivatives, the cyclodienes, and the hexachlorocyclohexanes. Some of these chemicals (e.g., DDT) were introduced in the 1940s and were widely used in agricultural and health programs. This was because of their relatively low acute toxicity and their persistence, which reduced the need for repeated applications. However, the persistence was later recognized as a liability rather than an asset.

Both DDT and methoxychlor are chlorinated ethane derivatives, but methoxychlor is much less toxic and less persistent than DDT. The cyclodiene insecticide endrin is extremely toxic, aldrin and dieldrin somewhat less toxic, and chlordane, heptachlor, and mirex even less toxic. Lindane is the gamma isomer of hexachlorocyclohexane (HCH) that is in use. It is highly toxic but less cumulative. Consequently, lindane is used much more widely than HCH.

Botanical and Other Insecticides   These include nicotine from tobacco. Nicotine is extremely toxic acutely and acts on the nervous system. Pyrethrum is obtained from the flowers of *Chrysanthemum cinerariaefolium*. An enzyme inhibitor, piperonyl butoxide, is often used in combination with this insecticide as a synergist. Pyrethrum has a low toxicity in mammals but is allergenic to sensitive individuals, causing contact dermatitis. It is also a neurotoxicant. Rotenone is extracted from roots of the plant *Derris elliptica*. It also has a low toxicity in mammals but is more toxic to insects and fish. Many microorganisms are known to be pathogenic to insects. The ones being used are *Bacillus thuringiensis* and certain insect baculoviruses. They are not known to be pathogenic to humans.

Herbicides

There are several types of herbicides. Some retard the growth of weeds by inhibiting photosynthesis, respiration, cell division or synthesis of protein or lipids. Others act as growth stimulants, thereby disturbing the normal growth (Ecobichon, 1993).

Chlorophenoxy compounds are exemplified by 2,4-D (2,4-dichlorophenoxyacetic acid) and 2,4,5-T (2,4,5-trichlorophenoxyacetic acid). They act in plants as growth hormones. Their toxicities in animals are relatively low. However, chloracne, the main toxic effect of 2,4,5-T in humans, seems attributable to the contaminant 2,3,7,8-tetrachlorobenzo-*p*-dioxin (TCDD). For additional information on this contaminant, see chap. 21, Persistent Organic Chemicals subsection.

Bipyridyl herbicides, such as paraquat and diquat, have been widely used. They exert their toxicity via the formation of free radicals. The toxicity of paraquat is characterized by its pulmonary effects not only after exposure via inhalation but also by the oral route, as noted on page 166.

Other herbicides include dinitro-*o*-cresol (DNOC), amitrole, the carbamates propham and chloropropham, and a number of other chemicals.

Fungicides

Mercury compounds such as methyl- and ethylmercury are very effective fungicides and had been widely used to preserve seed grains. However, several tragic accidents, involving numerous deaths and permanent neurologic damage, occurred with their use (chap. 1, Appendix 1-2). This fact has deterred their further use.

Dicarboximides include the dimethylthiocarbamates (ferbam, thiram, and ziram) and the ethylenebisdithiocarbamates (maneb, nabam, and zineb). These compounds have relatively low acute toxicity and have hence been widely used in agriculture. However, there is concern about their carcinogenic potential (see chap. 7 and in this chapter, the Carcinogenicity subsection).

Phthalimide derivatives such as captan and folpet have very low acute and chronic toxicity. However, captan has been shown to reduce body weight of pups of treated rats and folpet induced keratosis of the gastrointestinal tract (FAO, 1990).

Substituted aromatics such as pentachlorophenol (PCP) have been widely used as wood preservatives. PCP increases metabolic rate through uncoupling of oxidative phosphorylation. It has a low LD_{50} but its technical grade is more toxic, indicating greater toxicity of its contaminants. Pentachloronitrobenzene (PCNB) has been used as a fungicide in treating soil. It is somewhat less toxic acutely than PCP, but may be carcinogenic.

Other fungicides include certain *N*-heterocyclic compounds such as benomyl and thiobendazole. These chemicals have very low toxicity and have been widely used in agriculture. Hexachlorobenzene has been used as a seed treatment agent but has caused mass poisoning (chap. 1, Appendix 1-2).

Rodenticides

Warfarin is an anticoagulant by acting as an antimetabolite to vitamin K, thereby inhibiting the formation of prothrombin. It has been widely used because its toxicity is observed only after repeated ingestion, a circumstance unlikely to occur among children and pets.

Thioureas such an ANTU (α-naphthylthiourea) are extremely toxic to rats but only moderately toxic to humans. Their main toxicity is pulmonary edema and pleural effusion.

Sodium fluoracetate ("1080") and fluoroacetamide ("1081") are extremely toxic and their use has hence been restricted to licensed personnel. They exert toxic effect through blockage of the citric acid cycle as described on pp. 38 and 49.

Other rodenticides include botanical products such as the alkaloid strychnine, a potent central nervous system (CNS) stimulant, and red squill, which contains the glycosides scillaren-A and -B. These glycosides, similar to digitalis, have cardiotonic and central emetic effects. Because of the latter effect, these substances are relatively nontoxic to most mammals but are potent poisons to rats, which do not vomit. Inorganic rodenticides include zinc phosphide, thallium sulfate, arsenic trioxide, and elemental phosphorus, acting through different mechanisms.

Fumigants

As the name implies, this group of pesticides includes a number of gases, liquids that readily vaporize, and solids that release gases by chemical reactions. In the gaseous form, they permeate storage areas and soil to control insects, rodents, and soil nematodes. Many fumigants, such as acrylonitrile, chloropicrin, and ethylene dibromide, are reactive chemicals and are also used widely in the chemical industry; some of them are described in chap. 21.

TOXICOLOGICAL PROPERTIES

Toxicity on the Nervous System

The organochlorine (OC) insecticides stimulate the nervous system and induce paresthesia, susceptibility to stimulation, irritability, disturbed equilibrium, tremor, and convulsions. Aldrin, dieldrin, and lindane induce facilitation and hyperexcitation at synaptic and neuromuscular junctions, resulting in repetitive discharge in central, sensory, and motor neurons. DDT exerts its toxic effect in the nervous system by adversely affecting the axon membrane (Doherty, 1979; Narahashi, 1980).

The organophosphate (OP) and carbamate insecticides inhibit acetylcholinesterase. Normally, the neurotransmitter acetylcholine (ACh) is released at the synapses. Once the nerve impulse is transmitted, the released ACh is hydrolyzed to acetic acid and choline by the acetylcholinesterase (AChE) at the site. Upon exposure to OP and carbamate insecticides, AChE is inhibited, resulting in an accumulation of ACh. The accumulated ACh in the CNS will induce tremor, incoordination, convulsion, etc. In the autonomic nervous system it will cause diarrhea, involuntary urination, bronchoconstriction, miosis, etc. Its accumulation at the neuromuscular junction will lead to contraction of the muscles, followed by weakness, loss of reflexes, and paralysis. The inhibition of AChE induced by the carbamate is readily reversible, whereas that following exposure to OP compounds is generally less readily so. In fact, certain OP compounds, such as DFP (diisopropyl fluorophosphate), cause irreversible inhibition; recovery only follows synthesis of new AChE.

Several OP compounds, including DFP, tri-o-cresyl phosphate (TOCP), leptophos, mipafox, and trichlorofon, cause "delayed neurotoxicity." For the mechanism of action and testing procedures, see chap. 16.

The two types of pyrethroid insecticides also act on the nervous system. Type I pyrethroids (e.g., permethrin) interact with sodium channel on nerve fibers, inducing hyperexcitation, ataxia, tremor, etc. Type II pyrethroids (e.g., cypermethrin) induce depolarization block of sensory nerve membrane; human exposure results in a tickling sensation (Abou-Donia, 1992).

Interactions

The most notable type of interaction is the potentiation observed between certain organophosphorus insecticides. Frawley and co-workers (1957) reported marked potentiation of the toxicity of EPN [o-ethyl-o-(4-nitrophenyl) phenyl phosphonothioate] and malathion. Combinations of a number of OP insecticides have since been tested. Some showed additive effects, others were less than additive, and still others were synergistic. The most pronounced potentiation (about 100-fold increase) was observed between malathion and TOCP (tri-o-cresyl phosphate). The mechanism of the potentiation has been attributed to the inhibition of enzymes, such as carboxylesterase and amidases, which are responsible for the detoxication of certain OP compounds such as malathion and its more toxic metabolite malaoxon (Murphy, 1969).

Carcinogenicity

The organophosphate insecticides are in general not carcinogenic, with the exception of compounds that contain halogens such as tetrachlorvinphos. These chemicals evidently possess this property of the organochlorine insecticides (discussed later). The carbamate insecticides per se are not carcinogenic either. But carbaryl has been shown to form, in the presence of nitrous acid, nitrosocarbaryl, which is carcinogenic. A number of other pesticides are also nitrosatable under extreme conditions, and their products are carcinogenic and mutagenic (IARC, 1983). However, because of the unrealistic conditions required for such nitrosation to take place, the health concern arising from this type of reaction is questionable.

On the other hand, the organochlorine insecticides tested have all been shown to induce hepatoma in mice (Secretary's Commission on Pesticides,

1969; IARC, 1983). The pesticide that has aroused most controversy has been DDT. It showed no carcinogenicity in rats, nor in hamsters and several other species of animals. Furthermore, epidemiological findings are essentially negative, and so are the short-term mutagenesis tests. For these reasons the WHO Expert Committee on Pesticide Residues reaffirmed the acceptable daily intake (ADI) for DDT and several other organochlorine insecticides (WHO, 1974; FAO, 1985). Similar conclusions were reached by other groups such as the Task Force of Past Presidents of the Society of Toxicology (Task Force of Past Presidents, 1982) and the Nutrition Foundation (1983). A comprehensive review of the toxicological data and their interpretations on DDT was provided by Coulston (1985). Nevertheless, its use has been restricted or suspended in several nations based partly on this potential health hazard and partly on its ecological impact. The only pesticide for which there is some epidemiological evidence of carcinogenicity is hexachlorocyclohexane (Wang et al., 1988). The results, however, need confirmation.

The fumigants EDB (ethylene dibromide) and DBCP (1,2-dibromo-3-chloropropane) have been found to produce highly malignant squamous-cell carcinoma in the stomach of rats and mice (IARC, 1977). However, their use has not been restricted or suspended, because the fumigated foods, upon aeration, contain negligible residue.

Amitrole (aminotriazole), a herbicide, produces thyroid tumors apparently through an indirect mechanism (Steinhoff et al., 1983; McClain, 1992). Thyroid peroxidase normally oxidizes iodine to an oxidized form, which then conjugates with tyrosine to form thyroxine. Amitrole inhibits this enzyme, thus lowering the thyroxine level. This lowered level, through a biofeedback mechanism, stimulates the pituitary gland to release more thyroid-stimulating hormone (TSH). TSH in turn stimulates the thyroid gland to become hyperplastic and eventually to form tumors. Amitrole is thus a "secondary carcinogen." Similarly, the ethylenebisdithiocarbamate fumigants (mancozeb, maneb, nabam, and zineb) have also been reported to produce thyroid tumors. This action is evidently mediated through the major breakdown and metabolic product ethylenethiourea. The Joint FAO/WHO Meeting on Pesticide Residues assessed these fungicides and recommended maximum residue limits in foods (FAO, 1993).

Teratogenicity and Effects on Reproductive Functions

In the late 1960s, several articles appeared reporting a variety of teratogenic and reproductive effects of carbaryl in dogs. Summaries of these reports have been included in a monograph (WHO, 1970). A comprehensive study in rats given carbaryl in the diet at doses of 100 mg/kg and 200 mg/kg showed no effect on various reproductive functions and no teratogenic effects. Some effects were observed in rats given carbaryl by gavage (Weil et al., 1972). The authors attributed the effects in rats to the gavage method of administering the pesticide and the effects in the dog to its routes of biotransformation of cabaryl being different from those in humans and several other species.

Other pesticides reported as having teratogenic effects include the dithiocarbamate fungicides. Such effects are likely due, at least partly, to their breakdown product ethylenethiourea (WHO, 1974). In addition, abamectin, dinocap, glyphosate, and procymidone induced cleft palate, defects in the neural tube, renal defects, and hypospadia, respectively (see Lu, 1995).

Other Adverse Effects

Certain renal effects of carbaryl were reported in a group of human volunteers ingesting carbaryl at a daily dose of 0.12 mg/kg for 6 wk. There was an increase in the ratio of urinary amino acid nitrogen to creatinine, compared to those taking placebo. This was interpreted as an indication of a decrease in the ability of the proximal convoluted tubules to reabsorb amino acids. This effect was not observed in individuals taking carbaryl at 0.06 mg/kg daily (Wills et al., 1968).

Paraquat produces pulmonary edema, hemorrhage, and fibrosis (Smith and Heath, 1976) following either inhalation or ingestion, but the closely related herbicide diquat does not (see also chap. 11). However, both chemicals are toxic to cultured lung cells. Since paraquat is retained in the lung whereas diquat is not, it is evident that the difference between those two herbicides in their pulmonary toxicity is related to the special affinity of paraquat for certain pulmonary cells (type II cells). For additional details see Clark et al. (1966), and Rose et al. (1976).

Hypersensitivity reactions to pyrethrum have been reported. The most common form is contact dermatitis. Asthma has also been reported. Several cases of anaphylactic reactions have been reported, but are very rare (Hayes, 1982).

Organochlorine insecticides, such as DDT, chlorodecone, and mirex, are hepatotoxic, inducing liver enlargement and centrolobular necrosis. They are also inducers of microsomal monooxygenases, thereby affecting the toxicity of other chemicals.

A number of organophosphorus, carbamate, and organochlorine insecticides, the dithiocarbamate fungicides, and herbicides alter various immune functions. For example, malathion, methylparathion, carbaryl, DDT, paraquat, and diquat have been shown to depress antibody formation, impair leukocyte phagocytosis, and reduce the germinal centers in spleen, thymus, and lymph nodes (Koller, 1979; Street, 1981).

Bioaccumulation and Biomagnification

These properties per se do not necessarily represent adverse biological effects. They are generally associated with substances that are lipophilic and resistant to breakdown. The organochlorine pesticides in general are more persistent in the environment and tend to be stored in the fat depot. However, the bioaccumulation is more marked with some chemicals than others. For example, DDT is stored in the body fat for a much longer time than methoxychlor. The half-lives of these insecticides in rats are 612 mo and 12 wk, respectively.

Their persistence in the environment may create ecological problems. DDT and related chemicals in the environment enhance the metabolism of estrogens in birds. In the egg-laying and nestling cycle of certain birds, this disturbance of hormones adversely affects reproduction and survival of the young (Peakall, 1970).

Biomagnification is the result of bioaccumulation in the organism alone or in conjunction with persistence in the environment also. For example, DDT is lipophilic, and thus occurs in the fat portion of body fluids including milk. While a mother's daily intake of DDT may be 0.5 μg/kg, her breastfed baby's might be 11.2 μg/kg. This magnification results from the fact that DDT is stored in the human body at 10- to 20-fold chronic daily intake level and the baby consumes essentially only the milk. Furthermore, the caloric intake per kilogram body weight is higher in babies compared to adults. The significance of the much greater intake of DDT by babies is not clear because of the relatively short duration of this greater level of intake and the remarkable insensitivity of the young versus the adult (Lu et al., 1965; see also p. 61).

The biomagnification is even more marked in carnivorous animals. DDT and methylmercury can accumulate through a series of plankton, small fish, large fish, and birds and result in a magnification of the concentration amounting to several hundredfold (Woodwell, 1967). The decision to suspend the use of DDT was partly based on its adverse ecological impact, as noted earlier.

TESTING, EVALUATION, AND CONTROL

Categories of Data Required

Various categories of data are required in the evaluation of pesticides. The basic data required are essentially the same as those listed for food additives (see chap. 18). However, a number of specific toxicological problems have been encountered with pesticides as outlined in the preceding section. The additional studies for certain pesticides include the following.

LD_{50} and Short-Term Toxicity Because of the greater acute toxicity of most pesticides, the LD_50 is usually determined more precisely. Furthermore, in view of the fact that certain occupational workers, such as manufacturers, formulators, and applicators, may be exposed through the skin and respiratory tract, the dermal LD_{50} and the LC_{50} by inhalation are generally required. Furthermore, as occupational workers are likely to be exposed for some lengths of time, the toxicity of repeated exposure through dermal and inhalation is generally ascertained (see chaps. 11 and 14).

Delayed Neurotoxicity (Peripheral Axonopathy) This type of toxicity has been observed with a number of organophosphorus insecticides. The appropriate test is performed on new chemicals of this group to exclude this potential hazard (see chap. 16).

Interaction Marked interaction exists between certain pairs of organophosphorus insecticides. The potential health hazard is assessed using LD_{50}s of the individual chemicals alone and in combination.

Toxicological Evaluation

As discussed in chap. 22, there are two approaches to the evaluation of the safety/risk of toxicants.

The acceptable daily intake (ADI) involves assessing the database for completeness and relevance, determining a no-observed-adverse-effect level in terms of milligrams per kilogram body weight (NOAEL), and selecting an appropriate safety factor to extrapolate to an acceptable daily intake for humans, also in terms of milligrams per kilogram body weight. A list of the ADIs of the 230 pesticides that have been evaluated and reevaluated by the WHO Expert Committtee on Pesticide Residues since 1965, along with the NOAELs, safety factors, and critical effects, is included in a recent review article (Lu, 1995).

While all pesticides are toxic, they vary in the nature and magnitude of toxicity. Certain pesticides have an inherent potential for specific toxic effects. The presence of such properties must be assessed by conducting appropriate tests as discussed earlier, before determining a NOAEL. The size of the safety factor will depend on a number of factors as discussed in chap. 22.

The second approach, risk assessment, is generally applied to genotoxic carcinogens. However, pesticides that have been shown to be genotoxic carcinogens are prohibited from agricultural use. Nongenotoxic carcinogens and pesticides with dubious carcinogenesis data are generally evaluated by the ADI procedure. For example, amitrole acts through a hormonal imbalance mechanism that has a threshold dose, and DDT induces hepatoma in mice, the significance of which to humans is dubious. These problems were addressed by the Joint FAO/WHO Meeting of Experts on Pesticide Residues (WHO, 1974). That international group allocated to these pesticides acceptable daily intakes that were reaffirmed at subsequent meetings.

Standards

Tolerances   To protect the health of the consumer, standards are formulated. The standards, in the form of "tolerances" (also known as "maximum residue limits"), are established. The standards provide maximum permitted levels in each food commodity in which the pesticide may leave residues following its use. A pesticide may be used during any one or more stages of the preplanting, growth, harvesting, handling, and storage of the food crop.

Dietary Intakes   Several procedures are used to ensure that the total intake of each pesticide from its residues in all food commodities does not exceed its ADI. One procedure involves chemical analysis of the residue levels in food represented in the "total diet" and the calculation of the "dietary intake" of each pesticide by adding the products of the residue levels and the per capita consumption of each of these foods. The latest survey by the U.S. FDA shows the dietary intakes of all the pesticides analyzed were considerably lower than the corresponding ADIs (FDA, 1987).

The other procedure, which is much simpler, involves calculating the "potential daily intake" and comparing it with the corresponding ADI. The former figure is obtained by adding the products of the tolerance levels in each of the foods and the per capita consumption of these foods. Details are given in a WHO report (WHO, 1970). Evidently the potential daily intake represents an overestimation. First, a pesticide is not necessarily used in all the food commodities in which there are tolerances. Furthermore, in a vast majority of the cases, the actual residue levels are much lower than the tolerances. Nevertheless, this procedure offers distinct advantages. Apart from a few industrialized countries, figures for dietary intakes of pesticides are not available; for them the potential daily intakes provide a ready yardstick for assessing the health hazards to the consumer posed by the dietary intake of pesticides. The overestimation may also compensate for differences in dietary habits in different parts of the world and for variations in the levels of pesticide residues in certain foods. According to actual analysis, the residue levels may, although infrequently, exceed the tolerances (see also chap. 22).

Apart from assessing the potential hazard of pesticides, the dietary intake figures, obtained by analysis or calculation, are also used in assessing, and possibly in recommending modification of the agricultural use of these chemicals. Where the residue levels appear too high, they may be lowered, for example, by a reduction of the rate of application or by an increase of the interval between the last application and harvesting of the food crop.

Figure 19-1 depicts the relationships between the research community, "regulatory agencies," and the consumer, as applied at an international level (Lu, 1988). Similar relationships exist at a national level in many countries.

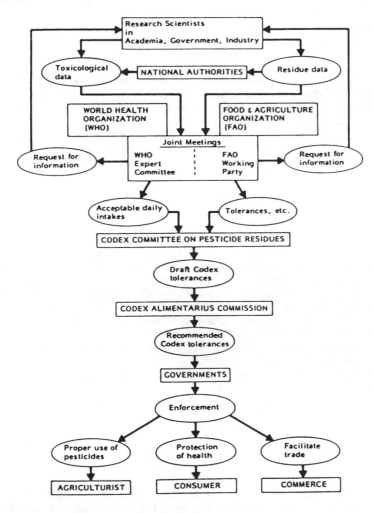

RELATIONSHIP BETWEEN THE VARIOUS ORGANIZATIONS CONCERNED
WITH THE EVALUATION AND CONTROL OF PESTICIDE RESIDUES

Figure 19-1 The relationship among research scientists, the Joint Meeting on Pesticide Residues, the Codex Alimentarius Commission, and the national authorities, as well as their impact on the consumer and others (Lu, 1988).

REFERENCES

Abou-Donia, M. B. 1992. Pesticides. In *Neurotoxicology*, ed. M. B. Abou-Donia, pp. 437–478. Boca Raton, FL: CRC Press.

Clark, D. G., McElligot, T. F., and Hurst, E. W. 1966. The toxicity of paraquat. *Br. J. Ind. Med.* 23:126–132.

Coulston, F. 1985. Reconsideration of the dilemma of DDT for the establishment of an acceptable daily intake. *Regul. Toxicol. Pharmacol.* 5:332–383.

Doherty, J. D. 1979. Insecticides affecting ion transport. *Pharmacol. Ther.* 7Z:123–151.

Ecobichon, D. J. 1993. Toxic effects of pesticides. In *Casarett and Doull's toxicology*, eds. M. O. Amdur, J. Doull, and C. D. Klaassen, pp. 565–622. New York: McGraw-Hill.

Food and Drug Administration. 1987. *Residues in Foods, 1987*. Washington, DC: FDA.

Food and Agricultural Organization of the United States. 1990. Pesticide Residues in Food—1990. *Report of the FAO and WHO Groups of Experts on Pesticide Residues.* FAO Plant Production and Protection Paper No. 102. Rome: FAO.

Food and Agriculture Organization of the United Nations. 1993. Pesticide Residues in Food—1993. FAO Plant Production and Protection Paper No. 122. Rome: FAO.

Food and Agriculture Organization of the United Nations. 1985. Pesticide residues in food—1984 evaluation. FAO Plant Production and Protection paper No. 67. Rome: FAO.

Frawley, J. P., Fuyat, H. N., Hagen, E. C., Blake, J. R., and Fitzhugh, O. G. 1957. Marked potentiation in mammalian toxicity from simultaneous administration of two anticholinesterase compounds. *J. Pharmacol. Exp. Ther.* 121:96–106.

Gaines, T. B. 1969. Acute toxicity of pesticides. *Toxicol. Appl. Pharmacol.* 14:515–534.

Hayes, W. J., Jr. 1982. *Pesticides studied in man*. Baltimore: Williams & Wilkins.

International Agency for Research in Cancer. 1977. *Monographs on the evaluation of carcinogenic risk of chemicals to man*, vol. 15. *Some fumigants, the herbicides 2,4-D and 2,4,5-T, chlorinated dibenzodioxins and miscellaneous industrial chemicals.* Lyon, France: IARC.

International Agency for Research on Cancer. 1983. *Monographs on the evaluation of carcinogenic risk of chemicals to man*, Vol. 30. *Miscellaneous pesticides.* Lyon, France: IARC.

Koller, L. D. 1979. Effects of environmental contaminants on the immune system. *Adv. Vet. Sci. Comp. Med.* 23:267–295.

Lu, F. C. 1988. Acceptable daily intake: Inception, evolution and application. *Regul. Toxicol. Pharmacol.* 8:45–60.

Lu, F. C. 1995. A review of the acceptable daily intakes of pesticides assessed by WHO. *Regul. Toxicol. Pharmacol.* 21:352–364.

Lu, F. C., Jessup, D. C., and Lavalle, A. 1965. Toxicity of pesticides to young versus adult rats. *Food Cosmet. Toxicol.* 5:591–596.

McClain, R. M. 1992. Thyroid gland neoplasia: non-genotoxic mechanisms. *Toxicol. Lett.* 64/65:307–408.

Murphy, S. D. 1969. Mechanisms of pesticide interactions in vertebrates. *Residue Rev.* 25:201–221.

Narahashi, T. 1980. Nerve membrane as a target of environmental toxicants. In *Neurotoxicology*, eds. P. Spencer and H. H. Schaumberg. Baltimore: Williams & Wilkins.

Nutrition Foundation. 1983. Report of the International Expert Advisory Committee on the Relevance of Mouse Liver Hepatoma to Human Carcinogenic Risk. Washington, DC: Nutrition Foundation.

Peakall, D. B. 1970. Pesticides and the reproduction of birds. *Sci. Am.* 222:72–78.

Rose, M. S., Lock, E. A., Smith, L. L., and Wyatt, I. 1976. Paraquat accumulation: Tissue and species specificity. *Biochem. Pharmacol.* 25:419–423.

Secretary's Commission on Pesticides, U.S. Department of Health, Education and Welfare 1969. Report of the Secretary's Commission on Pesticides and Their Relationship to Environmental Health. Washington, DC: U.S. Government Printing Office.

Smith, P., and Heath, D. 1976. Paraquat. *CRC Crit. Rev. Toxicol.* 4:411–445.

Steinhoff, D., Weber, H., Mohr, U., and Boehme, K. 1983. Evaluation of amitrole (aminotria-zole) for potential carcinogenicity in orally dosed rats, mice and golden hamster. *Toxicol. Appl. Pharmacol.* 69:161–169.

Street, J. C. 1981. Pesticides and the immune system. In *Immunologic considerations in toxicology*, ed. R. P. Sharma, pp. 45–66. Boca Raton, FL: CRC Press.

Task Force of Past Presidents. 1982. Animal data in hazard evaluation. Paths and pitfalls. *Fundam. Appl. Toxicol.* 2:101–107.

Wang, X. Q., Gas, P. Y., Lin, Y. Z., and Chen, C. 1988. Studies on hexachlorocyclohexane and DDT contents in human cerumen and their relationship to cancer mortality. *Biomed. Environ. Sci.* 1:138–151.

Weil, C. S., Woodside, M. D., Carpenter, C. P., and Smyth, H. F., Jr. 1972. Current status of tests of carbaryl for reproductive and teratogenic effects. *Toxicol. Appl. Pharmacol.* 21: 390–404.

Wills, J. H. 1972. The measurement and significance of changes in the cholinesterase of erythrocytes and plasma in man and animals. *CRC Crit. Rev. Toxicol.* 2:153–202.

Wills, J. H., Jameson, E., and Coulston, F. 1968. Effects of oral doses of carbaryl on man. *Clin. Toxicol.* 1:265–271.

Woodwell, G. M. 1967. Toxic substances and ecological cycles. *Sci. Am.* 216(3):24.

World Health Organization. 1970. Pesticide Residues in Food. WHO Tech. Rep. Ser. 458. Geneva: WHO.

World Health Organization. 1974. Pesticide Residues in Food. Report of the 1973 Joint FAO/WHO Meeting. Tech. Rep. Ser. 545. Geneva: WHO.

Appendix 19-1   Toxicological Findings and Evaluation on Certain Insecticides

Pesticides	LD$_{50}$ (mg/kg)	NOAEL (mg/kg)			ADI (mg/kg)
		Rat	Dog	Human	
Azinphosmethyl	13	0.45	0.74	0.3	0.005
Chlorfenvinphos	15	0.05	0.05		0.002
Diazinon	108	0.02	0.02	0.025	0.002
Dichlorvos	80			0.04	0.004
Dimethoate	215	0.4		0.2	0.02
Disulfoton	6.8	0.06	0.03	0.01	0.0003
Malathion	1375	5.0		0.2	0.02
Mevinphos	6.1	0.02	0.025	0.014	0.0015
Parathion	13			0.05	0.005
Parathion-methyl	14	0.1	0.375	0.3	0.02
Trichlorfon	630	2.5	1.25		0.01
Aldicarb	0.8	0.125	0.25	0.025	0.003
Carbaryl	850	10		0.06	0.01
Propoxur	83	12.5	50		0.02
DDT	113	0.05		0.25	0.02
Aldrin/dieldrin	40	0.025	0.025		0.0001
Chlordane	335	0.25	0.05		0.0005
Endrin	18	0.05	0.025		0.002
Heptacholor	100	0.25	0.025		0.0001
Lindane	88	1.25	1.75		0.008
Methoxychlor	6000	10			0.1

Source: LD$_{50}$s from Gaines (1969), and other data from various WHO reports, summarized in Lu (1995).

Toxicity of Metals

CHAPTER 20 CONTENTS

INTRODUCTION

Metals are a unique class of toxicants. They occur and persist in nature, but their chemical form may be changed because of physicochemical, biological, or anthropogenic activities. Their toxicity may be drastically altered as they assume different chemical forms. Most of them have some value to humans because of their uses in industry, agriculture, or medicine. Some are essential elements, required in various biochemical/physiological functions. On the other hand, they may pose health hazards to the public because of their presence in food, water, or air, and to workers engaged in mining, smelting, and a variety of industrial activities.

Occurrence

Most of the metals and "metalloids" occur in nature, dispersed in rocks, ores, soil, water, and air. However, their distribution is grossly uneven. In general, their levels are relatively low in soil, water, and air. These levels may be increased by such geological activities as degassing, which releases, for example, 25,000–125,000 tons of mercury a year. Anthropogenic activities such as mining of mercury contribute about 10,000 tons a year.

It must be noted that anthropogenic activities may be more significant in relation to human exposure because they increase the levels of the metals at the site of the human activities.

Uses and Human Exposure

In ancient times, certain metals such as copper, iron, and tin were used to make utensils, machinery, and weapons. Mining and smelting were undertaken to supply such demands. These activities increased their environmental levels. In addition, as the ores often contain other metals, such as lead and arsenic, the levels of these "contaminants" were also increased.

In later years, a greater variety of metals has found uses in industry, agriculture, and medicine. For example, mercury is used extensively in the chlor-alkali industry as the cathode in the electrolysis of salt in water to produce chlorine and sodium hydroxide, both of which are important raw materials in the chemical industry. Lead is used in the storage batteries and cable industry. However, the use of various lead compounds as insecticides, fuel additives, and pigments in paints has gradually been discontinued.

More recently, the aerospace industry and medico-dental profession require materials that have strength, resistance to corrosion, and nonirritant properties. Alloys of titanium and other metals are becoming even more important.

These human activities have increased the extent of exposure not only to occupational workers but also to the consumers of these products. In addition, the toxicity of a metal may be significantly altered by changes of its chemical form. For example, inorganic mercury compounds are toxic primarily to the kidney, whereas methylmercury is a central nervous system (CNS) toxicant.

CERTAIN COMMON FEATURES

Metals have a wide range of toxicity. Some, such as lead and mercury, are very toxic; others are almost nontoxic, such as titanium. They also possess a variety of toxic properties. Nevertheless, there are a number of toxicological features that are shared to some extent by many metals.

Site of Action

Enzymes A major action of toxic metals is the inhibition of enzymes. This action usually occurs as a result of the interaction between the metal and the SH group of the enzyme. An enzyme may also be inhibited by a toxic metal through displacement of an essential metal cofactor of the enzyme. For example, lead may displace zinc in the zinc-dependent enzyme δ-aminolevulinic acid dehydratase (ALAD).

Another mechanism by which metals interfere with the functions of enzymes is by inhibiting their synthesis. For example, nickel and platinum inhibit the δ-aminolevulinic acid synthetase (ALAS), thereby interfering with the synthesis of heme, which is an important component of hemoglobin and cytochrome (Maines and Kappas, 1977). The enzymes can be protected from toxic metals by the administration of "chelating agents," such as dimercaprol (BAL), that form stable bonds with the metals.

Enzymes differ in their susceptibility to metals. Figure 20-1 depicts the synthesis of heme and the various enzymes involved, most of which may be inhibited by lead. However, they differ in susceptibility (see section on lead). Inhibition of ALAD occurs at a blood lead level (Bl-Pb) of 10 μg/dl or lower. As a result, δ-aminolevulinic acid (ALA) will not be processed to become porphobilinogen and thus will be spilled over into urine at a Bl-Pb of 40 μg/dl, and anemia will only occur at a Bl-Pb of about 50 μg/dl (WHO, 1977).

Subcellular Organelles In general, the toxic effects of metals result from reactions between them and intracellular components. For a metal to exert its toxic effect on a cell, it must enter the cell. The entry across the membrane is facilitated if it is lipophilic, such as methylmercury. When it

Figure 20-1 Schematic diagram representing the reactions involved in heme synthesis. Large arrows indicate steps that are inhibited by Pb. ALAS, δ-aminolevulinic acid synthetase; ALAD, δ-aminolevulinic acid dehydratase; UROD, uroporphyrinogen decarboxylase; CO-PROD, coproporphyrinogen oxidase; and HS, heme synthetase (adapted from Jaworski, 1978). For further explanation, see text subsection on Lead, Toxicity.

is bound to a protein, it is absorbed by endocytosis. Passive diffusion is another form of entry of metals such as lead.

After their entry into the cell, metals may affect different organelles. For example, the endoplasmic reticulum contains a variety of enzymes. These microsomal enzymes are inhibited by many metals, such as cadmium, cobalt, methylmercury, and tin. Toxic metals also disrupt the structure of the endoplasmic reticulum. The lysosomes are another site of action of metals such as cadmium (as a conjugate of metallothionein). Cadmium is accumulated in the lysosomes of renal proximal tubular cells. In the lysosomes, the cadmium complex degrades and releases Cd^{2+}. The cadmium ion inhibits the proteolytic enzymes in the lysosomes and causes cell injury. The mitochondria, because of their high metabolic activity and rapid membrane transport, are also a common target of metals. The respiratory enzymes in these organelles are readily inhibited by metals. A number of metals enter the nucleus and may form inclusion bodies. For example, chronic exposure to lead can induce inclusion bodies in the nuclei of renal proximal tubular cells. It also stimulates DNA, RNA, and protein synthesis. The lead-induced renal adenocarcinoma has been attributed to this mechanism (Goering et al., 1987).

It is therefore evident that the subcellular organelles either enhance or impede the movement of metals across these biological membranes, thereby affecting their toxicity. In addition, certain proteins in cytosol, lysosomes, and nuclei may bind with toxic metals, such as Cd, Pb, and Hg, thereby reducing their availability for toxic effects on sensitive organelles and metabolic sites (Fowler et al., 1984).

Factors Affecting Toxicity

Levels and Duration of Exposure   As with other toxicants, the toxic effects of metals are related to the level and duration of exposure. In general, the higher the level and the longer the duration, the greater the toxic effects. However, apart from these quantitative differences, changes in the level and duration of exposure may alter the nature of the toxic effects. For example, ingestion of a single, large dose of cadmium induces gastrointestinal (GI) disturbances. Repeated intakes of smaller amounts of Cd result in renal dysfunction.

Chemical Form   A notable example of a toxicant with multiple chemical forms is mercury. Its inorganic compounds are essentially renal toxicants, while methylmercury and ethylmercury compounds are more toxic to the nervous system. The latter mercury compounds are lipophilic and thus readily cross the blood–brain barrier. Similarly, tetraethyllead readily enters the myelin sheath and affects the nervous system.

Metal–Protein Complexes   Perhaps as protective mechanisms, various metal–protein complexes are formed in the body. For example, the complexes formed with lead, bismuth, and mercury–selenium are microscopically visible as "inclusion bodies" in the affected cells. Iron may combine with protein to form ferritin, which is water soluble, or hemosiderin, which is not. Cadmium and several other metals (e.g., zinc) combine with metallothionein, a low-molecular-weight protein. The Cd complex is less toxic than Cd^{2+}. However, in the renal tubule cells, the cadmium–metallothionein is broken down by the cysteine protease in lysosomes to release Cd^{2+} and cause toxic effects (Squibb and Fowler, 1984; Min et al., 1992).

Host Factors   As with most other toxicants, young and old animals are in general more susceptible than young adults to metals (chap. 5). Young children appear to be especially susceptible to lead because of the generally greater sensitivity and the greater extent of GI absorption. Furthermore, they have, on a unit body weight basis, a greater intake of food, which is the main source of lead.

Dietary factors such as deficiencies of protein and vitamins C and D enhance the toxicity of lead and cadmium.

Certain metals, such as lead and mercury, can cross the placenta, thus affecting the fetus. There is evidence that prenatally exposed children are affected more severely than their mothers: It was found in a study that the median dose that caused ataxia in the mothers was 2.7 ± 0.18 mg/kg, whereas that in the prenatally exposed children was 1.23 ± 0.87 (Clarkson, 1981).

Biological Indicators / Biomarkers

Exposure to metals can usually be quantitatively assessed. Some of the indicators reveal the extent and the approximate time of exposure. Others are early signs of biological effects.

The presence and level of the metal in blood and urine are often used as indicators of recent exposure. As the metal compounds are distributed, stored, or excreted, the levels in blood and urine will diminish.

Many metals are accumulated in hair and nail. Their levels generally bear a relationship with those in blood at the time when the hair and nail are formed. Therefore hair, which grows at a relatively constant rate, has been used to determine the level of exposure at various times in the past. For example, this procedure has been used extensively to ascertain the intake of methylmercury among the inhabitants in the areas where methylmercury poisoning was reported. Using different approaches, a fairly reliable conversion factor has been established. Thus the level of methylmercury in hair is about 250 times of that in blood, and their relation to the daily intake, after a steady state is reached, is as follows: 0.2 μg/g in blood = 50 μg/g in hair = 3 μg/kg body weight per day (WHO, 1976).

Such biological indicators are useful in assessing the average blood level of selenium of inhabitants. In areas where there was selenosis it was 3.2 mg/L; where there was Se deficiency syndrome, it was 0.021 mg/L; and in an area where there was neither overexposure nor deficiency, it was 0.095 mg/L (WHO, 1987).

Minimal inhibition of δ-aminolevulinic acid dehydrase by lead represents a special type of "indicator of exposure" in that this biological effect does not seem to indicate an adverse effect.

Certain Common Toxic Effects

Carcinogenicity   A number of metals have been shown to be carcinogenic in humans or animals or both. As listed in Appendix 7-1, arsenic and its compounds, certain chromium compounds, and nickel and its compounds have been shown to be human carcinogens. Beryllium, cadmium, and cisplatin are probable human carcinogens. Certain other metals may be carcinogenic, but the available information is insufficient to confirm this suggestion.

The aforementioned metals as well as several others might be carcinogenic through multiple mechanisms of action such as the substitution of Ni^{2+}, Co^{2+}, or Cd^{2+} for Zn^{2+} in finger-loops of transforming proteins (Sunderman and Barber, 1988) and injury to the cytoskeleton by certain metals (Chou, 1989), which affects fidelity of the polymerase involved in DNA biosynthesis.

Immune Function Exposure to certain metals may result in inhibition of immune functions (chap. 10, Immunodysfunction subsection). Other metals such as beryllium, chromium, nickel, gold, mercury, and platinum and zirconium may induce hypersensitivity reactions. The clinical manifestations and mechanisms of action are listed in Table 20-1.

Nervous System Because of its susceptibility, the nervous system (NS) is a common target of toxic metals. However, even with the same metal, its physicochemical form often determines the nature of the toxicity. As noted earlier, metallic mercury vapor and methylmercury readily enter the NS and induce toxic effects. Inorganic mercury compounds are unlikely to enter the NS in significant amounts and thus usually are not neurotoxic. Similarly, the organic compounds of lead are mainly neurotoxic, whereas inorganic lead compounds affect the synthesis of heme first. But at much higher levels of exposure, they may induce encephalopathy, and in young children a moderate level of exposure to these compounds may result in a

Table 20-1 Hypersensitivity Reactions to Metals

Metal	Type of reaction	Clinical features	Mechanism of reactions
Platinum, beryllium	I	Asthma, conjunctivitis, urticaria, anaphylaxis	IgE reacts with antigen on mast cell/basophil to release vasoreactive amines
Gold, salts of, mercury	II	Thrombocytopenia	IgG binds to complement and antigen on cells, resulting in their destruction
Mercury vapor, gold	III	Glomerular nephritis, proteinuria	Antigen, antibody, and complement deposit on epithelial surface of glomerular basement
Chromium, nickel	IV	Contact dermatitis	Sensitized T cells react with antigen to cause delayed hypersensitivity reaction
Beryllium, zirconium		Granuloma formation	

deficit of mental functions. Other neurotoxic metals include copper, trie-thyltin, gold, lithium, and manganese. For additional information, see Bondy and Prasad (1988).

Kidney   The kidney, as the main excretory organ in the body, is also a common target organ. Cadmium affects the renal proximal tubular cells, causing urinary excretion of small-molecule proteins, amino acids, and glucose. In addition, inorganic mercury compounds, lead, chromium, and platinum also induce kidney damage, mainly on the proximal tubules (see chap. 13).

Respiratory System   The respiratory system is the primary target or-gan of most metals following occupational exposure. There are several types of responses. Many cause irritation and inflammation of the respi-ratory tract; the parts affected depend on the metal and the duration of exposure. With acute exposures, chromium affects the nasal passage, ar-senic the bronchi, and beryllium the lungs. Prolonged exposure may cause fibrosis (aluminum, iron), carcinoma (arsenic, chromium, nickel), or gran-uloma (beryllium). These effects are included in Appendix 11-1.

METALS OF MAJOR TOXICOLOGICAL CONCERN

Lead, mercury, and cadmium are metals of major health concern because of their impact on large numbers of people resulting from environmental pollution as well as the serious nature of their toxic effects. Several other metals also pose serious toxicological problems.

Mercury

General Considerations   The elemental form of mercury (Hg) exists in liquid form. It is released from the earth crust through degassing. It is also present in the environment as inorganic and organic compounds. El-emental Hg may become inorganic compounds by oxidation and revert to elemental Hg by reduction. Inorganic Hg may become organic Hg through the action of certain anaerobic bacteria, and it degrades to inorganic Hg slowly.

A variety of anthropogenic activities may raise its levels in the envi-ronment. Among these are mining, smelting (to produce metals from their sulfide ores), burning of fossil fuel, and production of steel, cement, and phosphate. Its principal users include the chlor-alkali plants, paper-pulp industry, and electrical equipment manufacturers. These uses fortunately have decreased in recent years.

The Hg level in the ambient air is extremely low. The level in water in unpolluted areas is about 0.1 μg/L, but it may be as high as 80 μg/L near Hg ore deposits. Its level in food, except fish, is very low, generally in the range of 520 μg/kg. Most fishes contain higher levels; the levels in tuna and swordfish usually range from 200 to 1000 μg/kg.

Toxicity   Because of the massive outbreaks of poisoning from consuming grain treated with mercury fungicide or fish contaminated with methylmercury (chap. 1, Appendix 1-2), extensive investigations have been carried out. The populations studied ranged from "normal" subjects to those fatally poisoned. Table 20-2 lists some of these population groups. The "fishermen" were exposed to higher than normal levels but showed no signs of poisoning. Those involved in the Niigata episode were exposed to smaller intakes than those in the Iraq episode, and hence the latency in Niigata was generally 2–3 yr whereas that in Iraq was 23 mo.

These studies have revealed that the toxic effects are related to the nervous system, which is extremely sensitive to this toxicant and readily invaded by it. Paresthesia is usually the earliest symptom. Constricted visual field is pathognomonic. At higher levels of exposure, ataxia, dysarthria, deafness, and eventually death occur. Figure 20-2 shows graphically the dose-response and dose-effect relationships. Pathologically the major damage is atrophy in the occipital lobe, the cerebellar folia, and the calcarine cortex. There are also degenerative changes in the axons and myelin sheaths of peripheral nerves.

From these studies it was concluded that methylmercury poisoning would be unlikely if the daily intake corresponds to a blood level of 20 μg/dl and a hair level of 50 μg/g (WHO, 1976). More recent studies indicate that fetal brain is much more susceptible to methylmercury than that of adults. This difference is due to the ease of transport across the placenta, the preferential uptake by the fetal brain, and the inhibitory action on cell division and cell migration, both of which are essential in the proper development of fetal brain (Clarkson, 1991).

Elemental Hg vapor constitutes a hazard virtually only in occupational settings. Its target organ is also the CNS. The usual symptoms are objective tremors and mental disturbances. Among workers exposed to Hg vapor the triad of excitability, tremor, and gingivitis has long been observed (Goldwater, 1972). After a continual exposure to a time-weighted air concentra-

Table 20-2   Daily Intake of Methylmercury by Certain Populations

Population	Daily intake (μg)	
	Average	Range
"Normal"	—	1–20
Fisherman	300	Up to 1000
Niigata	1500	250–5000
Iraq	4500	Up to 12,000

MAXIMUM HAIR CONC. (ppm)

Figure 20-2 The frequency of signs and symptoms of methylmercury poisoning in adult victims in Iraq plotted according to the estimated maximum hair concentration. Hair samples were not available for all patients and are estimated based on the patient's history of exposure, observed blood levels, and blood half-times and a hair-to-blood concentration ratio of 250 to 1 (from Clarkson, 1987).

tion of 0.05 mg Hg/m^3, sensitive workers may exhibit nonspecific (neurasthenic) symptoms, and at a concentration of 0.1–0.2 mg/m^3, they may have tremors (WHO, 1976).

Inorganic Hg salts are either monovalent or divalent. The divalent mercuric chloride, the "corrosive sublimate," is corrosive on contact. After ingestion, it causes abdominal cramps and bloody diarrhea, with corrosive ulceration, bleeding, and necrosis of the GI tract. These effects are followed by *renal* damage, mainly necrosis and sloughing off of the proximal tubular cells, thereby blocking the tubules and causing oliguria, anuria, and uremia. It may also damage the glomerulus, possibly as a result of disturbed immune function. The monovalent salt calomel, the mercurous chloride, is less corrosive and less toxic. But mercurous chloride may cause the "pink disease," characterized by *dermal* vasodilation, hyperkeratosis, and hypersecretion of the sweat glands. This effect is probably a hypersensitivity reaction, since it is not dose related.

Lead

General Considerations Lead is more ubiquitous than most other toxic metals. The environmental levels have been increasing because of lead mining, smelting, refining, and various industrial uses.

Generally Pb levels in soil range from 5 to 25 mg/kg, in groundwater from 1 to 60 μg/L and somewhat lower in natural surface water, and in air under 1 $\mu g/m^3$, but may be much higher in certain workplaces and areas with heavy motor traffic.

The major industrial uses, such as fuel additives, and lead pigments in paints, which contributed greatly to the Pb levels in the environment, have been gradually phased out. However, its uses in storage batteries and cables have not been significantly reduced. Drinking water may be appreciably contaminated by Pb from the use of lead and polyvinyl chloride (PVC) pipes. Glazed ceramic foodware is another source of Pb, as noted in chap. 18. For most people, the major source of their Pb intake is food, which contributes generally 100–300 μg per day.

Infants and young children are likely exposed to a greater extent than adults, because of their habit of licking, chewing, or eating foreign objects, such as soil and flakes of old paints from the wall.

Toxicity The hematopoietic system is extremely sensitive to the effect of Pb. The main component of hemoglobin is heme. It is synthesized from glycine and succinyl coenzyme A (CoA), with pyridoxal phosphate as cofactor. After a number of steps, it finally combines with iron to form heme. The initial and final steps take place in the mitochondria, with the intermediate steps in the cytoplasm as shown in Fig. 20-1. Among the enzymes involved in these steps, five are susceptible to the inhibitory effect of Pb. δ-Aminolevulinic acid dehydratase (ALAD) and heme synthetase (HS) are the most susceptible, whereas δ-aminolevulinic acid synthetase (ALAS), uroporphyrinogen decarboxylase (UROD), and coproporphyrinogen oxidase (COPROD) are less sensitive to inhibition by Pb. Only two of them are not affected, namely, porphobilinogen deaminase and uroporphyrinogen cosynthetase.

While clinical anemia is evident only when there is moderate exposure to Pb, with its level in blood around 50 $\mu g/dl$, a number of other effects may be observed at much lower levels of exposure. For example, ALAD inhibition becomes perceptible at a blood Pb level just over 10 $\mu g/dl$ and free erythrocyte porphyrins (FEP) at 20–25 $\mu g/dl$. ALAD inhibition, and possibly FEP, may be considered as an indicator of exposure rather than an indicator of toxicity. The impaired heme synthesis may result in anemia that is hypochromatic and microcytic. The anemia may be due partly to the greater fragility of the erythrocyte membrane (WHO, 1977).

The nervous system is also a main target organ of Pb. After high levels of exposure, with blood Pb level over 80 $\mu g/dl$, encephalopathy may occur. There are damages to the arterioles and capillaries, resulting in cerebral edema, increased cerebrospinal fluid pressure, neuronal degeneration, and glial proliferation. Clinically this condition is associated with ataxia, stupor, coma, and convulsion. In children, this clinical syndrome may occur with a blood Pb level of 70 $\mu g/dl$. At still lower levels (40–50 $\mu g/dl$), children may exhibit hyperactivity, decreased attention span, and a slight lowering of IQ scores (Ernhardt et al., 1981). These subtle manifestations may be a result of impairment of the function of neurotransmitters and calcium ion. Peripheral neuropathy is characterized by wrist-drop and foot-drop, signs of damage to the motor nerves. Lead causes degeneration of Schwann cells followed by demyelination and possibly axonal degeneration. This syndrome occurs mainly among occupational workers.

Lead generally affects the kidney insidiously, resulting in chronic renal failure after long-term exposure. The proximal tubule is the main target. An early sign of lead toxicity on the kidney is the excretion of the lysosomal enzyme N-acetyl-B-D-glucosaminidase (Verschoor et al., 1987). One characteristic of lead poisoning is the presence of lead "inclusion bodies" in the nucleus of tubular cells. These bodies consist of fibrillary lead–protein complexes.

Other Effects Carcinogenicity of Pb has been demonstrated in kidneys of rodents, but there is little human data in this respect (IARC, 1980). Pb also adversely affects reproductive functions, mainly through its gametotoxicity in both male and female animals, resulting in sterility, abortion, and neonatal deaths. Young children are likely to be exposed to higher levels of Pb, as noted earlier. Furthermore, they and unborn fetuses are also more sensitive to the toxicity of this metal.

Organic lead compounds such as tetraethyllead and tetramethyllead are readily absorbed after inhalation and dermal exposures and rapidly enter the central nervous system (CNS) with ensuing encephalopathy. This hazard concerns essentially occupational workers, but not the general public, because the small amounts emitted from automobile exhaust readily degrade.

Cadmium

General Considerations Cadmium occurs in nature mainly in lead and zinc ores. It is thus released near the mines and smelters of these metals. It is used as a pigment (such as in ceramics), in electroplating, and in making alloys and alkali storage batteries. Its level in the air is usually in the range of nanograms per cubic meter, but may amount to several milligrams per cubic meter in certain workplaces. The level in water is very low (around 1 μg/L) except in contaminated areas. Most foods contain trace amounts of cadmium. Grains and cereal products usually constitute the main source of Cd.

While meat, poultry, and fish have relatively low levels of Cd, liver, kidney, and shellfish have much higher levels. The environmental levels are raised by smelting and industrial uses. An additional source is the use of sludge as a food crop fertilizer.

Apart from these environmental sources, humans may be exposed to Cd through cigarette smoking: A pack a day may double the Cd intake. Extensively decorated and improperly fired ceramic foodware is another source of Cd (see chap. 18). Occupational exposure occurs mainly in smelteries.

Toxicity   The acute effects of Cd exposure result mainly from local irritation. After ingestion, the clinical manifestations are nausea, vomiting, and abdominal pain; after inhalation, the lesions include pulmonary edema and chemical pneumonitis.

Cadmium is only very slowly excreted, with a half-life of about 15–30 years. After long-term exposure, kidney lesions predominate. The primary site of action is the proximal tubules. Damages to these tubules generally occur when the Cd level in the kidney reaches 200 $\mu g/g$, the "critical concentration." These tubular damages result in their inability to reabsorb small-molecule proteins, the major one of which is B_2-microglobulin. Other proteins include retinol-binding protein, lysozyme, ribonuclease, and immunoglobulin light chains (Lauwerys et al., 1979). Similarly, aminoaciduria is another result of damage to tubular cells that normally reabsorb the amino acids filtered through the glomeruli. Other related effects are glycosuria and decreased tubular reabsorption of phosphate.

At later stages, there may be hypercalcinuria, which, probably in conjunction with altered bone metabolism, may lead to osteomalacia. However, the connection between Cd and itai-itai disease, characterized by chronic renal disease and bone deformity, reported in Toyama, Japan, where the Cd level in rice was high, has not been firmly established (Nomiyama, 1980).

Effects on the respiratory system result from inhalation exposure. Chronic bronchitis, progressive fibrosis of the lower airway, and rupture of septae between alveoli lead to emphysema.

Other effects include hypertension, which may be the result of sodium retention, vasoconstriction, and hyperreninemia. Carcinoma of the prostate has been reported among occupational workers (Kipling and Waterhause, 1967).

OTHER METALS

Arsenic

Although arsenic is a ubiquitous metalloid, its levels in water and ambient air are generally low. The major source of human exposure is food, which contains somewhat less than 1 mg/kg. However, its level in seafood may reach 5 mg/kg.

In certain parts of Taiwan and South America, the water may contain hundreds of milligrams of arsenic per liter. In these areas, the inhabitants may suffer from dermal hyperkeratosis and hyperpigmentation. A more serious condition is gangrene of lower extremities, the black-foot disease (Tseng, 1977), resulting from peripheral endarteritis.

Cancer of the skin is also observed in those areas, as well as among patients who had been taking Fowler's solution ($KAsO_2$) as a therapy for leukemia. Cancer of the lung may occur among workers exposed to As in copper smelteries and plants that manufacture As-containing pesticide (Pinto et al., 1978; Enterline et al, 1987; Viren and Silvers, 1994). Unlike other human carcinogens, As has not been shown to be carcinogenic to laboratory animals. Furthermore, mutagenesis tests have been essentially negative.

Other effects include toxicity to liver parenchyma, resulting clinically in jaundice in early stages and in cirrhosis and ascites later. Acutely, very large doses of As compounds induce GI damage with vomiting and bloody diarrhea, muscular cramps, and cardiac abnormality (WHO, 1981).

Beryllium

Beryllium is released into the environment mainly through combustion of fossil fuel. It is used in ceramic plants and in making alloys. Beryllium and its alloys have a number of applications in nuclear, space, and other industries.

The major toxic effect is berylliosis, resulting from long-term inhalation exposures. This disease of the lung is characterized by granulomas, which in time become fibrotic tissues. These lesions reduce the number of alveoli and consequently the pulmonary function.

After dermal contact, beryllium produces hypersensitivity reactions of the skin. The reaction is cell mediated and therefore delayed (type IV allergy). The soluble compounds of Be induce papilovesicular lesions, whereas the insoluble compounds induce granulomatous lesions.

Beryllium has been shown to be carcinogenic to several species of animals. Epidemiological data suggest that Be is a potential human carcinogen (Kuschner, 1981).

Chromium

Chromium occurs in ores. Mining, smelting, and industrial uses tend to increase its environmental levels. It is used in making stainless steel, various alloys, and pigments. Fossil-fuel-powered plants and cement-producing plants are also sources of environmental pollution. However, chromium levels in air, water, and food are generally very low. The major human exposure is occupational.

Chromium is a human carcinogen, inducing lung cancers among workers exposed to it. The carcinogenicity is generally attributed to the hexavalent Cr^{6+}, which is corrosive and water insoluble. It has been suggested that Cr^{6+}, which is more readily taken up by cells, converts to Cr^{3+} intracellularly. The trivalent Cr ion, which is more active biologically, binds with nucleic acid and initiates the carcinogenesis process. The Cr^{6+} is corrosive and causes ulceration of the nasal passages and skin. It also induces hypersensitivity reactions of the skin. Acutely, it induces renal tubular necrosis.

Nickel

Nickel occurs in ores. Smelting and industrial uses tend to increase its levels in the environment. Its many industrial uses include storage batteries, electrical contacts and similar devices, electroplating, and as catalysts. It is also emitted from coal gasification.

Nickel is a human carcinogen among occupational workers. Nasal cancer appears to be the predominant type of neoplasm. But Ni also induces cancer of the lung, larynx, stomach, and possibly also the kidney.

It is one of the most common causative agents of dermal hypersensitivity reactions among the general public. The reactions usually follow contact with Ni-containing metal objects such as coins and jewelry.

RISK / BENEFIT CONSIDERATIONS

The metals discussed in the previous section offer certain benefits because of their industrial and minor medical uses. However, they pose serious toxicological risks either to the population at large or specific occupational workers. On the other hand, there are two groups of metals that are more valuable. One group, the essential metals, is required in certain physiological functions, and the other is used for a variety of medical purposes. These three groups of metals are different in risk/benefit considerations.

Toxic Metals

The general population is at risk to these metals mainly through food. Tolerances, or equivalents, are established for various foodstuffs to ensure that the total intake will not exceed the amount that is considered acceptable from a toxicological point of view.

However, more targeted action is taken in certain cases. For example, the main source of methylmercury is fish. The levels in swordfish range from about 0.5 to 1.2 ppm and in tuna from 0.2 to 0.5 ppm, whereas those in most other kinds of fish are 0.1 ppm or lower. The permissible levels for methylmercury set by most nations range from 0.4 to 1.0 ppm. Assuming a daily consumption of 200 g fish, the intake of methylmercury would not exceed 0.2 mg. An intake at this level is considered unlikely to induce methylmercury toxicity (WHO, 1976). The safety is provided by the fact that most of the fish samples contain much less methylmercury than the 1.0 ppm permitted. The Joint FAO/WHO Expert Committee on Food Additives and Contaminants established a "tolerable intake" of 0.2 mg/wk, thus allowing a safety factor of 7, which the Committee considered adequate in this case (WHO, 1972). The rationale was the availability of the exceptionally extensive data obtained from populations exposed to the full gamut of intake levels, ranging from "normal" to questionably poisoned, minimally poisoned, seriously poisoned, and fatally poisoned (Table 20-2), as well as the fact that most of the investigations were thoroughly conducted and properly reported. Second, fish was considered as an important source of nutrients, which should not be discarded for minimal or nonexistent risks. The intake was set on a weekly basis because fish is consumed, in many parts of the world, once a week.

Similarly, targeted action has been taken with respect to Cd in rice in Japan, where rice is the main source of this contaminant. Permissible levels of release of Pb and Cd from ceramic foodware have been established internationally (WHO, 1979) and in many nations.

There are also tolerances for toxic metals such as As, Cd, and Pb in water and foods for the protection of the health of consumers.

Occupational workers are likely exposed to higher levels of toxic metals in mining, smelting, manufacture, and similar occupations. The main routes of entry to the body are the skin and respiratory tract. For their protection, threshold limit values of toxicants in air are established. For additional information, see chap. 21.

Essential Metals

Selenium is a typical element that is toxic at high levels of intake and induces a deficiency syndrome when the intake is too low.

Human overexposure to Se has been observed in China as well as in a few isolated regions in the Americas. The clinical manifestations include hair loss, nail pathology, and tooth decay. In animals overexposure induces more severe ill effects including retarded growth, liver necrosis, enlargement of spleen and pancreas, anemia, and various disorders of reproductive function.

Deficiency of Se results in muscular dystrophy in sheep and cattle, exudative diathesis in chicken, and liver necrosis in swine and rats. In rats it may also cause reproductive failures, vascular changes, and cataracts. Selenium is a component of glutathione peroxidase, which is responsible for the destruction of H_2O_2 and lipid peroxides. Its function is therefore closely related to that of vitamin E, the biological antioxidant. This close relation is reflected in the fact that the minimal intake of Se in rats is 0.01 mg/kg, but if there is also a vitamin E deficiency, an intake of 0.05 mg/kg will be needed.

It was only in the late 1970s that Se was recognized as an essential element in humans also. In certain regions in China where the Se levels were low in soil and food, a special type of cardiomyopathy was noted. It was known as Keshan disease because it was first observed there. The Se levels in the blood, urine, and hair of the inhabitants were low. As expected, the blood glutathione peroxidase activity was also low. When they were given a sodium selenite supplement, the incidence of this endemic cardiopathy dropped sharply. There is also an endemic osteoarthropathy observed in China. It is known as Kashin-Beck disease, and is believed to be due to Se deficiency. However, the evidence on its etiology is not as strong. Selenium deficiency associated with muscular pain has been reported from New Zealand.

For the general population, Se exposure is essentially from food, especially cereals. The average daily intake of Se of inhabitants in areas where there were cases of Keshan disease was about 0.011 mg, whereas in areas where there were cases of selenosis it was about 5 mg. It has been estimated that there is about a 100-fold margin between the highest no-toxic-effect level and the lowest level at which deficiency syndrome is avoided. However, this margin is subject to the influence of various modifying factors. For example, vitamin E deficiency increases the toxicity as well as the physiological requirements of Se, thus effectively reducing the margin. Methylmercury increases the effect of Se deficiency, whereas inorganic mercury increases the toxicity of methylated Se compounds. A hypothetical dose-response (all effects) relationship of Se is depicted in Fig. 4-1, which shows that ill effects are induced when the dose is too low (curve A), whereas other ill effects are induced when the dose is too high (curve B). Furthermore, because of the great individual variations in susceptibility resulting from host and environmental factors, it is not clear whether there is a dose that can be considered as devoid of deficiency as well as toxic effect on a population basis.

Additional details on various aspects of the Se problem and reference citations may be found in a WHO document (WHO, 1987).

Cobalt, copper, and *iron* are all essential metal elements required in the proper development of erythrocytes. Iron is a component of hemoglobin, and Cu facilitates the utilization of Fe in the synthesis of hemoglobin. Thus deficiency of either metal results in hypochromatic, microcytic anemia. Cobalt is a component of vitamin B_{12}, which is required in the development of erythrocyte. Its deficiency results in pernicious anemia.

Excessive intake of Co results in polycythemia, an overproduction of erythrocytes, and cardiomyopathy. The heart lesion was observed under special conditions, as discussed in chap. 22. Excess Cu storage in the body is not a result of overexposure to Cu but rather a genetic disorder (Wilson's disease). Copper is accumulated in brain, liver, kidney, and cornea. Clinical manifestations are thus related to disorders of these organs. Overexposure to Fe may result from excessive intake of Fe or frequent blood transfusion. The excess Fe is deposited as hemosiderin mainly in liver, causing liver dysfunction.

Occupational exposure to Co induces respiratory irritation and dermal hypersensitivity reactions. Certain Fe industry workers have been reported as having pneumoconiosis and increased lung cancer incidence. Acute oral poisonings have been reported after consuming improperly canned vegetable juices containing excessive amounts of Cu and after taking large doses of Fe supplement medications. The clinical manifestations relate mainly to GI irritation.

Other essential metals include manganese and molybdenum, which are cofactors in a number of enzyme systems such as phosphorylase, xanthine oxidase, and aldehyde oxidase. However, these metals are so plentiful in the human diet that no cases of deficiency syndrome have been reported. These metals have a variety of industrial uses, notably in making high-temperature-resistant steel alloys. Occupational exposure to Mn results in pneumonitis acutely, and encephalopathy chronically. Overexposure to Mn in animals orally induces GI disturbances followed by fatty degeneration of liver and kidney.

Zinc is the cofactor in scores of metalloenzymes and is therefore an essential element. Deficiency of Zn thus induces a great variety of effects on the nervous system, hematopoietic system, skin, liver, eye, testis, etc. Zinc is readily excreted, and excessive intake by the oral route is thus unlikely to induce toxic effects. Occupational exposure to Zn_2O_3 fume results in "metal fume fever" (Goyer, 1993).

Metals Used in Medicine

Therapeutic Agents   A number of metal compounds have been used in medicine. For example, compounds of Hg have been used as diuretics. Because of their toxicity, their uses have been discontinued. Those that are less toxic include compounds of aluminum as antacid, bismuth as astringent, gold for rheumatoid arthritis, lithium for mental depression, platinum complexes as antitumor agents, and thallium as depilatory. They may produce toxic effects on the nervous system (e.g., Al, Bi, Li, Th), kidneys (e.g., Bi, Au, Li), skin (e.g., Au, Pt), and cardiovascular and gastrointestinal systems (e.g., Li, Th). Although used as antitumor agents, Pt complexes may induce tumors.

Other Uses   Aluminum in hemodialysis for chronic renal failure has resulted in fatal neurologic syndrome. The use of barium and gallium, in conjunction with x-rays, as a radiopaque agent and radioactive tracer has proved to be relatively safe. However, accidental ingestion of soluble Ba salts has resulted in serious gastrointestinal, muscular, and cardiovascular disturbances. Therapeutic use of radiogallium has resulted in disease conditions related to radioactivity. Of special interest is titanium. It is inert and resistant to corrosion and thus has been used widely in surgical and dental implants. It is present in trace amounts in a variety of foods of plant origin, and titanium dioxide has been used as a color additive because of its low toxicity.

REFERENCES

Bondy, S. C., and Prasad, K. N. 1988. *Metal neurotoxicity*. Boca Raton, FL: CRC Press.

Chou, I. N. 1989. Distinct cytoskeletal injuries induced by As, Cd, Co, Cr, and Ni compounds. *Biomed. Environ. Sci.* 2:358–365.

Clarkson, T. W. 1981. Dose-response relationships for adult and prenatal exposures to methyl mercury. In *Measurements of risks*, eds. G. G. Berg and H. D. Maillie, pp. 111–130. New York: Plenum Press.

Clarkson, T. W. 1987. Metal toxicity in the central nervous system. *Environ. Health Perspect.* 75:59–64.

Clarkson, T. W. 1991. Methyl mercury. *Fundam. Appl. Toxicol.* 16:20–21.

Enterline, P. E., Henderson, V. L., and Marsh, G. M. 1987. Exposure to arsenic and respiratory cancer: A reanalysis. *Am. J. Epidemiol.* 125:929–938.

Ernhardt, C. B., Landa, B., and Schnell, N. B. 1981. Subclinical levels of lead and developmental deficits: A multivariate follow-up reassessment. *Pediatrics* 67:911–919.

Fowler, B. A., Abel, J., Elinder, C. G., et al. 1984. Structure, mechanism and toxicity. In *Changing metal cycles and human health*, ed. J. Nriagu, pp. 391–404. New York: Springer-Verlag.

Goering, P. L., Mistry, P., and Fowler, B. A. 1987. Mechanism of metal toxicity. In *Handbook of toxicology*, eds. T. J. Haley and W. O. Berndt, pp. 384–425. New York: Hemisphere.

Goldwater, L. J. 1972. *Mercury: A history of quicksilver.* Baltimore: York Press.

Goyer, R. A. 1993. Toxic effects of metals. In *Casarett and Doull's toxicology,* Eds. M. O. Amdur, J. Doull, and C. D. Klaassen, pp. 624–680. New York: McGraw-Hill.

International Agency for Research on Cancer. 1980. *Monograph on the evaluation of the carcinogenic risks of chemicals to humans*, vol. 23, *Some metals and metallic compounds*. Lyon, France: IARC.

Jaworski, J. K. 1978. *The effects of lead in the Canadian environment*. Ottawa, Canada: National Research Council Canada.

Kipling, M., and Waterhause, J. 1967. Cadmium and prostatic carcinoma. *Lancet* i:730–731.

Kuschner, M. 1981. The carcinogenicity of beryllium. *Environ. Health Perspect.* 40:101–106.

Lauwerys, R. R., Roels, H. A., Poncket, J. P., Bernard, A., and Stanerscu, D. 1979. Investigations on the lung and kidney function in workers exposed to cadmium. *Environ. Health Perspect.* 28:137–146.

Maines, M. D., and Kappas, A. 1977. Metals as regulators of heme metabolism. *Science* 198:1215–1221.

Min, K.-S., Nakatsubo, T., Fujita, Y., Onosaka, S., and Tanaka, K. 1992. Degradation of cadmium metallothionein in vitro by lysosomal proteases. *Toxicol. Appl. Pharmacol.* 113:299–305.

Nomiyama, K. 1980. Recent progress and perspectives in cadmium health effects studies. *Sci. Total Environ.* 14:199–232.

Pinto, S. S., Henderson, V., and Enterline, P. E. 1978. Mortality experience of arsenic exposed workers. *Arch. Environ. Health* 33:325–331.

Squibb, K. S., and Fowler, B. A. 1984. Intracellular metabolism of circulating cadmium-metallothionein in the kidney. *Environ. Health Perspect.* 54:31–35.

Sunderman, F. W., Jr., and Barber, A. M. 1988. Fingerloops, oncogenes and metals. *Ann. Clin. Lab. Sci.* 18:267–288.

Tseng, W. P. 1977. Effects and dose-response relationships of skin cancer and blackfoot disease with arsenic. *Environ. Health Perspect.* 19:109–119.

Verschoor, M., Wibowo, A., Herber, R., Van Hammen, J., and Zielhuis, R. 1987. Influence of occupational low-level lead exposure on renal parameters. *Am. J. Ind. Med.* 12: 341–351.

Viren, J. R., and Silvers, A. 1994. Unit risk estimates for airborne arsenic exposure: An updated view based on recent data from two copper smelter cohorts. *Regul. Toxicol. Pharmacol.* 20:125–138.

World Health Organization. 1972. Evaluation of Certain Food Additives and the Contaminants Mercury, Lead and Cadmium. Tech. Rep. Ser. 505. Geneva: WHO.

World Health Organization. 1976. Mercury. Environmental Health Criteria 1. Geneva: WHO.

World Health Organization. 1977. Lead. Environmental Health Criteria 3. Geneva: WHO.

World Health Organization. 1979. Ceramic Foodware Safety. Document HCS/79.7. Geneva: WHO.

World Health Organization. 1981. Arsenic. Environmental Health Criteria 18. Geneva: WHO.

World Health Organization. 1987. Selenium. Environmental Health Criteria 58. Geneva: WHO.

Industrial Chemicals and Environmental Pollutants

CHAPTER 21 CONTENTS

GENERAL CONSIDERATIONS

A large number of substances are manufactured and used in various industries. The major groups include food additives, pesticides, metals and their compounds, and a variety of organic chemicals including organic solvents. The first three groups of substances have been described in chaps. 18, 19, and 20. The toxicological problems of other industrial chemicals such as organic solvents are described here.

In addition to these intentionally manufactured chemicals, there are substances whose production is unintentional or unavoidable. Nevertheless, some of them are potentially hazardous to the general population. They may enter the human body via food, such as mycotoxins and other contaminants (chap. 18), or via water. The latter includes pesticides as runoff from treated farms and industrial chemicals discharged as liquid effluent or leached into groundwater from waste dumps. The ambient air is also an important environmental medium. A variety of air pollutants may result from factory and power plant emissions and automobile exhaust.

ORGANIC SOLVENTS

Solvents comprise a variety of organic chemicals such as aromatic hydrocarbons (e.g., benzene), aliphatic hydrocarbons (e.g., n-hexane), chlorinated aliphatic hydrocarbons (e.g., chloroform, CCl_4), alcohols, or glycols and their ethers. These chemicals are used extensively in paints, inks, thinners, adhesives, pharmaceuticals, cosmetics, etc. Some solvents are used mainly for dry-cleaning clothes and degreasing machinery.

Their manufacture and use in industry may pose health hazards to occupational workers. In addition, some of them become components of household products, thereby constituting potential health hazards to the consumer. Finally, the general public as noted earlier may be exposed through these substances contaminating the environmental media.

General Effects

Most of the solvents exert certain nonspecific effects. These include irritation at the site of contact, and depression of the central nervous system (CNS).

Irritation   At room temperature solvents are in the liquid form. When they are in contact with skin, irritation may occur. As they are volatile, inhalation of their vapors may cause irritation of the respiratory tract, and they may also cause eye irritation.

CNS Depression   At sufficiently high levels of exposure, a consistent effect of solvents is CNS depression. The clinical manifestation begins with disorientation, giddiness, and euphoria. The last-named effect is responsible for abuse of some of these chemicals. The syndrome may progress to paralysis, unconsciousness, and convulsion. Death may ensue.

The mechanism of action is not clear, but over half a century ago, Meyer (1937) observed that the narcosis (CNS depression) was related to the solubility of these substances in lipid and not related to their chemical structure, and hence suggested that narcosis resulted from CNS cell dysfunction following solubilizing of the solvents in the cell membrane.

Interaction   As noted earlier, most solvents may undergo biotransformation and may elevate the activities of cytochrome P-450 isozymes. Since solvents are often present in mixtures, interaction between them may occur. For example, a solvent, such as benzene, may potentiate the toxic effects of others by enhancing their bioactivation. On the other hand, the toxicity may also be decreased with certain mixtures. For example, toluene may reduce the toxicity of benzene by competitively inhibiting the bioactivation enzyme systems (Andrews et al., 1977).

Specific Effects

Apart from the general effects described already, a variety of specific effects may follow exposure to solvents. The diversity of these effects is a result of different reactive metabolites being formed. Some of the specific effects are described next.

Liver   As noted in chap. 12, ethanol is a common cause of fatty liver and liver cirrhosis. These effects likely result from the direct toxicity of ethanol plus nutritional deficiency commonly present among alcoholics. Various chlorinated hydrocarbons may cause a variety of liver damages. These include fatty liver as well as liver necrosis, cirrhosis, and cancer. The liver lesions are induced by reactive metabolites of these solvents. For example, the likely metabolite of carbon tetrachloride is trichloromethyl radical, that of chloroform is phosgene, and those of halogenated aromatic hydrocarbons, such as bromobenzene, are their epoxides (Reid and Krishna, 1973). However, the recurrent cytotoxicity and chronic tissue regeneration may be the cause of the carcinogenicity.

Kidneys   As noted in chap. 13, certain chlorinated hydrocarbons, such as chloroform and carbon tetrachloride, are nephrotoxic in addition to being hepatotoxic. At lower levels of exposure, the renal effects are related to tubular functions, such as glycosuria, aminoaciduria, and polyuria. At higher levels, there may be cell death along with elevated blood urea nitrogen (BUN) and anuria. In humans, CCl_4 affects mainly kidney when the route of exposure is inhalation, whereas liver is the major target organ when the chemical is ingested. Ethylene glycol is nephrotoxic because of its direct cytotoxicity as well as the blocking of the proximal tubules by the crystals of its metabolite, calcium oxalate.

Nervous System   Apart from their effects on CNS, as noted already, aliphatic hydrocarbons and certain ketones such as *n*-hexane and methyl *n*-butyl ketone affect also the peripheral nervous system. The clinical manifestation of this polyneuropathy begins with numbness and paresthesia, as well as motor weakness of both hands and feet. These effects then involve both arms and legs. Pathologically it is characterized by distal axonopathy (chap. 16). The reactive metabolite of these two solvents is 2,5-hexanedione (Krasavage et al., 1980).

Hematopoietic System   Benzene is an outstanding example of a solvent affecting this system. It depresses bone marrow in animals and humans, thereby decreases the circulating erythrocytes, leukocytes, and thrombocytes. In humans exposed to benzene, however, leukemia has been reported (Aksoy and Erdem, 1978). Leukemia has not been observed in treated animals. However, animals given benzene have developed solid tumors (Maltoni et al., 1989).

Carcinogenesis   As noted earlier, a number of chlorinated hydrocarbons are known to produce liver tumors, and benzene is carcinogenic in animals and produces leukemia in humans. In addition, dioxane is also a liver carcinogen and has produced nasopharyngeal cancers (Andrews and Snyder, 1993).

Diethylene glycol induced bladder tumors in rats fed large doses of the solvent. In all the tumor-bearing rats, there were bladder stones that were composed of calcium oxalate, a metabolite of this chemical. None of the rats that did not have bladder stones had bladder tumors (Fitzhugh and Nelson, 1946). This solvent has thus been considered a secondary carcinogen (chap. 7).

Other Effects   Testicular degeneration and cardiovascular (CV) malformation have been observed in animals exposed to ethylene glycol monoethyl ether. Methanol may damage the retina through its metabolite and affect mainly the part that is responsible for central vision. Methylene chloride causes CNS depression and irritation to the eye and skin as do many other solvents. However, it also induces carboxyhemoglobinemia because CO is formed in the biotransformation (WHO, 1984). Chloroform may induce cardiac arrhythmia, probably as a result of sensitization of the myocardium to epinephrine. This is one of the reasons why chloroform has been discontinued as a general anesthetic.

It should be noted that certain solvents are practically nontoxic. For example, propylene glycol has low toxicities, with LD_{50} values of 32 and 18 ml/kg in rats and rabbits, respectively, and rats fed this solvent at 1.8 ml/kg for 2 years showed no adverse effects. This chemical has thus been used as a food additive (WHO, 1964).

Exposure Limits

The major group of population at risk is the occupational workers engaged in the manufacture and use of solvents. Limits for their exposure are recommended and updated from time to time in some countries. In the United States, a yearly booklet listing the threshold limit values (TLV) is published by the American Conference of Governmental Industrial Hygienists (AC-GIH, 1995). The limits refer to airborne concentrations of substances and are based on relevant data from industrial experience, controlled studies in humans, and experimental animal studies. They represent conditions under which "nearly all workers may be repeatedly exposed day after day without adverse effects." The list includes solvents, pesticides, metals, and their compounds. There are three categories of TLV:

1   TLV-TWA refers to the time-weighted average concentration for a normal 8-h workday and a 40-h work week.
2   TLV-STEL refers to the short-term exposure limit to which workers may be exposed. It is defined as a 15-min time-weighted average exposure. This limit is set mostly to avoid irritation and narcosis, but also to avoid chronic or irreversible tissue damage.
3   TLV-C refers to the ceiling that should not be exceeded during any part of the working exposure.

These limits are expressed in terms of ppm and/or milligrams per cubic meter. Since 1 mole of an ideal gas at 25° C and 760 mm Hg occupies 24.45 L, the following equation can be used to convert the limits: parts of vapor/million parts air (ppm) = $(mg/m^3) \times 24.45/$(molecular weight of the solvents).

AIR POLLUTANTS

Introduction

Past Disasters   Several episodes of severe air pollution affecting the health and lives of large numbers of people have been reported. The notable ones occurred in the Meuse Valley, Belgium (December 1930); Donora, Pennsylvania (October 1948); London, England (December 1952); Los Angeles, California (August or September 1942, 1952, 1955); and Piscataway,

New Jersey (September 1971). These episodes fell into two categories. One type occurred in winters, especially during the night, when domestic burning of coal was an important source of pollution, and the other occurred in summers and during daytime when photooxidation of automobile exhaust was the major source of pollutants. In either case, the meteorological conditions, low wind and high barometric pressure, kept the pollutants at the ground level. The major effects were related to distress of respiratory and, to a lesser extent, cardiovascular systems. A number of deaths were reported, mainly from strains on preexisting diseases or deficiencies in these systems (Waldbott, 1978).

As a result of these tragic events, measures have been taken to reduce the extent of air pollution. Nevertheless, the health problem remains, although somewhat abated.

Sources   Natural sources of air pollution include eruptions of volcanoes and decay of organic matter. Their contribution to the total air pollution is greater than the anthropogenic sources, but the latter are concentrated near human communities and thus have greater effects on human health.

The most important anthropogenic sources in many developed nations are automobiles. Other sources include combustion (coal, natural gas, fuel oil, incineration of refuse), metallurgical industry (see chap. 20), and chemical industry (solvents, chemical intermediates, etc.).

Reducing-Type Pollutants

Composition and Sources   The major pollutants are sulfur oxides and suspended particulate matter. The former include sulfur dioxide, sulfuric acid, and sulfates; the latter includes finely divided solids and liquids. Particles of 0.1–10 μm in diameter settle very slowly, with a velocity of 8×10^{-7} to 3×10^{-3} m/s, while larger particles (1000 μm in diameter) settle at a velocity of 3.9 m/s (Fuchs, 1964). Thus, particles smaller than 10 μm are suspended in air and are inhalable, as noted in chap. 2.

The main sources of these pollutants are domestic burning of coal and other fuel for heating and cooking and industrial combustion of these fuels to generate energy. Smelting of ores also generates these and other pollutants.

Toxic Effects SO_2 is very soluble, and hence it is readily absorbed in the nose and upper respiratory tract, where it induces irritation. This is followed by thickening of the mucous layer in trachea and hypertrophy of goblet cells.

The irritation causes cough, expectoration, dyspnea, and bronchoconstriction. Respiratory functions are impaired, manifesting as decreased tidal volume, increased pulmonary resistance, and increased respiratory rate. Among exposed individuals, there is an increase of the incidence of respiratory tract infections, which may be attributable in part to an interference with the respiratory tract clearance mechanism. Under normal conditions, this mechanism is responsible for removing bacteria and other particles from the tract. Aerosols of sulfuric acid, formed from SO_3, are even more irritant than sulfur dioxide, which forms sulfurous acid (Amdur, 1993).

The effects of these sulfur pollutants are enhanced by the presence of suspended particulate matter. Ozone also exerts a synergistic effect. Exposure to very high concentrations of sulfur dioxide and smoke (suspended particulate matter) can cause deaths, especially among the elderly and those with preexisting diseases of the respiratory tract and heart, as those in Belgium (1930), Pennsylvania (1948), and London (1952).

Even at lower concentrations (e.g., $SO_2 \mp 500$ kg/m^3 and smoke $\mp$ 500 μg/m^3), there is likely to be excess mortality among the elderly and the chronically sick. When exposure to these pollutants takes place at half of these concentrations, there is likely to be a worsening of existing respiratory diseases (WHO, 1979).

Photochemical Oxidants

Composition and Sources This group of air pollutants consists of nitrogen dioxide (NO2), ozone, and a number of other oxides of nitrogen (N_2O, NO, NO_2, N_2O_3, N_2O_4, and N_2O_5). N_2O is the most abundant among these chemicals, but it is generated by anaerobic processes in the soil and in the surface layer of the oceans, and hence is not an important air pollutant, as far as human health is concerned. The last three oxides of nitrogen can be formed from NO and/or NO_2. However, their levels are very low and are not known to have any harmful effects.

NO is the main oxide formed from man-made sources. However, after its discharge from the sources to the atmosphere, it reacts with O_2 to form NO_2. This reaction is facilitated in the presence of ozone.

Ozone is the most ubiquitous photochemical oxidant. At times, it constitutes as much as 90% of the oxidants in smog. Ozone is also a natural constituent of the upper atmosphere, formed by the photolysis of oxygen. Atmospheric circulation carries some to the lower levels.

The main sources of photochemical oxidants are automobiles and industrial combustion. Domestic heating and power stations also generate significant amounts. Ozone is also produced by a variety of high-voltage electrical equipment. Formaldehyde, which is one of the photochemical oxidants, is discussed under Indoor Air Pollutants.

Toxic Effects In contrast to SO_2, NO_2 is not very water soluble. It therefore passes through the upper respiratory tract to the terminal bronchioles and alveoli, where it forms nitric and nitrous acids. These acids are irritant and corrosive. Acute exposure causes pulmonary edema and congestion. It damages ciliated epithelium and type I cells, which are then replaced by the less sensitive nonciliated epithelial cells and cuboidal type II cells. Chronic exposure causes emphysema. Resistance to bacterial and viral infections is decreased (WHO, 1977).

After inhalation exposure, ozone reacts with organic matter in the respiratory tract. Similar to NO_2, its main effects are on the epithelial cells of the terminal bronchiles and alveoli, affecting the more susceptible ciliated epithelial cells and type I cells. The endothelia surrounding these structures are also damaged, resulting in pulmonary edema. Chronic exposure results in emphysema, atelectasis, focal necrosis, and sometimes bronchopneumonia. Resistance to bacterial and viral infection is decreased. Because of the oxidative activity of ozone, vitamin C decreases its toxicity whereas vitamin E deficiency has the opposite effect (WHO, 1978).

Apart from their toxic effects on the respiratory tract, these air pollutants also cause eye irritation (see chap. 15, Toxicants and Sites of Their Effects).

Indoor Air Pollutants

In recent years, the importance of indoor pollutants has become increasingly appreciated. The more efficient insulation of modern buildings, resulting in inadequate ventilation and in the use of certain insulation materials, has intensified the problem. The most common types of adverse effects of indoor air pollutants are irritating and allergic reactions of the respiratory tract. Some of the more important pollutants and reactions are described next. Additional details are provided in articles by Karol (1991) and Samet (1993).

Formaldehyde This organic chemical is a product of photooxidation of hydrocarbons. But it is more important as a component of urea formaldehyde foam insulation material, which has been widely used in mobile homes and, to a lesser extent, in conventional houses. Because of its volatility and its toxicity, it has been a significant indoor air pollutant.

Formaldehyde is irritant and very water soluble. It therefore irritates the eyes, nose, and upper respiratory tract. At higher concentrations, it also affects the bronchioles and alveoli, and induces pulmonary edema and pneumonia. The dose-effect relationship is listed in Table 21-1. In addition, it has been reported to cause nasal cancers in rodents (Albert et al., 1982). For a more detailed discussion on formaldehyde, see Gibson (1983).

Table 21-1   Acute Human Health Effects of Formaldehyde at Various Concentrations

Reported effects (ppm)	Formaldehyde concentration
None reported	0.0–0.5
Neurophysiologic effects	0.05–1.5
Odor threshold	0.05–1.0
Eye irritation[a]	0.01–2.0
Upper airway irritation	0.10–25
Lower airway and pulmonary effects	5–30
Pulmonary edema, inflammation, pneumonia	50–100
Death	>100

Source: Adapted from NRC, Committee on Aldehydes (1981).

[a]As measured by determination of optical chronaxy, electroencephalography, and sensitivity of dark-adapted eyes to light. The low concentration (0.01 ppm) was observed in the presence of other pollutants that may have been acting synergistically.

Asbestos   Asbestos is a naturally occurring silicate fiber. Because of its heat and electrical insulation properties, it has been widely used in houses, ships, automobiles, etc. Workers in certain occupations are the main population at risk. However, the general public may also be exposed to it through the air and, to a lesser extent, the drinking water (WHO, 1986).

After inhalation, it enters the alveoli and produces parenchymal asbestosis consisting of fibrosis and asbestos bodies. It may pierce the alveoli and cause pleural asbestosis. It also causes lung carcinoma, the incidence of which is significantly higher among cigarette smokers (see chap. 5, Chemical Interaction). Mesothelioma is a rare type of malignant tumor. It may originate from the pleural and peritoneal surfaces after inhalation and ingestion respectively.

The asbestos fibrosis appears to result from its entering the cells (macrophages and lymphocytes), breaking the lysosomal membrane, and releasing hydroxylases. It produces tumors either by carrying carcinogenic hydrocarbons into the body or by acting as a cocarcinogen (Selikoff and Hammond, 1979).

Others   CO (see chap. 17), NO_2, SO_2, and suspended particulate matters exist indoors as well as outdoors. In fact, this type of indoor air pollution may be more important than what exists outdoors. This is because people in general spend more time indoors and because domestic heating may be done by burning coal or other fuel indoors without adequate ventilation, as shown by a study carried out under the sponsorship of the World Health Organization (WHO) and the United Nations Environment Program (Wang et al., 1988).

Various volatile organic compounds are present in offices and homes, arising from paints, adhesives, cleaners, cosmetics, furnishings, and printed materials. In addition, there are many types of biological material such as bacteria, viruses, fungi, fungal spores, and dandruff. These substances may induce allergic reactions or "building-related illness." The latter is characterized by a variety of vague symptoms, which are aggravated by recirculation of air instead of ventilation and by humidification (Samet et al., 1988).

WATER AND SOIL POLLUTANTS

General Considerations

Various pollutants are discharged into environmental media. Those that predominate in the air are described in the preceding section. Others are discharged in wastewater as effluent or stored in dump sites. Generally these will contaminate both the water and soil.

Water and soil contaminants include pesticides and metals, which have been discussed in chaps. 19 and 20. Asbestos is also an important environmental pollutant. Its major health hazard is related to inhalation exposure as outlined in the preceding section. It is also present in water because of various mining, milling, and industrial uses, as well as its use in filter pads for wine, beer, etc.

A great variety of organic chemicals, including some solvents, has been detected in water, and most of these are present at extremely low levels. However, some of them are more persistent. In addition, a number of inorganic ions may also present health hazards. Both of these groups are described next.

Persistent Organic Chemicals

PCB Polychlorinated biphenyls (PCB) are manufactured by the progressive chlorination of biphenyl. Commercial products are mixtures of biphenyl with a different degree of chlorine substitution. These products have a variety of uses in electric insulators and rubber and paper industries, as plasticizers. They are stable, and hence persistent in the environment. Their levels in water range from 0.5 to 500 ppb, depending on the extent of contamination. They are lipophilic, and thus they bioaccumulate in aquatic organisms; fish caught from certain lakes contain 520 ppm PCB. Because of their extreme persistence and toxicity, many nations have suspended or restricted their use. However, they will remain in the environment for a long time.

PCB, being lipophilic, is stored in adipose tissue and is secreted in milk. It is a potent inducer of microsomal enzymes. As a result, it enhances the metabolism of steroids such as estradiol and androsterone, a fact that may account for some of its effects on reproductive function. Because of this effect on enzymes, it can modify the toxicity of other chemicals and act as a promoter of carcinogenesis.

It has a variety of toxic effects in animals. For example, it induces hepatic adenoma and carcinoma. Among the reproductive functions affected are lengthened estrus cycles and decreased frequency of implanted ova in mice, lowered fertility in mink and rhesus monkey, and reduced hatchability of eggs in birds. Acting on the immune system, it causes atrophy of lymphoid tissue in chickens and in rabbits. It suppresses a variety of humoral and cell-mediated immunity.

An outbreak of poisoning occurred in Japan in 1968 from consumption of rice oil contaminated with PCB. It affected more than 1000 people. The major clinical manifestations were chloracne, hyperkeratosis, and darkening of skin. Immunosuppression was also noted. Various subjective symptoms were reported, such as numbness of the limbs, coughing, expectoration, general fatigue, and eye discharge. There may also be an increase of liver and lung cancer among the male patients. Additional information and references to these topics are compiled in publications such as WHO (1993) and Japan–U.S. Joint Seminar (1985).

PBB Polybrominated biphenyls are used as fire retardants. They gained notoriety because of a large-scale contamination of cattle feed in Michigan in 1973. The beef was contaminated with PBB. They are similar to PCB in many aspects, such as biotransformation, storage, and effects on reproduction, carcinogenesis, immune system, and skin (chloracne).

TCDD 2,3,7,8-Tetrachlorodibenzo-*p*-dioxin attracted wide attention after its accidental release from a factory in Seveso, Italy, in 1976. While its level in water is low, it is important toxicologically because of its extreme potency. Furthermore, it is a contaminant of other chemicals, notably the herbicide 2,4,5-T, which was extensively used as a defoliant in Vietnam during the war there. It is extremely toxic, with LD_{50}s ranging from 0.0006 to 0.115 mg/kg in different species of animals (NRC, 1977).

TCDD is a potent inducer of microsomal enzymes, by binding to a specific receptor as described in chap. 4. It is a potent carcinogen (2 ppb in rats), inducing cancers in a variety of organs such as liver, respiratory tract, and oral cavity (Kociba et al., 1977). At somewhat higher doses, it is hepatotoxic, immunosuppressive, teratogenic, and fetotoxic. In humans, the predominant effect of TCDD is chloracne. It has not been reported to be carcinogenic in humans in spite of its extremely potent carcinogenicity in rats (Zack and Suskind, 1980; WHO,1989).

Other Organic Chemicals Phthalate esters are extensively used in plastics, and are widely distributed in the environment, especially water. Their acute toxicity is low, but DEHP [di(2-ethylhexyl) phthalate] has been shown to be carcinogenic and to adversely affect reproductive functions in animals (Conference on Phthalates, 1982). Trihalomethanes are formed through the chlorination of water. These chemicals comprise chloroform, bromodichloromethane, dibromochloromethane, and bromoform. They are found in drinking water from less than 0.1 to 311 ppb. Among them, chloroform had the highest concentration. These chemicals are hepatotoxic and may be carcinogenic (see Amdur, 1993).

Inorganic Ions

Nitrates　The increase of nitrates in soil and water results mainly from intensive application of fertilizers, but also from wastes (excreta) of humans and farm animals. They are converted to nitrites in soil, water, and the gastrointestinal tract through microbial action. Nitrites can induce methemoglobinemia, thus reducing the oxygen-carrying capacity of hemoglobin as noted in chap. 4. Furthermore, they may react with certain amines to form nitrosamines, most of which are carcinogenic (chaps. 7 and 18).

Phosphates　These substances arise mainly from fertilizers and detergents. They have very low toxicity, but their presence in a stagnant water body results in excessive growth of algae. The algae reduce the oxygenation of the water, resulting in fish kill. Certain "algae," the cyanobacteria, contain hepatotoxins which may act as promoters in hepatocarcinogenesis (Carmichael, 1994).

Fluoride　The natural level of fluoride in water varies greatly, depending on the location. Industrial activities may also raise its level. While fluoride has been added to water to about 1 ppm to reduce dental cavity formation, excessive levels in water (10 ppm) are likely to cause fluorosis. The enamel on the teeth is weakened, resulting in surface pitting. Changes in the bones, including osteosclerosis and exostoses, usually affect the spine and cause the knee deformity known as genu valgum. At lower levels of fluoride intake, chalky-white patches appear on the surface of the dental enamel. These patches are then stained yellow or brown and give rise to the characteristic "mottled" appearance.

REFERENCES

Aksoy, M., and Erdem, S. 1978. Follow-up study on the mortality and the development of leukemia in 44 pancytopenic patients with chronic exposure to benzene. *Blood* 52: 285–292.

Albert, R. E., et al. 1982. Gaseous formaldehyde and hydrogen chloride induction of nasal cancer in the rat. *JNCI* 68:597–603.

Amdur, M. O. 1993. Air pollutants. In *Casarett and Doull's toxicology*, eds. M. O. Amdur, J. Doull, and C. D. Klaassen, pp. 854–871. New York: McGraw-Hill.

American Conference of Governmental Industrial Hygienists. 1995. TLVs. Threshold Limit Values for Chemical Substances in Workroom Air. Cincinnati, OH: Publications Office, ACGIH.

Andrews, L. S., Lee, E. W., Witmer, C. M., Kocsis, J. J., and Snyder, R. 1977. Effects of toluene on metabolism, disposition, and hematopoietic toxicity of (^{3}H) benzene. *Biochem. Pharmacol.* 26:293–300.

Andrews, L. S., and Snyder, R. 1993. Toxic effects of solvents and vapors. In *Casarett and Doull's toxicology*, eds. M. O. Amdur, J. Doull, and C. D. Klaassen. New York: McGraw-Hill

Carmichael, W. W. 1994. The toxins of Cyanobacteria. *Sci. Am.* 270:78–86.

Conference on Phthalates. 1982. Proceedings of the Conference. *Environ. Health Perspect.* 45:11–51.

Fitzhugh, O. G., and Nelson, A. A. 1946. Comparison of the chronic toxicity of triethylene glycol with that of diethylene glycol. *J. Ind. Hyg. Toxicol.* 28:40–43.

Fuchs, N. A. 1964. *The mechanisms of aerosol*, p. 28. Oxford: Pergamon Press.

Gibson, J. E. 1983. *Formaldehyde*. Washington, DC: Hemisphere.

Japan–U.S. Joint Seminar. 1985. Toxicity of chlorinated biphenyls, dibenzhofurans, dibenzodioxins and related compounds. *Environ. Health Perspect.* 59:11–81.

Karol, M. H. 1991. Allergic reactions to indoor air pollutants. *Environ. Health Perspect.* 95:45–51.

Kociba, R. J., Keyes, D. G., Beyer, J. E., et al. 1977. Results of a two-year chronic toxicity and oncogenicity study of 2,3,7,8-tetrachlorodibenzo-*p*-dioxin in rats. *Toxicol. Appl. Pharmacol.* 46:279–303.

Krasavage, W. J., O'Donoghue, J. L., DiVincenzo, G. D., and Terhaar, C. J. 1980. The relative neurotoxicity of methyl *n*-butyl ketone, *n*-hexane and their metabolites. *Toxicol. Appl. Pharmacol.* 52:433–441.

Maltoni, C., Ciliberti, A., Cotti, G., Conti, B., and Belpoggi, F. 1989. Benzene, an experimental multipotential carcinogen: Results of the long-term bioassays performed at the Bologna Institute of Oncology. *Environ. Health Perspect.* 82:109–124.

Meyer, K. H. 1937. Contributions to the theory of narcosis. *Faraday Soc. Trans.* 33:1062–1064.

National Research Council. 1977. *Drinking water and health*. Washington, DC: National Research Council, National Academy of Sciences.

National Research Council, Committee on Aldehydes. 1981. *Formaldehyde and other aldehydes*. Washington, DC: National Academy Press.

Reid, W. D., and Krishna, G. 1973. Centrolobular hepatic necrosis related to covalent binding of metabolites of halogenated aromatic hydrocarbons. *Exp. Med. Pathol.* 18:80–99.

Samet, J. M. 1993. Indoor air pollution: A public health perspective. *Indoor Air.* 3:219–226.

Samet, J. M., Marbury, M. C., and Spengler, J. D. 1988. Health effects and sources of indoor air pollution. Part II. *Am. Rev. Respir. Dis.* 137:221–242.

Selikoff, I. J., and Hammond, E. C. 1979. Health hazards of asbestos exposure. *Ann. NY Acad. Sci.* 330:1–814.

Waldbott, G. K. 1978. *Health effects of environmental pollutants*. St. Louis, MO: C. V. Mosby.

Wang, J. N., Cao, S. R., Li, Z., Zhang, Y., and Li, S. M. 1988. Human exposure to carbon monoxide and inhalable particulate in Beijing, China. *Biomed. Environ. Sci.* 1:5–12.

World Health Organization. 1964. Seventh Report of the FAO/WHO Expert Committee on Food Additives. Tech. Rep. Ser. 281. Geneva: WHO.

World Health Organization. 1977. Oxides of Nitrogen. Environmental Health Criteria 4. Geneva: WHO.

World Health Organization. 1978. Photochemical Oxidants. Environmental Health Criteria 7. Geneva: WHO.

World Health Organization. 1979. Sulfur Oxides and Suspended Particulate Matter. Environmental Health Criteria 8. Geneva: WHO.

World Health Organization. 1984. Methylene Chloride. Environmental Health Criteria 32. Geneva: WHO.

World Health Organization. 1986. Asbestos and Other Natural Mineral Fibers. Environmental Health Criteria 53. Geneva: WHO.

World Health Organization. 1989. Polychlorinated Dibenzo-*p*-Dioxins and Dibenzofurans. Environmental Health Criteria 88. Geneva: WHO.

World Health Organization. 1993. Polychlorinated Biphenyls and Terphenyls, 2nd ed. Environmental Health Criteria 140. Geneva: WHO.

Zack, J. A., and Suskind, R. R. 1980. The mortality experience of workers exposed to tetrachlorodibenzodioxin in a trichlorophenol process accident. *J. Occup. Med.* 22:1–114.

Toxicologic Evaluation: Assessment of Safety/Risk

CHAPTER 22 CONTENTS

INTRODUCTION

Importance and Reasonableness

Descriptions in prior chapters make it abundantly clear that chemicals differ greatly in the nature and potency of their toxicity. Since human exposure to chemicals is not always avoidable (it may even be desirable in certain cases), toxicological evaluation of many chemicals must be carried out to determine the level of exposure (or intake in the case of food and water) under which no risk is likely to occur. Because of the gaps in our knowledge, it is prudent to be conservative in assessing the safety/risk. But when undue caution is incorporated into the process, the public may be denied chemicals of great values and society may be burdened with unnecessary economic costs, such as pollution prevention measures and environmental cleanup. Therefore the most important function of toxicology is to establish the scientific basis for regulating the use (and disposal) of chemicals without undue human health hazards or undue cost.

Historical Development

Around the turn of the century, industrialization and urbanization prompted people to move from their farms to cities. Away from the farm, they had to consume stored and processed food. Food adulteration became a serious problem. In the United States, the first U.S. Food and Drug Act was enacted in 1906. Similar action was taken in several other countries. At that time, health hazards were based essentially on qualitative assessments; the mere presence of a toxic substance in food was considered adulteration, and "adulterated" food was banned outright.

To permit judicious use of food additives, Lehman and Fitzhugh of the U.S. Food and Drug Administration initiated in 1954 quantitative assessment by the use of a "100-fold margin of safety" approach. This assessment of food additives stipulates that "the chemical additive should not occur in the total human diet in a quantity greater than 1/100 of the amount that is the maximum safe dosage in long-term animal experiments" (Lehman and Fitzhugh, 1954).

While this margin of 100 seemed reasonable for food additives, it could not be applied to other chemicals, such as contaminants and pesticide residues, whose levels in food are not readily controllable. Furthermore, it would be impracticable on an international level: There would be marked differences among nations, both in dietary pattern and technological usage. The Joint FAO/WHO Expert Committee on Food Additives therefore coined, in 1961, the term *acceptable daily intake* (ADI). This term was later that year adopted by the Joint FAO/WHO Meeting on Pesticide Residues.

In 1977, the U.S. National Research Council (NRC) extended the concept to the assessment of contaminants in water, and the U.S. Environmental Protection Agency (EPA) extended it to pollutants in air, with slight variation in the terminology.

Later the Delaney Amendment (see chap. 18, Legal Definition of Food Additives) and the concept of "negligible residues" were introduced to regulate carcinogenic chemicals. As shown in subsequent sections, these measures were no panacea. Mathematical models were then devised to estimate doses that could be considered as virtually safe (Mantel and Bryan, 1961).

The National Research Council (NRC, 1983) divided the management of risk assessment into the following steps:

1 *Hazard identification*—scrutinizing all relevant toxicological and related data to identify the hazard associated with a chemical.

2 *Dose-response assessment*—determining the relationship between the magnitude of exposure and the probability of health effects.

3 *Exposure assessment*—determining the extent of human exposure.

4 *Risk characterization*—estimating the nature and magnitude of human risk, and the uncertainty of the estimate.

Major Approaches

At high enough doses, all chemicals exhibit toxic effects. As the dose is reduced the severity of the effects as well as the responses diminish. For a majority of the chemicals, there are threshold doses below which they will not elicit adverse effects. There are various reasons for the thresholds. The chemical in question may not reach the site of action because of its limited absorption and distribution or its prompt elimination. Metabolic detoxication often plays an important role. Furthermore, repair and regeneration of affected cells and excess functional capacity may overcome/overshadow any minute, temporary effects.

The "safety" of such chemicals can be estimated using the "acceptable daily intake" approach, which involves identification of the most sensitive, yet appropriate, indicator of adverse effect and the application of a suitable safety factor to the no-observed-adverse-effect level (NOAEL) to compensate for potential differences between animals and humans and between the relatively small number of test subjects and the large human population, which is more heterogeneous.

Genotoxic carcinogens, on the other hand, probably have no threshold doses. The rationale is that a cancer cell can be induced by a single change in the cellular genetic material, and the cancer cell has the capacity of self-replicating. Therefore, theoretically, a single molecule of such a chemical can induce a cancer.

In the absence of threshold doses, it would be impossible to identify a no-adverse-effect level, thus rendering the ADI approach impracticable. Mathematical models have been designed to estimate, from the dose-response relationship and a variety of assumptions, a "virtually safe dose," exposure to which would result in an extremely small risk, say 10^{-6} (one risk in a million).

ACCEPTABLE DAILY INTAKE

Definition and Usage

As noted earlier, the term *acceptable daily intake* (ADI) was coined by the Joint FAO/WHO Expert Committee on Food Additives in 1961 (WHO, 1962a). It has been adopted by the Joint FAO/WHO Meeting of Experts on Pesticide Residues (WHO, 1962b). This term has been used at all subsequent meetings of these two international expert bodies in their toxicologic evaluation, and reevaluation, of large numbers of food additives and pesticides that leave residues in food. The term has also been adopted by a number of other bodies in the toxicological evaluation of chemicals in food, water, etc. as a basis for setting standards (e.g., U.S. EPA; Cotruvos, 1988).

ADI is defined as "the daily intake of a chemical which, during an entire lifetime, appears to be without appreciable risk on the basis of all the known facts at the time. It is expressed in milligrams of the chemical per kilogram of body weight (mg/kg)." It is worth noting that the ADI is qualified by the expressions "appear to be" and "on the basis of all the known facts at the time." This caution is in keeping with the fact that it is impossible to be absolutely certain about the safety of a chemical and that the ADI may be altered in the light of new toxicologic data.

Toxicologic evaluations of food additives and pesticides, in terms of ADIs by these international expert bodies, have been used by the regulatory agencies in many countries as an important consideration in the formulation of national regulations. ADIs have also been used collectively by national authorities in the framework of the Codex Alimentarius Commission. The Commission is an intergovernmental body with more than 150 countries as members. Its principal function is to elaborate international food standards for the protection of the health of the consumer and to facilitate international food trade. These food standards contain provisions for food additives that are accepted by the Commission only when ADIs have been allocated by the Expert Committee on Food Additives. The latter goal is achieved through the removal of "noneconomic" trade barriers based on unjustified claims of health hazards alleged to be associated with a certain additive or pesticide. Additional details about the Codex Alimentarius Commission are given in an article by Lu (1988), as well as in chaps. 18 and 19.

There are a number of variations of the terminology. For instance, in dealing with food contaminants, the Joint FAO/WHO Expert Committee on Food Additives in 1972 coined the term *provisional tolerable weekly intake.* The procedure used in arriving at such intakes is identical to that for ADIs. The Committee, however, felt that, unlike food additives, which serve certain useful purposes, contaminants do not. Therefore they are not acceptable but merely "tolerable." Furthermore, the intakes were expressed in terms of "weekly" because the contaminants dealt with then (mercury, lead and cadmium) are cumulative, and vary (especially mercury) in their daily intake, but less so on a weekly basis.

Another variation is used by U.S. EPA, which assesses *reference doses* (RFD) instead of ADIs, using essentially the same procedure, except that the safety factor is called the *uncertainty factor* (Dourson and Stara, 1983). It might be noted that the term ADI is widely used on an international level as well as by regulatory agencies in many nations, including the U.S. FDA.

Procedure for Estimating ADIs

The following steps are involved in estimating ADIs:

1 Compile adequate relevant data.
2 Select a NOAEL.
3 Divide by a safety factor (SF) to obtain an ADI.

Adequate, Relevant Data   As noted in previous chapters, chemicals possess different toxicity. This is true even among chemically related substances. Consequently a great variety of studies must be done (see chaps. 18 and 19). Furthermore, pharmacokinetic studies facilitate the assessment of the effects on humans from findings obtained in experimental animals. In addition, the data must be obtained from relevant studies. For example, findings of epithelial hyperplasia in the forestomach of rats given an irritant fumigant by gavage have little, if any, bearing on the possible adverse effect on humans consuming food that has been fumigated by the fumigant (see Lu and Coulston, 1996).

The assessment of certain chemicals requires less data for establishing their ADIs. Examples are food additives obtained from edible animals, plants, and microbes. The extent of testing and the reasons thereof have been described by WHO (1987).

No-Observed-Adverse-Effect Level (NOAEL)   This is the maximum dose level that has not induced any sign of toxicity (adverse effect) in the most susceptible but appropriate species of animals tested, and using the most sensitive indicator of toxicity. As a rule, this level is selected from a long-term study. However, certain signs of toxicity, such as cataract, delayed neurotoxicity and effects on reproduction, are demonstrable in short-term studies. The NOAEL is not necessarily an absolutely no-effect level; rather it is a "no *observed* effect level," because the use of a more sensitive indicator of toxicity or a more susceptible animal species may reveal a lower NOAEL. In addition, an effect might well be demonstrable if a sufficiently large number of animals were used in the test. However, the general consensus is that there is an absolute NOAEL no matter how large the dose groups are (Lu and Sielken, 1991).

On the other hand, certain effects are generally considered as physiologic, adaptive, or otherwise "nontoxic." These effects are therefore excluded in establishing the NOAEL. For example, liver enlargement may result from stimulation in the activity of hepatic mixed-function oxidases and the de novo protein synthesis in the smooth endoplasmic reticulum. A decrease of body weight may follow reduced food consumption, which in turn may be a result of toxicity or unpalatability of the chemical. A reduction in liver glycogen or alteration in leukocyte count may not be indicative of a toxic effect but an adaptation to a stress situation. Feeding large amounts of inert substances such as mannitol and cellulose derivatives may cause diarrhea and malnutrition. However, before disregarding these effects in evaluating the toxicity of a chemical, care must be taken to ensure that these are not manifestations of toxicity. Additional studies may have to be done to elucidate the nature of the effect. These various points have been elaborated in several WHO reports and summarized in a review article (Lu, 1988).

Safety Factors   To extrapolate from the NOAEL in animals to an acceptable intake in humans, a safety factor of 100, originally proposed by Lehman and Fitzhugh (1954), is generally used. This factor is intended to allow for differences in sensitivity of the animal species and humans, to allow for wide variations in susceptibility among the human population, and to allow for the fact that the number of animals tested is small compared to the size of the human population that may be exposed (WHO, 1958, 1974a; NAS, 1970).

While the factor 100 is often used, the WHO expert committees have used figures that have ranged from 10 to 2000. The size of the safety factor is determined according to the nature of the toxicity. In addition, a larger figure is used to compensate for slight deficiencies of toxicity data, such as small numbers of animals on test. On the other hand, minimal, reversible, and inconsequential effects such as a slight inhibition of cholinesterase by an organophosphorus pesticide may justify the use of a smaller safety factor. In addition, available human data may warrant the use of a smaller figure since they obviate the need for interspecies extrapolation.

Biochemical data relating to the absorption, distribution, and excretion of the toxicant and its biotransformation (detoxication and bioactivation) in various species of animals and in humans are often useful in determining the size of the safety factor. These and other bases for altering the safety factor are elaborated in two WHO documents (WHO, 1987, 1990).

The reasons for the use of different safety factors by WHO in the evaluation/reevaluation of the 230 pesticides in the past three decades are noted and explained in a recent review (Lu, 1995).

Quantitative Assessment of Acceptability

Daily Intakes   The ADI is used as a yardstick to check the acceptability of the proposed uses. This is done by comparing the ADI with the "potential" daily intake (PDI), since the actual intake cannot be readily determined. PDI is the sum of the products of the amounts of the food (calculated on the basis of the average per capita consumption) and the permitted use levels of the additives in them.

PDI $= (F_1 \times L_1) + (F_2 \times L_2) + (F_3 \times L_3) + \ldots$ where $F_1, F_2, F_3,$ $\ldots$ are per capita consumption of food commodities and $L_1, L_2, L_3 \ldots$ are use levels of food additives or maximum residue levels of pesticide residues or other contaminants. If the potential daily intake exceeds the ADI, the use levels may be lowered or some of the uses may be deleted. The Commission follows the same procedure in accepting the maximum limits for pesticide residues in food. The use of the "potential daily intake" and other estimated intakes by WHO in assessing the acceptability of food additives and pesticides has been reviewed by Lu and Seilken (1991), and in some detail in a WHO document (1989).

Margin of Safety   The ADI approach is not designed to provide information on the risks involved at intakes higher than the ADI. This is because of the wide "gray area" between the NOAEL and the ADI. However, the margin of safety between the estimated intake (just discussed) and the ADI, or the NOAEL, is sometimes used to indicate the degree of confidence in the safety at a specified intake. It is also used to indicate the spread between the ED_{50} and LD_{50} or ED_{99} and LD_{01}.

MATHEMATICAL MODELS

As discussed in chap. 7, there are genotoxic and nongenotoxic carcinogens. It is generally agreed that there are probably no thresholds for genotoxic carcinogens. In view of the theoretical absence of threshold doses and in the absence of a reliable procedure to determine a threshold for a carcinogen for an entire population, estimating the levels of risk has been considered to be more appropriate.

Estimation of Risks

Definition Risk has been defined as the expected frequency of undesirable effects arising from exposure to a pollutant. It may be expressed in absolute terms as the risk due to exposure to a specific pollutant. It may also be expressed as a relative risk, which is the ratio of the risk among the exposed population to that among the unexposed (WHO, 1978).

The term was first adopted by the International Commission on Radiological Protection (ICRP, 1966) in evaluating the health hazards related to ionizing radiation. The use of this term stems from the realization that often a clear-cut "safe" or "unsafe" decision cannot be made.

Risks Levels and Virtual Safety Estimation of risks involves development of suitable dose-response data and extrapolation from the observed dose-response relationship to the expected responses at doses occurring at actual exposure situations. A number of mathematical models have been proposed for this purpose. Such models are also used to estimate the dose that is expected to be associated with a specific level of risk.

Mantel and Bryan (1961) first introduced the concept of virtual safety. The term was defined as a probability of carcinogenicity of less than $1/100$ million (10^{-8}) at a statistical assurance level of 99%. The U.S. Food and Drug Administration, however, found that the doses associated with such a low risk level were too small to be enforceable in most actual situations and thus adopted a risk level of 10^{-6} (FDA, 1977). These levels of risk are so low that the doses associated with them are referred to as virtually safe doses (VSD).

Commonplace Activities and Their Risks In order to place the risk levels in perspective, risks associated with certain commonplace activities and natural occurrences are sometimes cited. Table 22-1 includes a number of estimates of such risks.

Table 22-1 Estimated Risks for Certain Activities and Natural Occurrences

Activity	Risk[a]
Smoking (10 cigarettes/d)	1/400
All accidents	1/2,000
Driving (16,000 km/y)	1/5,000
All traffic accidents	1/8,000
Work in industry	1/30,000
Natural disasters	1/50,000
Being struck by lightning	1/1,000,000

Source: Adapted from Royal Commission on the Environment (1976), by permission of the Controller of Her Majesty's Stationery Office, London.

[a]Risk is expressed as probability of death of an individual for a year of exposure and is given in round figures.

The risks in Table 22-1, apart from lightning, are considerably greater than 10^{-6}. Estimates of risks associated with other common activities and occupations have been compiled by others, for example, Wilson (1980).

Apart from its magnitude, the acceptability of a risk depends on the nature of the activity. In general, risks associated with voluntary, pleasurable, and/or beneficial activities, such as smoking and driving, are more acceptable to the individual. On the other hand, risks associated with activities that are perceived as having no benefit and those that are not controllable by the individual tend to be rejected, such as food colors suspected of being carcinogenic.

Models for Estimating Risk/VSD

A number of mathematical models have been developed for this purpose. In general, they involve extrapolating from the observed dose response to either of the following:

1   The risks at a specific exposure level.
2   The *risk specified dose* (RSD). When the specified risk is low enough, such as 10^{-5} or 10^{-6}, the dose associated with it is known as the *virtually safe dose* (VSD).

Probability Models   As noted earlier, Mantel and Bryan (1961) first introduced the concept of virtual safety, and developed a model based on the assumption that the responses (tumor formation) will be the same as most other quantal (all-or-none) toxicologic responses, namely, normally distributed among the subjects.

This S-shaped dose-response curve can be straightened, as described in chap. 6, by plotting the points on a probit basis. Variations of this probit model include logit and Weibull.

These are also known as "tolerance models," as they are based on the probability of individuals in a population whose tolerances to the carcinogen will be exceeded.

Mechanistic Models   Several other models have been designed based on presumed mechanisms of action of carcinogenesis. The *one-hit* model assumes that a critical hit in a cell by a carcinogen may induce a cancer through initiation, promotion, and progression. On the other hand, the *multihit* model assumes that several hits are required for a response to occur. The *multistage* model is built on the assumption that the induction of a carcinogenic response follows random biological events, with the time rate of occurrence of each event being in linear proportion to the dose rate.

The conservativeness of these models is achieved through the use of upper confidence limits to responses on the risk estimated, shallow slopes, or the lower confidence limits on the VSD estimated. Figure 22-1 shows

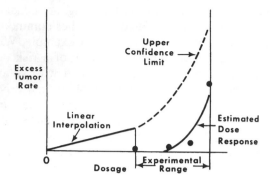

Figure 22-1 Linear extrapolation showing the observed responses, the upper confidence limit of the response at the lowest experimental dose, and the linear interpolation (from Gaylor and Kodell, 1980).

the observed responses, the upper confidence limit, and the linear interpolation.

Several U.S. regulatory agencies, including the U.S. EPA (1986), use the linearized multistage model (Anderson, 1986). With this model, it is presumed that no threshold dose exists, a multistage process is involved in chemical carcinogenesis, and the time rate of occurrence of each event is linearly proportional to the dose.

Based on a set of aflatoxin B_1 carcinogenesis data, low-dose extrapolation was done with various models. The marked difference among them is clearly visible in Fig. 22-2. The one-hit and multistage models yielded the most conservative estimates, whereas the probit model yielded the least conservative figure. According to the calculations of the Food Safety Council (1980), the VSDs at a risk of 10^{-6} are 3.4×10^{-5} ppb (one-hit), 7.9×10^{-4} (multistage), 4.0×10^{-2} (Weibull), 0.28 (multihit), and 2.5 (probit), respectively.

In addition, *physiologically based pharmacokinetic* (PB-PK) modeling has been developed to utilize toxicokinetic differences between the test animals and humans. For example, the target concentration of dichloromethane was about 150-fold higher in mice than in humans; these data provided a much lower, probably more realistic estimate of the risk of this toxicant (Andersen et al., 1987). For additional examples, see Andersen and Krishnan (1994) and Dallas et al. (1995). A modified version, the *biologically based pharmacodynamic* model, also incorporates data on the interaction of the toxicant with tissues and the response of the tissues (Conolly and Andersen, 1991). While such modeling has certain advantages, it involves complex mathematical equations, and the physiological parameters regarding various species and strains, disease states, and the like are often ill-defined (Klaassen and Rozman, 1993; Lu and Sielken, 1991).

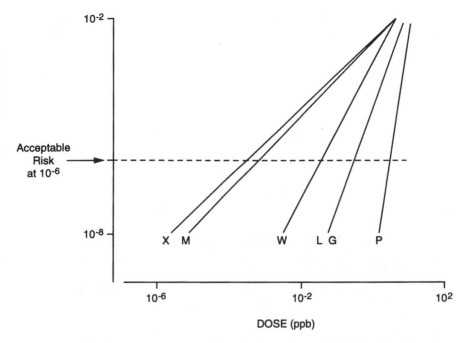

Figure 22-2 The low dose-response relationships based on a set of aflatoxin B_1 data, using different models: X = one-hit, M = multistage, W = Weibull, L = logit, G = multihit, and P = probit model (adapted from Krewski and Van Ryzin, 1981).

Other Variations The *time-to-response*, instead of the response itself, has also been proposed for use in the mathematical models (Chand and Hoel, 1974; Sielken, 1981). The importance of this approach has been pointed out by the SOT ED_{01} Task Force (1981). *Background responses*, that is, those occurring also among the unexposed, are often observed. They can also be incorporated into mathematical models (Hoel, 1980).

The response of an organism to a toxicant is related to the dose and the duration of exposure. It is also affected by *competing risks*. Kalbfleisch et al. (1983) proposed mathematical models that will take these three factors into account.

Since many carcinogens require bioactivation, the importance of incorporating *metabolic data* in evaluating their risks is obvious. For example, vinyl chloride is carcinogenic after bioactivation. Gehring et al. (1978) showed that the tumor incidence in rats exposed to various concentrations of this chemical was proportional to the metabolized amount rather than the exposure concentration (Table 22-2).

Risk Assessment

Risk assessment is done by estimating the risk associated with a toxicant at an ascertained level of exposure, using an appropriate mathematical

Table 22-2 Correlation Between Exposure Concentration of Vinyl Chloride (VC), Metabolism, and Induction of Hepatic Angiosarcoma in Rats

Exposure concentration (ppm of VC)	VC (µg / L air)	VC metabolized (µg)	Percentage liver angiosarcoma
50	128	739	2
250	640	2435	7
500	1280	3413	12
2500	6400	5030	22
6000	15360	5003	22
10,000	25600	5521	15

Source: Adapted from Gehring et al. (1978).

model as already described. Where the risk level is low, such as 10^{-6} or lower, the exposure might be considered acceptable. However, where the risk is higher, various risk management decisions may have to be taken. The options consist of lowering the exposure level, shortening the exposure duration, suspending the manufacture/use of chemical, and others.

OTHER PROCEDURES

Noncarcinogenic Chemicals

Not all chemicals require the whole gamut of toxicologic testing as described for estimating ADIs. For example, for chemicals to which humans are not likely to be exposed to an appreciable extent, such as indirect food additives and certain pesticides, a *toxicologically insignificant amount* may be estimated on the basis of toxicologic data that include at least 90-d feeding studies in two species of mammals and by the use of a larger safety factor (generally 1000) (NAS, 1965). Variations of this principle have been adopted by the U.S. FDA and EPA administratively.

Furthermore, a *decision to reject a chemical* may be made on much more limited data, especially in the course of developing new chemicals. Such data include extreme acute toxicity, positive response in short-term mutagenesis tests, or undesirable features in biochemical studies or short-term feeding studies in animals (see Fig. 22-3).

As discussed in the next section, most if not all nongenotoxic carcinogens should be assessed by the ADI approach.

Carcinogenic Chemicals

Chemicals with Questionable Data   The Joint FAO/WHO Expert Committee on Food Additives at its second meeting (WHO, 1958) recommended that "no proved carcinogen should be considered suitable for

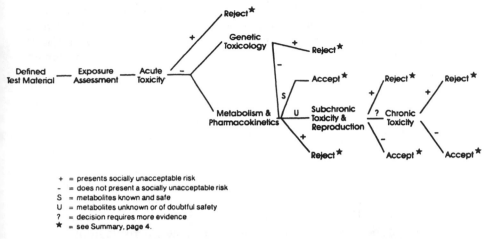

Figure 22-3 Safety decision tree (adapted from Food Safety Council, 1980).

use as a food additive in any amount." This principle has been followed at subsequent meetings of the Committee and at the Joint FAO/WHO Meetings on Pesticide Residues in not allocating ADIs to proved carcinogens. *Temporary or conditional ADIs*, however, have been estimated for chemicals with equivocal carcinogenicity data, such as nitrites and amitrole. On the other hand, discontinuation of the use of chemicals without essential functions has been recommended. The basis for the decisions on these and other such chemicals has been reviewed and summarized (Lu, 1979). This principle of considering both the soundness of the carcinogenesis data and the usefulness of the chemical is consistent with the policies of many national regulatory agencies (e.g., Somers, 1986).

Secondary and Nongenotoxic Carcinogens The concept of *secondary carcinogens*, which induce tumors only after certain noncarcinogenic effects, has been accepted by many toxicologists. For example, a WHO scientific group (WHO, 1974b) pointed out that the urinary bladder cancers in rats treated with Myrj 45 (polyoxyethylene monostearate) were caused by the bladder calculi rather than the chemical directly and that a NOEL can therefore be established. A variety of other types of nongenotoxic carcinogens have been discussed in chap. 7. Many investigators (e.g., Reitz et al., 1990) have suggested that the predominant mechanism whereby a chemical elicits a carcinogenic response should be considered in extrapolating laboratory data to humans. For examples of such carcinogens, see chap. 7.

Qualitative Assessment It is becoming more widely recognized that there are marked differences in the nature and extent of positive data among carcinogenic chemicals. Some chemicals, such as aflatoxin, consistently yield positive response in a variety of animals, with small doses and after a relatively short latent period, whereas others, such as saccharin, yield positive response inconsistently, and only with large doses and after long durations of treatment. Squire (1981) devised a ranking system to evaluate carcinogens, which are to be scored according to the following criteria: (1) number of species affected, (2) number of histogenetically different types of neoplasms in one or more species, (3) spontaneous incidence in appropriate control groups of neoplasms induced in treated groups, (4) dose-response relationships (cumulative oral dose equivalents per kilogram of body weight per day for 2 yr), (5) malignancy of induced neoplasms, and (6) genotoxicity, measured in an appropriate battery of tests. Using the total score for each carcinogen, the author ranked, for example, aflatoxin as I; 2-naphthylamine, II; chloroform, III; NTA (nitrilotriacetic acid), IV; and saccharin, V. This approach merits serious consideration in view of the widely different estimates derived from various mathematical modeling exercises.

COMMENTS ON THE TWO WIDELY
USED PROCEDURES

Acceptable Daily Intake

The widely adopted procedure for evaluating noncarcinogenic chemicals is to estimate their ADIs, based on the belief that there are threshold doses below which no adverse effects are expected from exposure to them. As noted earlier, many food additives, pesticides, and other chemicals have been so evaluated. This procedure has not excessively restricted the use of most of these chemicals and has failed only very rarely.

One such failure related to the myocardial effect, which was observed among heavy drinkers of beer that contained 1 ppm cobalt. Cobalt chloride was added to beer as a foam stabilizer and to prevent gushing. Cobalt salts have long been used in the treatment of anemia at doses of about 300 mg/d. No heart lesions have been reported from such treatment. The heavy beer drinkers drank about 10 L a day, containing therefore only one-thirtieth of the therapeutic dose of cobalt. Subsequent studies showed that the toxicity of cobalt was greatly enhanced by the malnutrition, especially the deficiency of certain amino acids, associated with a large caloric intake from the beer alone (Wiberg et al., 1969). The magnitude of potentiating effects of alcohol and malnutrition on cobalt was not expected and therefore was not taken into account in assessing the safety of cobalt in beer.

Another glaring failure in toxicologic evaluation resulted in the tragedy following the clinical use of thalidomide. This sedative/hypnotic was tested according to the then prevailing protocol and found to have a low toxicity. However, after its use in pregnant women, there appeared many cases of phocomelia from mothers who had taken this drug (Lenz and Knapp, 1962). This failure resulted, obviously, from a lack of appropriate prior testing for teratogenicity, a serious gap in toxicity testing which has since been remedied.

These two examples illustrate that toxicologic evaluations can be invalidated when there are significant, unexpected toxic effects or undetected but marked influences of modifying factors. They do not, however, signify an absence of threshold doses. Furthermore, the deficiency of biologic data is unlikely to be overcome by mathematical manipulations of the available dose-response data, such as the use of the "benchmark dose" proposed by Crump (1984). The WHO expert groups considered that the proposal needs further study. Furthermore, while the slope of the dose-response relationship is an important factor to consider, the available data are in general inadequate for this purpose (WHO, 1990).

Since it is impossible to be certain that all appropriate tests have been conducted on a chemical, a caveat must be included in any toxicologic evaluation. Apart from rigorous testing and cautious evaluation prior to the introduction of a new chemical to the human environment, it is prudent to monitor the exposed population for possible deleterious effects and to reassess its toxicologic implications in the light of new data and of improvements in toxicologic methodology (WHO, 1957), advice still valid today.

By the use of a sufficiently large safety factor, the ADI approach is designed to estimate the dose of a chemical in question that is safe/acceptable. It does not attempt to assess the risks involved when the intake is somewhat larger than the ADI, since there is too much uncertainty in the "gray area" between an intake that is safe and the one that is definitely toxic (see also Margin of Safety subsection).

Mathematical Models

Noncarcinogens Mathematical models have been used mainly in evaluating carcinogens, but they have also been proposed for use with noncarcinogens. This proposal was made because, according to certain toxicologists, an absolute NOAEL cannot be determined in view of the limitations on the number of animals that can be used and because the slope of the dose-response curve is not taken into account in the selection of a safety factor. Contrary to these views, it should be noted that the two points just mentioned are in fact considered by most toxicologists in deciding on the size of the safety factor, although only done according to "scientific judgment" rather than on a strict statistical basis. The validity of the use of the "apparent" NOAEL, the slope of the dose-response relationship, the preference of body weight instead of body surface, and the size of the safety factor as determined by the adequacy of data and by the seriousness of the effects are discussed in a number of WHO reports and summarized in two review articles (Lu, 1985; Lu and Sielken, 1991).

Mathematical models, which assume the absence of threshold, have been used by the Food Safety Council (1980) in estimating the VSD with respect to the lethal effect of botulinum toxin. This usage apparently ignores the fundamental difference between carcinogens and noncarcinogens. The effect of the former is not only irreversible but also capable of self-replicating, whereas the latter is not. In other words, a critical hit by a carcinogen theoretically can induce a cancer, but botulinum toxin cannot act in this way. For this toxin to cause death, or even respiratory distress, a huge number of myofibrils in the respiratory muscles must be paralyzed. Therefore, a dose that is too small to bind a sufficient number of the receptors on the nerve terminals supplying these muscles cannot cause death, no matter how sensitive an individual is.

Carcinogens   Even in considering carcinogens, cautious use of mathematical model is essential. In selecting the model to be used, the goodness of the fit of the data may be useful, but not decisive; it is more important to consider the metabolic data, as shown with the data in Table 22-2.

It is also worth noting that the estimated VSDs for the same chemical often differ by a factor of several orders of magnitude. This fact was illustrated by the FDA Panel on Carcinogenesis (FDA, 1971) and is also evident among VSDs compiled by the Food Safety Council (1980). An extreme example is provided by the calculations on saccharin. The National Academy of Sciences (NAS, 1979) estimated the expected number of cases of bladder cancer in the United States due to lifetime exposure to 120 mg saccharin per day to range from 0.001 to 5200 cases per million individuals, a difference of 5.2 million fold!

In assessing the risk of a toxicant, various assumptions are incorporated in the dose-response modeling. The degree of uncertainties of the estimated risk should be stated along with the estimated risk. A high degree of uncertainty of the estimated risk may be satisfactory in certain cases; where such estimates may prevent or restrict the use of a valuable chemical or impose enormous societal cost, the degree of uncertainty must be considered. It may be appropriate to conduct additional testing or to use better modelling. The importance of stating the degree of uncertainty, along with the estimated risk, as well as the value of the "best estimate" (the maximum likelihood estimate) have been elaborated in two review articles (Lu and Sielken, 1991; Sielken and Stevenson, 1994).

REFERENCES

Andersen, M. E., and Krishnan, K. 1994. Physiologically based pharmacokinetics and cancer risk assessment. *Environ. Health Perspect.* 102(suppl. 1):103–108.

Andersen, M. E., Clewell, H. J., Gargas, M. L., Smith, F. A., and Reitz, R. H. 1987. Physiologically based pharmacokinetics and risk assessment process for methylene chloride. *Toxicol. Appl. Pharmacol.* 87:185–205.

Anderson, P. 1986. *Ninth Symposium on Statistics and the Environment.* Washington, DC: National Academy of Sciences.

Chand, N., and Hoel, W. 1974. A comparison of models for determining safe levels of environmental agents. In *Reliability and biometry*, eds. F. Proschan and R. J. Serfling, p. 681. Philadelphia: SIAM.

Conolly, R. B., and Andersen, M. E. 1991. Biologically based pharmacodynamic models: Tools for toxicological research and risk assessment. *Annu. Rev. Pharmacol. Toxicol.* 31: 503–523.

Cotruvos, J. A. 1988. Drinking water standards and risk assessment. *Regul. Toxicol. Pharmacol.* 8:288–299.

Crump, K. S. 1984. A new method for determining allowable daily intakes. *Fundam. Appl. Toxicol.* 4:854–871.

Dallas, C. E., Chen, X. M., Muraledhara, S., Varkonyi, P., Tackett, R. L., and Bruckner, J. E. 1995. Physiologically based pharmacokinetic model useful in prediction of the influence of species, dose, and exposure route on perchloroethylene pharmacokinetics. *J. Toxicol. Environ. Health* 44:301–317.

Dourson, M. L., and Stara, J. F. 1983. Regulatory history and experimental support of uncertainty (safety) factors. *Regul. Toxicol. Pharmacol.* 3:224–238.

Food and Drug Administration. 1971. Food and Drug Administration Advisory Committee on Protocols for Safety Evaluation: Panel on Carcinogenesis report on cancer testing in the safety evaluation of food additives and pesticides. *Toxicol. Appl. Pharmacol.* 20:419–438.

Food and Drug Administration. 1977. Chemical compounds in food-producing animals: Criteria and procedures for evaluating assays for carcinogenic residues in edible products of animals. *Fed. Reg.* 42(35):10412–10437.

Food Safety Council. 1980. Proposed system for food safety assessment. *Food Cosmet. Toxicol.* 16(suppl. 2).

Gaylor, D. W., and Kodell, R. L. 1980. Linear interpolation algorithm for low dose risk assessment of toxic substances. *J. Environ. Pathol. Toxicol.* 4:305–312.

Gehring, P. J., Watanabe, P. G., and Park, C. N. 1978. Resolution of dose-response toxicity for chemicals requiring metabolic activation: Example vinyl chloride. *Toxicol. Appl. Pharmacol.* 44:581–591.

Hoel, D. G. 1980. Incorporation of background in dose-response models. *Fed. Proc.* 39:73–75.

International Commission on Radiological Protection. 1966. *Recommendations of the International Commission on Radiological Protection.* ICRP Publication No. 9. Oxford: Pergamon Press.

Kalbfleisch, J. D., Krewski, D., and van Ryzin, J. 1983. Dose-response models for time to response toxicity data. *Can. J. Stat.* 11:25–49.

Klaassen, C. D., and Rozman, K. 1993. Physiologically based toxicokinetic modelling. In *Casarett and Doull's toxicology*, eds. M. O. Amdur, J. Doull, and C. D. Klaassen, pp. 82–84. New York: McGraw-Hill.

Krewski, D., and Van Ryzin, J. 1981. Dose-response models for quantal response toxicity data. In *Statistical and related topics*, eds. J. Csorgo, D. Dawson, J. N. K. Rao, and E. Shileh. New York: Elsivier/North Holland.

Lehman, A. J., and Fitzhugh, O. G. 1954. 100-Fold margin of safety. *Q. Bull. Assoc. Food Drug Officials U.S.*, 18:33–35.

Lenz, W., and Knapp, K. 1962. Thalidomide embryopathy. *Arch. Environ. Health* 5:100–105.

Lu, F. C. 1979. Assessment at an international level of health hazards to man of chemicals shown to be carcinogenic in laboratory animals. In *Regulatory aspects of carcinogenesis and food additives: The Delaney clause*, ed. F. Coulston, pp. 315–327. New York: Academic Press.

Lu, F. C. 1985. Safety assessment of chemicals with thresholded effects. *Regul. Toxicol. Pharmacol.* 5:460–464.

Lu, F. C. 1988. Acceptable daily intakes: Inception, evolution and application. *Regul. Toxicol. Pharmacol.* 8:45–60.

Lu, F. C. 1995. A review of the acceptable daily intakes of pesticides assessed by WHO. *Regul. Toxicol. Pharmacol.* 21:352–364.

Lu, F. C., and Coulston, F. 1996. Safety assessment based on irrelevant toxicologic data. *Ecotoxicol. Environ. Safety* 33:100–101.

Lu, F. C., and Sielken, R. L. 1991. Assessment of safety/risk of chemicals: inception and evolution of the ADI and dose-response modeling procedures. *Toxicol. Lett.* 59:5–40.

Mantel, N., and Bryan, W. R. 1961. "Safety" testing of carcinogenic agents. *J. Natl. Cancer Inst.* 27:455–470.

Munro, I. C. 1988. Risk assessment of carcinogens: Present status and future directions. *Biomed. Environ. Sci.* 1:51–58.

National Academy of Sciences. 1965. *Report on "no residue" and "zero tolerance."* Washington, DC: National Academy of Sciences.

National Academy of Sciences. 1970. *Evaluation of the safety of food chemicals.* Washington, DC: National Academy of Sciences.

National Academy of Sciences. 1979. *Saccharin: Technical assessment of risks and benefits.* Washington, DC: National Academy of Sciences.

National Academy of Sciences. 1983. *Risk assessment in the Federal Government: Managing the process.* Washington, DC: National Academy of Sciences.

National Research Council. 1977. *Drinking water and health*, vol. 1. Washington DC: National Academy of Sciences.

Ramsey, J. C., and Gehring, P. J. 1980. Application of pharmacokinetic principles in practice. *Fed. Proc.* 39:60–65.

Reitz, R. H., Mendrala, A. L., Corley, R., Quast, A., Cargas, M. L., Andersen, M. E., Staats, D. A., and Conolly, R. B. 1990. Estimating the risk of liver cancer associated with human exposures to chloroform. *Toxicol. Appl. Pharmacol.* 105:443–459.

Royal Commission on the Environment. 1976. *Sixth report: Nuclear power and the environment.* London: Her Majesty's Stationery Office.

Sielken, R. L., Jr. 1981. Re-examination of the ED_{01} study: Risk assessment using time. *Fundam. Appl. Toxicol.* 1:88–123.

Sielken, R. L., Jr., and Stevenson, D. E. 1994. Another flaw in the linearized multistage model upper bonds on human cancer potency. *Regul. Toxicol. Pharmacol.* 19:106–114.

Somers, E. 1986. The weight of evidence: Regulatory toxicology in Canada. *Regul. Toxicol. Pharmacol.* 6:391–398.

SOT ED_{01} Task Force. 1981. Re-examination of the ED_{01} Study. *Fundam. Appl. Toxicol.* 1:26–128.

Squire, R. A. 1981. Ranking carcinogens: A proposed regulatory approach. *Science* 214:877–880.

U.S. Environmental Protection Agency. 1986. Guides for carcinogenic risk assessment. *Fed. Reg.* 51:3399234003.

Wiberg, G. S., Munro, I. C., Meranger, J. C., Morrison, A. B., and Grice, H. C. 1969. Factors affecting the cardiotoxic potential of cobalt. *Clin. Toxicol.* 2:257–271.

Wilson, R. 1980. Risk-benefit analysis for toxic chemicals. *Ecotoxicol. Environ. Safety* 4:370–383.

World Health Organization. 1957. General Principles Governing the Use of Food Additives. First Report of the Joint FAO/WHO Expert Committee on Food Additives. WHO Tech. Rep. Ser. No. 129. Geneva: WHO.

World Health Organization. 1958. Procedures for the Testing of Intentional Food Additives to Establish Their Safety in Use. Second Report. WHO Tech. Rep. Ser. No. 144. Geneva: WHO.

World Health Organization. 1962a. Evaluation of the Toxicity of a Number of Antimicrobials and Antioxidants. Sixth Report. WHO Tech. Rep. Ser. No. 228. Geneva: WHO.

World Health Organization. 1962b. Principles Governing Consumer Safety in Relation to Pesticide Residues. Report of a Joint FAO/WHO Meeting on Pesticide Residues. WHO Tech. Rep. Ser. No. 240. Geneva: WHO.

World Health Organization. 1974a. Toxicological Evaluation of Certain Food Additives with a Review of General Principles and of Specifications. 17th report. WHO Tech. Rep. Ser. No. 539. Geneva: WHO.

World Health Organization. 1974b. Assessment of the Carcinogenicity and Mutagenicity of Chemicals. Report of a WHO Scientific Group. WHO Tech. Rep. Ser. No. 546. Geneva: WHO.

World Health Organization. 1978. Principles and Methods for Evaluating the Toxicity of Chemicals. Environmental Health Criteria 6. Geneva: WHO.

World Health Organization. 1987. Principles for the Safety Assessment of Food Additives and Contaminants in Food. Environmental Health Criteria No. 70. Geneva: WHO.

World Health Organization. 1989. Guidelines for Predicting Dietary Intakes of Pesticide Residues. Geneva: WHO.

World Health Organization. 1990. Principles for the Toxicological Assessment of Pesticide Residues in Food. Environmental Health Criteria 104. Geneva: WHO.

ADDITIONAL READING

Lu, F. C., and Sielken, R. L. 1991. Assessment of safety/risk of chemicals: Inception and evolution of the ADI and dose-response modeling procedures. *Toxicol. Lett.* 59:5–40.

Chemical Index

Subject Index